OXFORD MEDICAL PUBLICATIONS

Thoracic Imaging

Oxford Specialist Handbooks in Radiology
Thoracic Imaging

Sujal R. Desai

Consultant Radiologist and Honorary Senior Lecturer,
King's College Hospital NHS Foundation Trust,
London, UK

Susan J. Copley

Consultant Radiologist and Reader in Thoracic Imaging,
Imperial College NHS Trust,
London, UK

Zelena A. Aziz

Consultant Radiologist,
Barts and The London NHS Trust,
London, UK

David M. Hansell

Consultant Radiologist and Professor of Thoracic Imaging,
Royal Brompton & Harefield NHS Foundation Trust,
London, UK

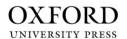
OXFORD
UNIVERSITY PRESS

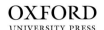

OXFORD
UNIVERSITY PRESS

Great Clarendon Street, Oxford, OX2 6DP,
United Kingdom

Oxford University Press is a department of the University of Oxford.
It furthers the University's objective of excellence in research, scholarship,
and education by publishing worldwide. Oxford is a registered trade mark of
Oxford University Press in the UK and in certain other countries

British Library Cataloguing in Publication Data

Data available

Library of Congress Cataloging in Publication Data

Library of Congress Control Number: 2012938383

ISBN 978–0–19–956047–9

Printed in Italy by
L.E.G.O S.p.A. — Lavis TN

Preface

There are several imaging tests available for the investigation of patients with lung disease and these include computed tomography, ultrasonography, magnetic resonance imaging, and fluorodeoxyglucose-positron emission tomography (PET). However, in the majority of cases, chest radiography and computed tomography suffice and this is reflected in their coverage in this book. The initial chapters deal with imaging techniques (including a review of radiation dose issues), anatomy, and radiological signs. Thoracic diseases are ordered and discussed according to the principal anatomical compartments that they affect (e.g. interstitium, mediastinum, pleura, etc), accepting that this is a somewhat arbitrary categorization as few diseases solely affect one compartment.

In a book of this size, we do not claim to have given a comprehensive account of all thoracic diseases. However, it is hoped that the majority of common and many of the less frequently encountered conditions have been covered. We also hope that this book will be come to be regarded as a useful aid and spend more of its time out of, rather than in, a pocket.

Sujal R. Desai
Susan J. Copley
Zelena A. Aziz
David M. Hansell

Acknowledgements

The authors would like to thank the following friends and colleagues from the UK and around the world for providing images:

Pamela Allen, Alexander A. Bankier, Sanjeev Bhalla, Philip M. Boiselle, Tomás Franquet, Fergus V. Gleeson, Siobhan Green, Thomas E. Hartman, Theresa C. McCloud, Nestor L. Müller, Martine Remy-Jardin, and Nicola Sverzellati.

Contents

Symbols and abbreviations

♂:♀	male/female ratio
~	approximately
≈	nearly equal to
±	with or without
°	degrees
📖	cross-reference to another section of this book
AAH	atypical adenomatous hyperplasia
ABPA	allergic bronchopulmonary aspergillosis
AIDS	acquired immune deficiency syndrome
AIP	acute interstitial pneumonia
ARDS	acute respiratory distress syndrome
CF	cystic fibrosis
COP	cryptogenic organizing pneumonia
COPD	chronic obstructive pulmonary disease
CT	computed tomography
CTD	connective tissue disease
CXR	chest X-ray
DIP	desquamative interstitial pneumonia
DPLD	diffuse parenchymal lung disease
FDG	fluorodeoxyglucose
HIV	human immunodeficiency virus
HP	hypersensitivity pneumonitis
HRCT	high-resolution computed tomography
HU	Hounsfield units
IIP	idiopathic interstitial pneumonia
ILD	interstitial lung disease
IPF	idiopathic pulmonary fibrosis
IV	intravenous
LCH	Langerhans' cell histiocytosis
LIP	lymphoid interstitial pneumonia
MDCT	multidetector CT
MDR	multi-drug resistant
MRI	magnetic resonance imaging
NSCLC	non-small cell lung cancer
NSIP	non-specific interstitial pneumonia

NTM	non-tuberculous mycobacteria
OB	obliterative bronchiolitis
OP	organizing pneumonia
PCP	*Pneumocystis jiroveci* pneumonia
PE	pulmonary embolism
PET	positron emission tomography
RB	respiratory bronchiolitis
RBILD	respiratory bronchiolitis-interstitial lung disease
SUV	standardized uptake value
TB	tuberculosis
TNM	Tumour-Nodes-Metastasis
UIP	usual interstitial pneumonia
US	ultrasound
V/Q	ventilation-perfusion

Chapter 1

Principles of imaging tests

Chest radiography

The chest radiograph (CXR) is the mainstay of radiological investigation in patients with suspected lung disease. Despite the considerable advances in radiographic technology, the key physical principles of chest radiography technique have not changed appreciably over 100 years.

Key aspects of conventional (film-screen) chest radiography

- The main components of a conventional x-ray imaging system include the following:
  - An x-ray tube which generates a collimated x-ray beam.
  - A grid to reduce scattered radiation reaching the x-ray film (detector).
  - The x-ray film-screen combination to 'capture' the energy of x-ray photons transmitted through the thorax.
  - The film cassette—houses the x-ray film-screen combination and shields it from light.
  - An automated film changer and processor.
- CXR projections that are used include:
  - **Postero-anterior** (Fig. 1.1): the standard projection for the CXR. The anterior chest is in contact with the film cassette. The elbows are flexed, the shoulders internally rotated and the hands are placed on the hips—these manoeuvres displace the scapulae laterally. The patient is asked to maintain a deep inspiratory effort; a suboptimal effort may lead to erroneous interpretations (e.g. bulky hila, cardiomegaly). Futhermore, in the optimal examination, the medial ends of the clavicles will be projected roughly equidistant from the line of the spinous process; suboptimal centring will lead to the spurious impression of abnormality on a CXR.
  - **Lateral** (Fig. 1.2): this projection is of value in *some* patients for localizing disease. For instance, loss of the normal retrosternal and retrocardiac lucency will localize disease to the mediastinum, and loss of clarity of the hemidiaphragm may indicate lower lobe pathology. In the era of CT, requests for lateral CXR have fallen.
  - **Antero-posterior:** this projection is used in patients unable to attend the radiology department (e.g. critically-ill, immobile patients); the projection is not optimal because the scapulae often overlap the lungs and the transverse diameter of the cardiac silhouette (an 'anterior' structure) may be magnified and appear enlarged.
  - **Lordotic** (Fig. 1.3): this projection is sometimes used when an apical abnormality is suspected but cannot be evaluated fully because of the presence of overlying bony elements (i.e. the clavicle, anterior ribs). Again, in the era before CT, this projection was sometimes used in patients with suspected pathology in the middle lobe.

Advantages of conventional chest radiography

- The radiation dose from CXR is very low (see ☐ Principles of imaging tests/Radiation dose, p19).
- Low cost.
- Portable equipment allows examination of patients unable to attend the x-ray department.

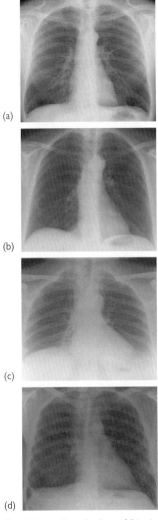

Fig. 1.1 (a) Normal frontal chest radiograph, taken at full inspiration and correctly centred. (b) and (c) Image pair in the same patient demonstrating the effect of a suboptimal inspiration: by contrast with the appearances in (b), in (c) the heart appears enlarged, the hilar structures are less distinct and the lungs more opaque (because of less air). (d) The effect of rotation: the medial ends of the clavicles are not equidistant from the spinous processes. The left lung appears more lucent than the right and this should not be interpreted as abnormal.

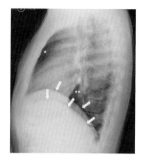

Fig. 1.2 Lateral CXR projection. The normal retrosternal (*) and retrocardiac (**) lucencies are clearly seen. Both hemidiaphragms are crisply delineated (arrows). Note the (normal) increasing lucency from top to bottom overlying the thoracic spine.

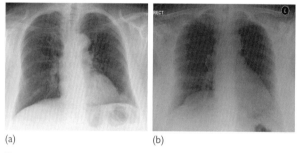

(a)   (b)

Fig. 1.3 A comparison of postero-anterior (PA) and lordotic projections. (a) PA projection demonstrating the normal overlap of the clavicle and anterior ribs at the lung apices. (b) Lordotic projection in which the clavicles no longer obscure the lung apices.

- Relative technical simplicity.
- Excellent spatial resolution (for conventional film-screen radiography systems).

Disadvantages of conventional radiography
- Anatomical superimposition hampers interpretation (cf. CT).
- Limited contrast resolution.
- Limited sensitivity, specificity, and diagnostic accuracy (compared with CT).

Alternative chest radiographic techniques
- Digital or computed radiography—have a linear dose-response to x-ray photons compared to the sigmoid dose-response of conventional film-screen radiography. Furthermore, digital data may be post-processed. The main disadvantage of these are the cost of the hardware.

Computed tomography (CT)

As with CXR, computed tomography (CT) imaging depends on the differential absorption of x-ray energy by tissues of differing physical densities. However, in contrast to CXR, images are constructed from multiple projections around the region of interest so that there is no anatomical superimposition. Moreover, because of the greater sensitivity to differences in the attenuation of x-ray energy by different tissues, the contrast resolution is significantly higher.

Key aspects of CT imaging

- The key components of a CT machine (see Fig. 1.4) include:
  - An x-ray source.
  - An array of detectors.
  - Sophisticated computer software.
  - A (sliding) scanning table.
- Reconstructing the CT image: The transmitted, attenuated x-ray energy is captured by detectors positioned opposite the x-ray tube. The detectors convert this energy into an electrical signal. The final image, of a particular body region, is generated from multiple x-ray projections of that region using a complex mathematical reconstruction technique. The axial image is viewed as if from the 'foot-end' of the patient (i.e. the patient's right side is to the viewer's left).
- Each CT image is made up of a matrix of small picture elements (termed 'pixels' [Fig. 1.4b]) each one of which represents the attenuation value within a volume element (voxel). The attenuation value in the voxel is a reflection of the average physical density in that specific region.
- The attenuation value in each voxel is assigned a numerical value (expressed in Hounsfield Units (HU) and grey-scale value. By convention, water has an attenuation (or Hounsfield) value equal to 0 HU, air a value of -1,000 HU and bone between 800 and 1000 HU. Other tissues have values in between the two extremes of air and bone.

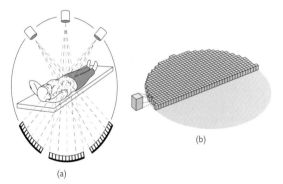

(a)   (b)

Fig. 1.4 Key aspects of CT. (a) The x-ray source and detector gantry are sited diametrically opposite and shown in three different positions in this illustration; attenuation data is gathered by the detectors from multiple different projections. (b) The CT image is made up of multiple 2D picture elements (pixels). The 'grey-scale' value of each is governed by the average density of tissue in the volume of the 3D voxel. A magnified voxel is shown.

Advantages of CT
- Superior contrast resolution gives exquisite detail of the various components of mediastinal anatomy (e.g. lymph nodes and vessels) and density differences (e.g. calcifications within a pulmonary nodule).

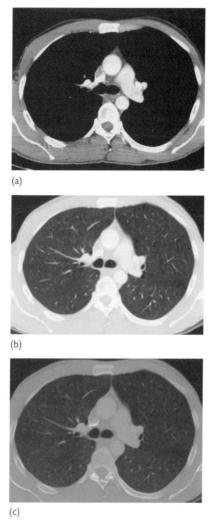

(a)

(b)

(c)

Fig. 1.5 CT of the chest on (a) mediastinal windows, (b) lung parenchymal windows and (c) bone windows.

- Because the image of a particular region is made up from multiple x-ray projections, there is no anatomical superimposition. This is a major advantage in comparison with two-dimensional chest radiography.
- On the same anatomical section, different image (window) settings allow the observer to view tissues of differing densities (i.e. soft tissue structures of the mediastinum, the aerated lung parenchyma and bony elements of the chest wall (Fig. 1.5).

Disadvantages of CT

- Increased radiation dose (see 📖 Principles of imaging tests/Radiation dose, p19).
- The cost of a CT machine (and particularly the newer generation of multidetector CT machines) is much higher than that of conventional x-ray equipment.
- The relative availability of CT (particularly machines of higher specification) may be restricted.
- Iodinated IV contrast administration may be contraindicated in some patients (e.g. renal failure) which may limit diagnostic utility.

Common indications for thoracic CT

- Investigation of an abnormal mediastinal or hilar contour on CXR.
- Investigation of a pulmonary nodule/mass detected on CXR.
- Follow-up of 'incidental' pulmonary nodule(s), particularly in smokers or patients with a known cancer.
- Staging of lung cancer.
- Investigation of haemoptysis.
- Diagnosis of pulmonary thromboembolism.
- Assessment of major thoracic or polytrauma.
- Detection of pulmonary disease in the context of a questionably abnormal CXR (e.g. diffuse interstitial disease or bronchiectasis).
- Guiding percutaneous needle biopsy (Fig. 1.6).

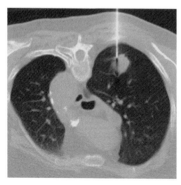

Fig. 1.6 Prone CT image of a percutaneous needle biopsy of a lung lesion.

High-resolution CT (HRCT)

High resolution computed tomography (HRCT; also known as thin-section CT) uses very thin collimation (1–2mm) and a high spatial frequency reconstruction algorithm to produce detailed images of the lung parenchyma. HRCT is the investigation of choice for patients with suspected or established diffuse lung disease; the essence of interspaced HRCT (i.e. with gaps between image sections) is that the lungs are 'sampled'. With the advent of helical and, more recently multidetector CT (MDCT), it is possible to obtain 'high-resolution' images without interspacing: the key point is that a 'volume' of data (without missing slabs of lung parenchyma) is acquired. The important drawback is the higher radiation burden of a volumetric acquisition.

Key aspects of HRCT

- Interspaced image slices typically with a gap (10–20mm) between images.
- HRCT enables resolution of sub-millimetre structures, demonstrating the subtle and sometimes complex morphology of interstitial and airway diseases with great clarity (Fig. 1.7).
- IV contrast is not routinely given.

Advantages of HRCT

- Increased sensitivity, specificity, and diagnostic accuracy compared to CXR for diffuse parenchymal lung disease (DPLD) and large and small airways diseases.
- HRCT correlates closely with the macroscopic appearances of pathological specimens in DPLD and may provide useful information about prognosis and response to treatment.
- CT 'samples' a greater volume of lung than lung biopsy and is therefore less prone to sampling error.
- Interspaced sections minimize radiation dose which is especially important in young patients.

Disadvantages of HRCT

- Small pulmonary nodules or endobronchial lesions may be missed on interspaced sections.

Indications for high-resolution CT

- Investigation of suspected diffuse lung diseases (interstitial, vascular or airways)
- Establishing a 'histospecific' diagnosis in some patients
- Identifying important co-existent disease (e.g. emphysema in patients with interstitial lung disease).
- As a guide to the optimal site for transbronchial/surgical lung biopsy.

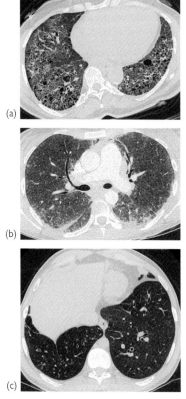

(a)

(b)

(c)

Fig. 1.7 HRCT patterns in three patients. (a) Image through the lower zones shows ground-glass opacification, a fine reticular pattern, and limited subpleural honeycombing caused by NSIP in a patient with mixed connective tissue disease; there is co-existent emphysema. (b) Diffuse ground-glass opacification in an HIV-positive patient with pneumocystis and (c) cylindrical bronchiectasis in both lower lobes.

Helical and multidetector CT (MDCT)

The key feature which differentiates helical and MDCT machines from earlier generations of scanners is that the scanner table moves throughout the x-ray exposure. The corollary is that scan acquisition times are markedly reduced. The principal advantage in the thorax is that the entire chest can now be imaged in a single breath-hold.

Key aspects of spiral/helical and MDCT

- Continuous rotation of the x-ray source and detectors around the patient while the table moves into the gantry (Fig. 1.8).
- MDCT is a more recent development where multiple rows of detectors rotate around the patient.
- MDCT acquires overlapping images from which volumetric data sets can be reconstructed.
- MDCT machines with up to 320-channels are now available.
- ECG gating allows detailed images of cardiac structures.

Advantages of MDCT

- Diagnostic quality images can be obtained in dyspnoeic patients and young children during quiet respiration.
- Allows accurate timing of IV contrast medium for optimum opacification of the pulmonary arteries (Fig. 1.9).
- Computer software can perform multiplanar two and three dimensional image reconstructions of volumetric data sets (Fig. 1.10).
- Evaluation of structures such as coronary arteries is increasingly feasible due to reduction in motion artefact and increased spatial resolution.

Disadvantages of MDCT

- Increased radiation dose.
- Availability may be limited in some countries.
- Large number of data sets increases the time needed for image interpretation.

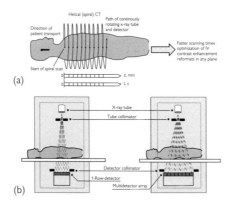

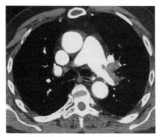

Fig. 1.8 Helical CT (a) Line drawing demonstrating the key principles of helical CT: there is continuous patient movement during scanning. In this way a volume of data is acquired. Reproduced with permission from Kalendar WA (2005) *Computed Tomography, Second Edition*, pg. 79, Wiley VCH. (b) Comparision of the arrangement of x-ray tube, collimators and detector gantry in a single-slice and a multidetector (8-channel) CT machine.

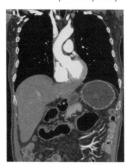

Fig. 1.9 Axial image from a contrast-enhanced CT pulmonary angiogram showing a pulmonary embolus within the left main pulmonary artery.

Fig. 1.10 Contrast-enhanced coronal MDCT image of the chest and upper abdomen.

Radionuclide imaging

Imaging with radiolabelled nuclides has widespread applications in clinical medicine. In broad terms, depending on the radiopharmaceutical used, radionuclide tests provide 'functional' information about tissues. A list of some of the tests which have applications in respiratory medicine is given in Table 1.1 and is followed by a discussion of ventilation-perfusion (V/Q) scanning and ^{18}fluorodeoxyglucose-positron emission tomography (^{18}FDG-PET).

Table 1.1 Radionuclide tests used in the investigation of thoracic disease

Radionuclide test	Principal indication(s)
• V/Q scintigraphy	Acute/chronic thromboembolism
	Differential lung 'function' (e.g. pre-pneumonectomy)
• ^{18}FDG-PET	Differentiation between malignant and benign disease
	Staging of lung cancer (locoregional/distant disease)
	Response evaluation following therapy
• Octreotide scanning	Diagnosis and staging of carcinoid tumour
• ^{99m}Tc-DTPA	Alveolar permeability/inflammation

Note: V/Q = ventilation/perfusion; ^{18}FDG-PET = ^{18}fluorodeoxyglucose-positron emission tomography; ^{99m}Tc-DTPA = ^{99m}Technetium diethylene triamine pentaacetic acid.

Miscellaneous radionuclide tests used in chest medicine

Ventilation/perfusion imaging

Ventilation-perfusion (V/Q) scintigraphy is a non-invasive technique which simultaneously assesses the distribution of pulmonary blood flow and alveolar ventilation. The most frequent reason for requesting V/Q imaging is in the patient with suspected pulmonary thromboembolic disease: a reduction in perfusion with maintenance of normal ventilation (the so-called 'mismatched perfusion defect') is the hallmark of acute pulmonary embolism (Fig. 1.11).

Key technical aspects

- Ventilation (V) imaging: this phase is performed using either radiolabelled aerosols or inert radioactive gases: agents that are in common use include:
  - Aerosols (^{99m}Tc-DTPA and ^{99m}Tc-technegas): imaging with these agents cannot be used simultaneously with the perfusion phase of scanning because the same radioactive 'label' ^{99m}Tc is used in both.
  - Inert gases (^{81m}Krypton and ^{133}Xenon): ^{81m}Krypton is the ideal agent because of the high energy photons and its short half-life but it is expensive to produce.
- Perfusion (Q) imaging: this phase of the test is performed after the IV injection of ^{99m}Tc-labelled protein microparticles which, because of their size (10–100µm diameter), lodge in the pulmonary vascular bed and create photopenic areas distal to the area of embolic occlusion.
- The standard projections are anterior, posterior, left posterior oblique, right posterior oblique. Right lateral, left lateral, right anterior, and left anterior oblique views may also be obtained.

V/Q lung scanning is part of the diagnostic algorithm in the investigation of patients with pulmonary embolism and (subject to availability) the current guidelines suggest that V/Q imaging may be considered the initial imaging investigation in patients with a normal CXR and/or in those with no evidence of concurrent cardiopulmonary disease (see 📖 Vascular diseases/Acute pulmonary embolism, p286).

Advantages of V/Q scanning

- A normal V/Q result, in a patient with a low clinical pre-test probability effectively rules out PE.
- The radiation dose is reasonably low.

Disadvantages of V/Q scanning

- Around two-thirds of studies are reported as showing intermediate probability of acute pulmonary embolism.
- In contrast to CT pulmonary angiography, V/Q scans do not identify alternative diagnoses which may have a similar clinical presentation.
- The majority of institutions do not offer an 'out-of-hours' (e.g. weekend) V/Q imaging service.

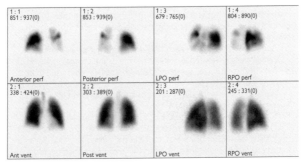

Fig. 1.11 V/Q scan: perfusion images (top row) demonstrate markedly reduced perfusion in the left lung with multiple perfusion defects in a segmental distribution. There are also small perfusion defects on the right. The ventilation images are normal. Appearances are those of a high probability of multiple PEs.

Positron emission tomography (PET)

The technique of PET relies on the principle that metabolically-active tissues (both benign and malignant) take up glucose. For most PET imaging, glucose is coupled with a positron-emitting radionuclide of fluorine (^{18}fluorodeoxyglucose [^{18}FDG]). The PET images provide a functional map of metabolically-active tissues.

Key aspects of PET

- ^{18}FDG is the most widely used isotope and is injected intravenously.
- Positron-emitting isotopes are neutron deficient and, because of this, tend to be unstable. To attain stability a proton must transmutate into a neutron and this process releases a positron and a neutrino. The positron interacts with an electron in an 'annihilation' reaction resulting in two gamma photons which travel at 180° to each other; the PET detectors (arranged around the patient) capture and map the site of origin of the two emitted gamma rays (Fig. 1.12).
- Early generations of PET machines are increasingly replaced by 'hybrid' PET-CT scanners in which the functional data from PET is fused with the more superior spatial/morphological information from CT (Fig. 1.13).

Advantages of ^{18}FDG-PET imaging

- By evaluating the standardized uptake values (SUVs), inactive or benign lesions may be distinguished from malignant lesions: in general the SUV of malignant masses is greater than that of benign lesions.
- PET imaging may identify otherwise cryptic distant disease in lung cancer staging.

Disadvantages of ^{18}FDG-PET imaging

- False positive results for malignancy may be caused by infection or inflammation, particularly granulomatous.
- False negative results with certain tumour cell-types (e.g. adenocarcinoma and carcinoid tumours) or in situations where the 'target' lesion is small (generally <1cm in diameter) and below the resolution limits of PET.
- Patients are required to lie still for some time during image acquisition; movement causes image degradation because of misregistration artefacts.
- Radiation dose (see 📖 Principles of imaging tests/Radiation dose, p19).

Positron Emission Tomography (PET)

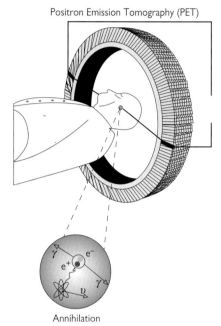

Annihilation

Fig. 1.12 Positron emission tomography (PET) produces a 3-D map of metabolically-active tissues in the body. Areas of higher metabolic activity take up more of the ^{18}FDG-PET. The inset demonstrates the decay of a nucleus which releases a positron (e+) and a neutrino (υ). The positron interacts with an electron (e−) in an annihilation reaction producing two gamma rays (γ) which travel at 180° to each other. These are detected by the PET detectors. Image courtesy of Wikimedia Commons.

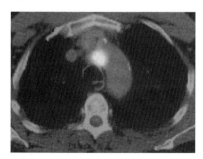

Fig. 1.13 Fused axial PET-CT image showing increased uptake in a pre-tracheal lymph node (SUV 13). The node was sampled at mediastinoscopy and found to contain metastatic lung adenocarcinoma.

Magnetic resonance imaging

The technique of magnetic resonance imaging (MRI) makes use of the phenomenon of nuclear magnetic resonance (NMR). A detailed discussion of NMR is not possible but a brief review is warranted to explain the principal limitations and the potential advantages of lung MRI.

Key aspects of magnetic resonance imaging

MR imaging of biological tissues is dependent on four key elements:

- Hydrogen atoms—the most abundant and magnetic element in biological tissues.
- A strong external magnetic field—the external field aligns the hydrogen atoms along the direction of that field and magnetizes them.
- A radiofrequency (RF) pulse—which momentarily tips the aligned hydrogen atoms (and thus, the net magnetization) into a perpendicular plane to the external field. When the RF pulse is switched off, the net magnetization 'relaxes'. This relaxation creates an electrical current. In lung, the relaxation is very rapid and the magnitude of the signal is very small.
- Detector (receiver) coils—which detect the electrical (MR) signal when the RF pulse is switched-off and the hydrogen atoms return ('relax') to the previously aligned state.

The electrical signal is converted into an image by assigning a 'grey-scale' value proportional to the strength of the signal. Hydrogen atoms in different tissues relax at different rates and this provides the exquisite tissue contrast seen on MR images.

Advantages of MR imaging

- No ionizing radiation.
- Multiplanar imaging—less of an advantage since the advent of multi-detector CT (see 📖 Principles of imaging tests/Helical and multidetector CT (MDCT), p10).
- Novel imaging 'sequences' allow tissue characteristics (e.g. fat, fluid, blood) to be enhanced; this facility may be of particular value when evaluating mediastinal lesions.

Disadvantages of MR imaging

There are three basic problems which limit the role of lung MR in clinical practice:

- Low proton density—lung has the lowest proton density of any organ in the body.
- Magnetic susceptibility artifact—in essence the MR signal from lung is very heterogeneous, relaxes too rapidly, and is of small magnitude.
- Movement—respiratory motion and cardiac pulsation degrade the MR image of the lung.

Ultrasound

High frequency sound waves do not traverse air and are reflected at interfaces between soft tissue and air. The use of ultrasound in the chest is therefore limited because of normally aerated lung. However, fluid can be readily detected and the main use of transthoracic ultrasound is for the localization of pleural effusions.

Key aspects of thoracic ultrasound

- High frequency sound waves are emitted by an ultrasound transducer and, depending on the acoustic 'reflectivity' of different tissues (and their components), the reflected sound energy is detected by the same ultrasound probe.
- The received sound signal is then converted into a grey scale (black and white) real-time image.
- An aqueous gel is required to form an acoustic interface between the probe and skin of the chest wall.

Typical indications for performing thoracic ultrasound

- Identification of pleural fluid and differentiation from consolidation.
- Detection of septations in pleural effusions.
- Evaluation of pleural thickening.
- Assessment of diaphragmatic dysfunction.
- Guidance for pleural fluid aspiration and/or drainage.
- Guidance for biopsy of chest wall/pleural lesions, some peripheral lung lesions or mediastinal masses abutting the pleura.

Advantages of thoracic ultrasound

- No ionizing radiation.
- Readily available and can be performed at the bedside.
- Rapid and inexpensive.
- 'Real-time' image guidance for thoracic intervention (see above).
- Colour Doppler imaging may be useful to identify, and thus avoid, large vessels during thoracic intervention.
- Superior to CT for the detection of septations in pleural fluid.

Disadvantages of thoracic ultrasound

- It may not be possible to image small lesions beneath bony structures.
- In patients with empyema, ultrasound appearances do not indicate the stage (see 📖 Infectious/parapneumonic effusions and empyema, p370), nor do they predict the presence of pus in the pleural space.
- Operator-dependent.
- Sound waves do not penetrate normally aerated lung.

Radiation dose

All ionizing radiation is potentially damaging and there is no threshold below which harmful effects do not occur. The contribution of medical radiation exposures to the overall population radiation burden has been increasing steadily and a large component of this can be attributed to the increasing dependence on CT imaging in medicine. Efforts to minimize radiation exposure are of paramount importance. One of the principal concerns is the excess risk of cancer. It has been estimated that around 2% of all cancer deaths may be attributable to ionizing radiation: as a rough guide, every 10mSv of exposure to ionizing radiation is believed to result in a 0.05% excess cancer deaths. The risks are higher in younger individuals.

Measures of radiation exposure

The radiation burden associated with medical imaging tests can be expressed or quantified in different ways:

- Radiation exposure (measured in Coulombs/kg): the simplest measure of radiation dose but this does not take into account the sensitivities of the tissues being exposed or the sources of radiation (i.e. x-ray energy versus γ- or α-radiation). Thus, this measure has little practical clinical value.
- Absorbed dose (measured in Grays or milliGrays): this is a measure of the radiation energy absorbed per unit mass which takes into account the tissue being exposed but, like radiation exposure, does not allow for the differing radio-sensitivities of tissue.
- Equivalent dose (measured in Sieverts or milliSieverts): this is derived from the absorbed dose and allows for comparison between different sources of ionizing radiation by applying a radiation 'weighting factor' that adjusts for the type of radiation source (eg, x-rays, γ-radiation). For x-rays (including CT), the radiation weighting factor is 1.
- Effective dose (measured in Sieverts or milliSieverts): probably the best expression of radiation burden. The effective dose is derived from the absorbed dose and not only takes into account the radiosensitivity of the exposed tissues (e.g. the female breast versus bones versus the lungs) but also the nature of the radiation source (e.g. background radiation versus x-ray versus γ-radiation).

Typical radiation doses for some lung imaging tests are listed in Table 1.2.

Table 1.2 Typical radiation doses for imaging tests used in the investigation of lung disease

Imaging tests	Effective dose (mSv)
CXR	0.02
HRCT (1mm sections every 10mm)	0.9–1.2
CT Chest (spiral single detector)*	8.0–10
CT Chest (multidetector)*	3.0–11
Ventilation-perfusion scintigraphy	1.5
^{18}FDG-PET	5–8
^{18}FDG-PET/CT	11–18

*A large variation in CT scanning parameters exists in chest CT. The tube voltage and current for a typical standard chest CT protocol ranges from 120 to 140 kVp and 100 to 500 mAs respectively.

Ways of reducing radiation dose from CT

Steps to reduce radiation dose to the population are the responsibility of clinicians and radiology staff alike.

What can requesting clinicians do?

- Ensure that the indications for a CT examination are appropriate (see Common indications for CT, 📖 Principles of imaging tests/Computed tomography, p7). Thus, before requesting the examination, clinicians should be in the habit of asking 'Is the CT really justified?'.
- In circumstances where a CXR or an alternative examination—such as ultrasound—would be satisfactory (e.g. in the follow-up of a known resolving pneumonia or in the evaluation of a pleural effusion), CT should not be requested.
- In patients referred to tertiary centres, CT examinations may already have been performed at the referring hospital. In such circumstances, every effort must be made to obtain all radiological examinations and the temptation to re-request recently undertaken CT should be strongly resisted.
- Accurate clinical details should be provided so that only the appropriate examination and, more importantly, only the necessary body regions are exposed.

What can radiologists and radiographers do?

- Reduction of tube current (measured in milliAmpere-seconds (mAs)) is one of the simplest methods for decreasing radiation dose. Low dose CT examinations of the lungs can be used in the follow-up of patients with a known abnormality (e.g., interstitial lung disease, a solitary pulmonary nodule).
- Reduce the number of image sections as in high-resolution CT imaging (see 📖 Principles of imaging tests/High-resolution CT (HRCT), p8) of diffuse interstitial lung diseases. With greater spacing between image slices it is possible to dramatically reduce dose.
- Reduce 'pitch'. In essence the pitch is a measure of the amount of 'coverage' (of whichever body region) for each rotation of the x-ray tube/detectors. Put simply, an increase in pitch shortens the total scanning time and decreases the radiation dose. Against this a higher pitch generally leads to increased image 'noise'. In fact, some MDCT scanner models compensate automatically for the increase in noise by increasing mAs thereby negating any potential benefit from increasing the pitch.
- Use the automatic exposure system which dynamically adjusts the tube current. Tube current is adjusted to achieve consistent image quality between patients and within a single patient. Three types of automatic exposure control operate: exposure adjustment to the overall body habitus, exposure adjustment along the craniocaudal axis of the patient (so-called 'z-axis' modulation), and exposure adjustment during gantry rotation (angular modulation).
- Use imaging filters to improve image quality by reducing noise and artefacts.
- Reduce the scanned volume strictly to the region of interest.

Chapter 2

Key radiological anatomy

Radiological anatomy

The accurate interpretation of radiological tests must be built on a sound knowledge of anatomy and specifically on normal anatomy (and its common variants) as seen at imaging.

Frontal (PA) CXR

Despite the increasing use of cross-sectional imaging, the CXR remains the first line of investigation in most patients with suspected or established lung disease. The normal anatomic landmarks/structures which should be visible on a CXR are listed below and illustrated in Fig. 2.1:

- 1 Trachea—on a well centred film, the trachea is a midline tubular lucency which normally bows slightly to the right at the level of the aortic arch.
- 2 Aortic arch.
- 3 Lateral margins of manubrium.
- 4 Descending thoracic aorta.
- 5 Right and 6 left hilar points—referring to the roughly v-shaped points, on a frontal chest radiograph, at which the upper lobe pulmonary vein crosses the basal pulmonary artery. The right hilar point is generally easier to see and may lie at the same level (but no more than 1.5cm lower than the left hilar point).
- 7 Carina—the normal branching angle at the carina is ~60–75 degrees.
- 8 Border of the right atrium.
- 9 Border of the left ventricle.
- 10 Right and 11 left hemidiaphragm.
- 12 Superior vena cava.
- 13 Aortopulmonary window—a small space between the aortic arch and the pulmonary artery that contains the ligamentum arteriosum, the recurrent laryngeal nerve, lymph nodes, and fatty tissue. The aortopulmonary window is a common location for mediastinal lymph node enlargement and 'filling in' of the AP window often reflects the presence of enlarged nodes (Fig. 2.2).

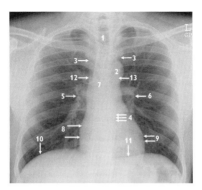

Fig. 2.1 Normal anatomical structures on a frontal (PA) chest radiograph.

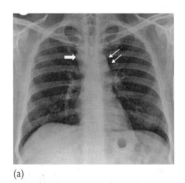

(a)

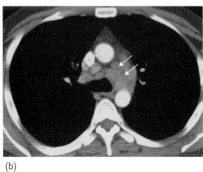

(b)

Fig. 2.2 (a) CXR shows an abnormal contour of the superior mediastinum (thick arrow) with 'filling-in' of the aortopulmonary (AP) window (thin arrows). (b) CT in the same patient confirms extensive lymph node enlargement in the AP window (arrows).

Lateral CXR

The lateral CXR (Fig. 2.3) is now less commonly requested. However, an awareness of the normal anatomical landmarks on a lateral projection is useful:

- Retrosternal/retrocardiac spaces—these regions should be lucent. A loss of the normal translucency in these regions indicates local pathology (e.g. a thymic or nodal mass).
- Thoracic vertebral bodies—progressive translucency in the cranio-caudal direction is the norm and loss of this feature may indicate pathology in the lower lobes or a posterior mediastinal mass (e.g. a neurogenic tumour).
- Hemidiaphragms—both are visible on a normal lateral CXR; anteriorly the left hemidiaphragm is not seen because of the absence of aerated lung (due to the heart) against it. This feature and the presence of a gastric air bubble (under the left hemidiaphragm) helps to identify—i.e. right versus left—the hemidiaphragms on a lateral projection.
- Posterior costophrenic angles—these should appear sharp (acute angle). Obliteration of the costophrenic angles indicates pleural fluid or thickening.
- Fissures—the oblique fissure can be followed forward from the level of T4/5, 'passing through' the hilum. The left oblique fissure tends to be steeper. The horizontal fissure arises at the hilum and ends at the anterior chest wall.

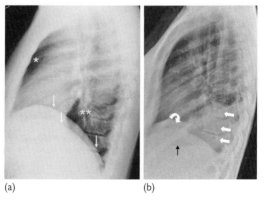

(a)   (b)

Fig. 2.3 (a) Normal and (b) abnormal lateral CXRs in two patients. (a) The normal retrosternal (*) and retrocardiac (**) lucencies and both hemidiaphragms (arrows) are clearly seen. There is also transradiancy overlying the spine which increases cranio-caudally. (b) A patient with right lower lobe pneumonia; there is loss of the retrocardiac lucency and the normal increasing transradiancy over the spine (block arrows). The posterior half of the right hemidiaphragm (curved arrow) is not seen; the gastric air bubble (black arrow) is just visible under the left hemidiaphragm.

Mediastinal anatomy

The key mediastinal landmarks that can be appreciated on a CXR are listed below (see Figs. 2.4 and 2.5).

- 1 Lateral border of the superior vena cava—this is increasingly difficult to trace towards the apex.)
- 2 Azygos vein—draining into the superior vena cava and seen as an ovoid opacity in the trancheobronchial angle
- 3 Lateral border of the right atrium
- 4 Left main pulmonary artery
- 5 Left atrial appendage
- 6 Lateral border of the left ventricle

Miscellaneous points about mediastinal anatomy on CXR

- The left atrium and right ventricle are the most posterior and anterior (respectively) chambers of the heart. On a frontal CXR, these chambers are not 'border-forming' and not normally visible on a chest radiograph.
- The left atrium may enlarge superiorly, elevating the left main bronchus and causing a widened subcarinal angle or may also enlarge to the right resulting in a double right heart border.
- Left atrial appendage enlargement occurs early in left atrial enlargement and can be seen as a fullness beneath the pulmonary artery.

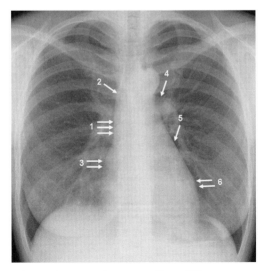

Fig. 2.4 Mediastinal contours and structures visible on a CXR.

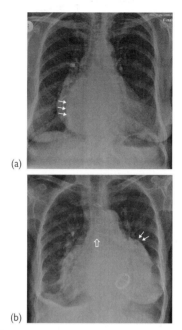

(a)

(b)

Fig. 2.5 Two different patients with mitral stenosis. (a) Note the double right heart border. The right lateral margin (arrows) of the enlarged left atrium is clearly seen. (b) Marked left atrial appendage enlargement (arrows) and a widened carina (open arrow) caused by an enlarged left atrium.

Mediastinal 'lines and stripes' on CXR

On frontal and lateral CXRs, there are a number of useful lines and stripes whose absence, displacement, or distortion may indicate otherwise subtle intrathoracic pathology. In essence, the various lines and stripes are generated at the interfaces between aerated lung and mediastinal components; depending on the relative thickness, a line or stripe is generated when structures of different densities (for example, air and soft tissue) abut one another. The key lines and stripes visible on CXR are discussed below (Figs. 2.6–2.8).

Right paratracheal stripe
- The right lateral wall of the trachea 'outlined' by air in the trachea and air in the adjacent right lung extends inferiorly to the right tracheobronchial angle.
- Maximum normal thickness 3–4mm.
- Different pathologies (e.g. right paratracheal lymph node enlargement, thyroid, or tracheal carcinoma) may cause it to disappear or thicken.

Aortopulmonary stripe

- The aortopulmonary stripe represents a mediastinal reflection formed by the pleura of the anterior left lung coming in contact with, and tangentially reflecting over, the mediastinal fat anterolateral to the left pulmonary artery and aortic arch.
- The stripe is straight or slightly convex and crosses laterally over the aortic arch and the main pulmonary artery.

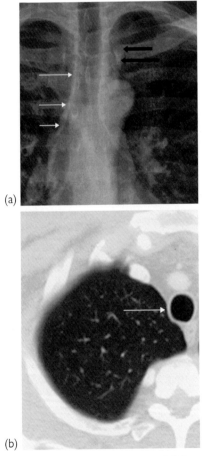

(a)

(b)

Fig. 2.6 (a) The right paratracheal stripe demonstrated on CXR (line arrows). The faint outline of the left subclavian artery (black arrows) is also visible. (b) Normal right paratracheal stripe on CT (arrow).

- Anterior mediastinal disease such as thyroid or thymic masses or prevascular lymph node enlargement may alter the normal appearance of the stripe, causing increased convexity laterally.

Azygo-oesophageal line

- The azygo-oesophageal line is generated by the interface between the (aerated) right lower lobe and soft tissues in the posterior mediastinum (which include the oesophagus and azygos vein).
- The azygo-oesophageal line is visible on a good quality PA CXR in the midline, projected over the spine; the line has a roughly inverted 'hockey stick' configuration as the upper few centimetres of the line are concave towards the right lung.
- Pathology in the sub-carinal region/posterior mediastinum (commonly nodal enlargement) may obscure or displace the line.

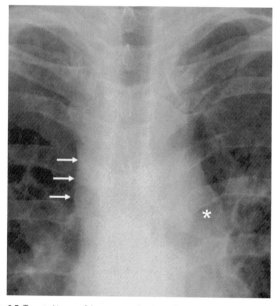

Fig. 2.7 Targeted image of the upper mediastinum shows widening of the right paratracheal stripe (arrows) caused by lymph node enlargement in a patient with sarcoidosis. There is also enlargement of lymph nodes in the aortopulmonary window (asterisk) causing a bulge in this region.

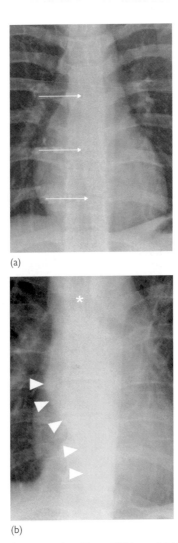

(a)

(b)

Fig. 2.8 (a) Normal azygo-oesophageal line on CXR (arrows). (b) Deviation of the azygo-oesophageal line (arrowheads), in the same patient as in Fig. 2.7, caused by subcarinal lymph node enlargement. Note that there is no splaying of the carina (asterisk).

The mediastinum on CT

Mediastinal anatomy is optimally evaluated on axial CT images. The normal mediastinal CT landmarks are illustrated in the following series of images (Fig. 2.9; also see the key on p33).

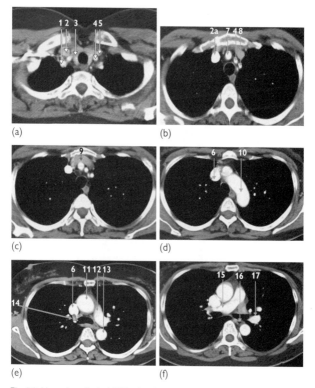

Fig. 2.9 Normal mediastinal CT landmarks.

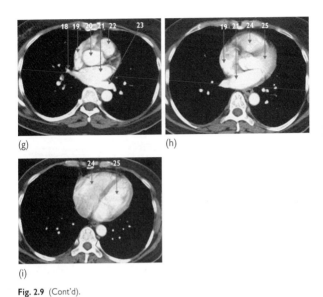

(g) (h)

(i)

Fig. 2.9 (Cont'd).

Key

1 Right subclavian artery	13 Descending aorta
2 Right internal jugular vein	14 (Partially-opacified) azygos vein
2a Right brachiocephalic vein	15 Right main pulmonary artery
3 Right lobe of thyroid	16 Oesophagus
4 Left common carotid artery	17 Left descending pulmonary artery
5 Left internal jugular vein	18 Right superior pulmonary vein
6 Superior vena cava	19 Right atrium
7 Brachiocephalic (innominate) artery	20 Aortic root
8 Left subclavian artery	21 Left atrium
9 Left brachiocephalic vein	22 Pulmonary outflow tract
10 Aortic arch	23 Left superior pulmonary vein
11 Ascending aorta	24 Right ventricle
12 Left main pulmonary artery	25 Left ventricle

Airways and vessels

Airway and vessel anatomy on CXR

- The central airways (i.e. trachea and right and left main bronchi) are usually visible on CXR; however, in general, the lobar and more distal (segmental/subsegmental) bronchi are only optimally visible on CT. The one exception is the anterior segmental bronchus of the upper lobes which, due to its 'end-on' orientation relative to the x-ray beam, is readily seen on a frontal CXR (Fig. 2.10).

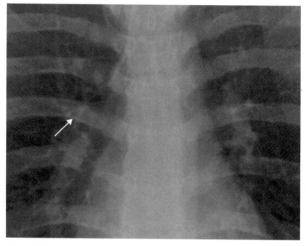

Fig. 2.10 The anterior segmental bronchi of the right upper lobe (arrow) on CXR.

- Vessels are seen as linear branching structures in the lungs. Vessels are rendered visible on CXR by the presence of air in adjacent alveoli.
- In the erect position, blood flow to the bases is greater than that to the apices; accordingly, the diameter of vessels at the lung base is greater than at the apex.
- Pulmonary vessels (arteries and veins) taper gradually from the centre to the periphery. It is usually not possible to distinguish arteries from veins in the outer two-thirds of the lungs on a CXR. However, because the arteries are coupled with airways in bronchovascular bundles, this distinction is straightforward on CT.
- Centrally, arteries and veins have a different orientation which can be recognized on a frontal CXR. In the upper lobes, both arteries and veins show a vertical orientation, but the upper lobe veins lie lateral to the arteries.

Airway anatomy at CT

The central and peripheral (segmental and subsegmental) airways are well demonstrated at CT.

Trachea

- The trachea extends from the inferior margin of the cricoid cartilage to the carina and is comprised of C-shaped cartilages.
- The cartilages are connected posteriorly by the membranous wall of the trachea, which lacks cartilage. During forced expiration, there is normal anterior bulging of the posterior membrane (Fig. 2.11). On axial CT images, taken at full inspiration, the normal tracheal lumen most commonly demonstrates a round or oval shape.
- The trachea is generally midline in position, but it is often displaced slightly to the right at the level of the aortic arch.

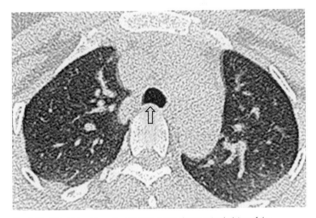

Fig. 2.11 CT obtained in end-expiration shows the anterior bulging of the posterior tracheal membrane (open arrow).

Anatomical variants of the central airways
- Tracheal or pig bronchus (Fig. 2.12).
  - A segment of the right upper lobe or the entire right upper lobe bronchus arises from the right tracheal wall above the carina.
  - Incidence ranges between 0.1 and 5%.
  - Usually an incidental finding but recognized associations include other bronchopulmonary anomalies, tracheal stenosis and Down's syndrome.
- Common origin of the right upper and middle lobe bronchi.
- Accessory cardiac bronchus.
  - A supernumerary bronchus arising from the medial aspect of the right main or intermediate bronchus proximal to the origin of the right apical segmental airway of the lower lobe.
  - Passes inferiorly and medially towards the heart.
  - The anomalous airway may be blind-ending or supply a small ventilated lobule.
  - An important anomaly because it is a rare cause of haemoptysis (when the small 'sump' becomes infected).
- Bridging bronchus.
  - A right lower lobe bronchus arising from the left main bronchus which crosses the mediastinum to reach the right lung.
  - Very rare.

Main bronchi
- The main bronchi arise from the trachea at the level of the carina and course obliquely to the axial plane.
- The right main bronchus is relatively short and usually about 1.1cm in length, compared with 5cm for the left main bronchus.
- On axial images, the shape of the left main bronchus is typically elliptical.

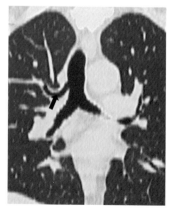

Fig. 2.12 Coronal CT illustrating a tracheal bronchus (arrow).

Segmental and subsegmental bronchi
- Segmental bronchial anatomy is readily identified on axial and multiplanar CT (Fig. 2.13 [see 'Key', page 39]).
- Normal subsegmental airways are not visible in the peripheral 2cm of the lung.

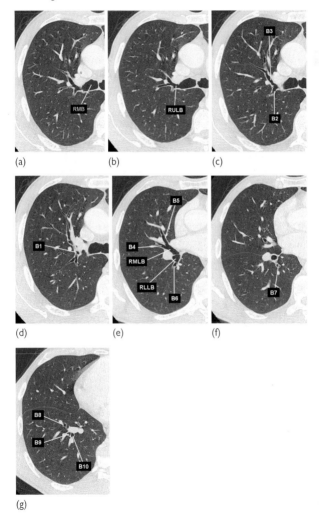

Fig. 2.13 Segmental bronchial anatomy on CT: (a–g) airways in the right lung and (h–p) showing airways in the left lung.

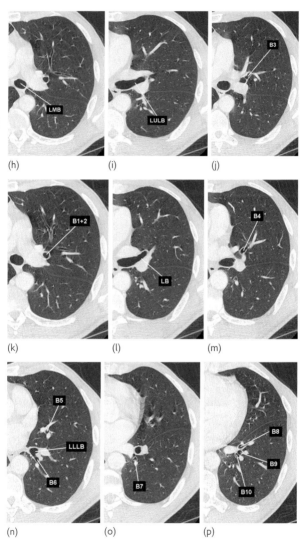

(h)

(i)

(j)

(k)

(l)

(m)

(n)

(o)

(p)

Fig. 2.13 (Cont'd).

Key:

Trachea (T)

Right-sided bronchial anatomy	Left-sided bronchial anatomy
(RMB) Right main bronchus	(LMB) Left main bronchus
(RULB) Right upper lobe bronchus	(LULB) Left upper lobe bronchus
(B1) Apical segmental bronchus	(B1 and B2) Apicoposterior segmental bronchus
(B2) Posterior segmental bronchus	(B3) Anterior segmental bronchus
(B3) Anterior segmental bronchus	
(RMLB) Right middle lobe bronchus	(LB) Lingular bronchus
(B4) Lateral segmental bronchus	(B4) Superior segmental bronchus
(B5) Medial segmental bronchus	(B5) Inferior segmental bronchus
(RLLB) Right lower lobe bronchus	(LLLB) Left lower lobe bronchus
(B6) Apical segmental bronchus	(B6) Apical segmental bronchus
(B7) Medial basal segmental bronchus	*(B7) Medial basal segmental bronchus
(B8) Anterior basal segmental bronchus	*(B8) Anterior basal segmental bronchus
(B9) Lateral basal segmental bronchus	(B9) Lateral basal segmental bronchus
(B10) Posterior basal segmental bronchus	(B10) Posterior basal segmental bronchus

*B7 and B8 are often combined into a single bronchus supplying the anteromedial segment of the left lower lobe.

Small bronchi and bronchioles

- The segmental bronchi divide into progressively smaller airways until after 6–20 divisions they become bronchioles. The last of the purely conducting airways is known as the terminal bronchiole. Beyond the terminal bronchiole are the acini, the gas exchange units of the lungs.

Pleura

- The pleura is a serosal membrane that envelopes the lung and lines the costal surface, diaphragm, and mediastinum. Pleural anatomy is considered in detail, see 📖 Pleural diseases/Pleural anatomy, p358.
- The pleural cavity has two layers: the visceral and parietal pleura that 'meet' at the hilum.
- The normal pleura is not visible on CXR (except in the fissures). On CT, the normal pleura appears as a 1–2mm smooth stripe lining the intercostal spaces between adjacent ribs (Fig. 2.14). This 'intercostal stripe' comprises the two pleural layers, extrapleural fat, the endothoracic fascia, and the innermost intercostal muscles (Fig. 2.14). The normal pleura is not visible where rib cortices are seen in parallel; the implication is that when pleura is visible, it is abnormally thickened.

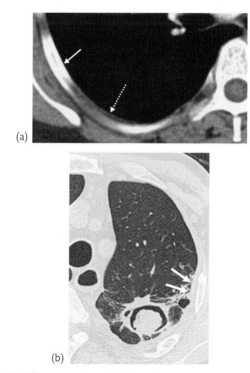

(a)

(b)

Fig. 2.14 (a) The intercostal stripe (dashed arrow) is seen in the intercostal spaces between adjacent ribs. Where the ribs cortices are in parallel (solid arrow), the pleura is not visible. (b) Targeted CT shows pleural thickening in a patient with a left apical aspergilloma; there is pleural thickening seen along the inner aspect of the rib where its cortices are in parallel (arrows).

Fissures

- Fissures consist of a double layer of visceral pleura. The fissures are demonstrated on CXR only when they are oriented tangential to the x-ray beam, appearing as 'hairlines' of soft tissue density.
- The major/oblique fissure separates the upper lobe from the lower lobe on the left, and the upper and middle lobes from the lower lobe on the right.
- The oblique fissures are seen on a lateral CXR where they are projected over each other and not always seen in their entirety (Fig. 2.15). The major fissures are well seen on HRCT, appearing as well-defined lines, extending to the chest wall.
- The minor or horizontal fissure extends forward and laterally from the right hilum and separates the right upper from the middle lobe. The fissure is visible as a thin line on frontal (Fig. 2.16) and lateral CXRs. On axial CT images, depending on its orientation to the plane of section and section thickness, there may be a curvilinear line or an ill-defined avascular band denoting the fissure.
- The azygos fissure is the most common accessory fissure and contains the azygos vein in its lower margin. The fissure results from failure of normal migration of the azygos vein from the chest wall through the right upper lobe to its position in the tracheobronchial angle. The invaginated visceral and parietal pleura persist to form a fissure. The fissure produces a curvilinear opacity which extends from the chest wall, crossing the right upper lobe obliquely to its normal position in the angle between the trachea and the right main bronchus (Fig. 2.17). The lung 'encapsulated' by the azygos fissure is termed the azygos lobe.

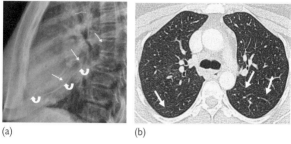

(a)   (b)

Fig. 2.15 (a) Oblique fissures on a lateral CXR. The left oblique fissure (straight line arrows) is steeper than the right. The right oblique fissure (curved arrows) terminates more anteriorly. (b) Oblique fissures seen on CT at the level of the carina (arrows) separating the upper lobes from the apical segments of the lower lobes.

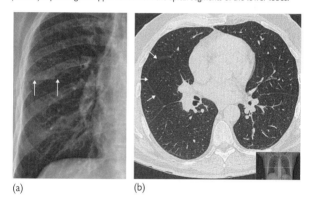

(a)   (b)

Fig. 2.16 (a) Horizontal fissure—seen clearly because of a patch of consolidation above the fissure (arrows) in the anterior segment of the upper lobe. (b) On CT, in a different patient, part of the horizontal fissure is seen (arrows).

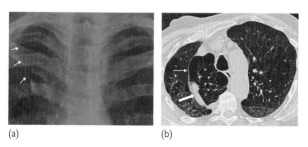

(a)   (b)

Fig. 2.17 (a) CXR shows an azygos fissure (arrows). (b)The azygos vein on CT (thick arrow) ultimately drains into the superior vena cava and is seen in the azygos fissure (thin arrow). The vein is distended in this patient with cardiac failure (thick arrow).

Diaphragm

- On a frontal CXR, taken at full inspiration, the top of the right hemidiaphragm is at the level of the anterior sixth rib and is usually no more than 1.5–2.5cm higher than the left.
- Partial incomplete muscularization (eventration) of the diaphragm is relatively common and usually regarded as a normal variant. Eventration typically affects the anteromedial portion of the right hemidiaphragm. Radiographically, there is elevation of the affected part of the diaphragm, with a smooth 'hump' of the contour of the diaphragm (Fig. 2.18). Partial eventrations are more common on the right whereas complete eventration is more often seen on the left.

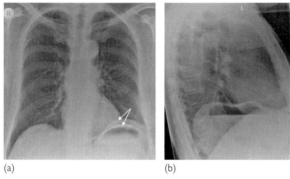

(a)   (b)

Fig. 2.18 (a) CXR demonstrating a double contour to the outline of the left hemidiaphragm (arrows). (b) The lateral view confirms this to be an eventration.

Pulmonary interstitium

The lung is supported by a network of connective tissue fibres termed the interstitium. The interstitium is organized into three fibre systems as follows:

- Peribronchovascular
- Subpleural
- Intralobular

Together these form a continuous fibre skeleton that serves to support lung parenchyma from the hila centrally to the pleural surfaces peripherally.

Peribronchovascular interstitium

A system of fibres that surrounds bronchi and pulmonary arteries and supports the core structures of the lungs. In the parahilar regions, the peribronchovascular interstitium forms a strong connective tissue sheath that surrounds large bronchi and arteries. The peribronchovascular interstitium extends to the lung periphery investing centrilobular arteries and bronchioles and continues to the level of the alveolar ducts and sacs.

Subpleural interstitium

Located beneath the visceral pleura and enveloping the lung in a fibrous sac from which connective tissue (interlobular) septa penetrate the lung parenchyma (see pulmonary lobule). These septa are most often seen in areas where they are best developed (i.e. at the apices anteriorly, along the mediastinal pleural surfaces and over the surfaces of the diaphragm).

Intralobular interstitium

A network of thin fibres forming a fine connective tissue mesh in the walls of the alveoli and bridging the gap between the peribronchovascular interstitium and the interlobular septa and subpleural interstitium.

Pulmonary lobule

The smallest lung unit bounded by interlobular septa (Fig. 2.19):

- Pulmonary lobules are irregularly polyhedral in shape and vary in size, measuring from 1–2.5cm in diameter.
- Each lobule is supplied by a small bronchiole and its accompanying pulmonary arterial branch. The lobule is marginated by connective tissue interlobular septa in which run the pulmonary veins and lymphatics.
- On HRCT, a linear, branching, or dot-like opacity is seen in the centre of a lobule or within 1cm of the pleural surface representing the centrilobular artery branch (Fig. 2.19). The complete septal margins of a few pulmonary lobules may be visible in the normal lung on HRCT.

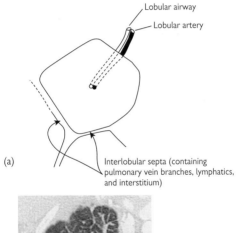

(a)

Lobular airway

Lobular artery

Interlobular septa (containing pulmonary vein branches, lymphatics, and interstitium)

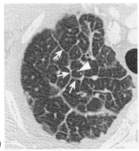

(b)

Fig. 2.19 (a) Diagramatic representation of the secondary lobule showing the central position of the lobular artery and airway with the veins and lymphatics running in the periphery within interlobular septa. (b) Targeted HRCT through the right upper lobe in a patient with lymphangitis carcinomatosis (caused by breast cancer). There are thickened interlobular septa (thin arrows). The centrilobular artery (arrowhead) is visible as a dot at the centre of the lobule but the accompanying airway is not seen because the thin-wall is not resolved.

Importance of the pulmonary lobule in diagnosis of lung disease

Knowledge of the anatomy of the pulmonary lobule and specifically, the distribution of disease in relation to the components of the lobule is of considerable value in CT diagnosis. Examples of conditions that highlight the anatomy of the pulmonary lobule are shown (Figs. 2.20–2.26). The lobular distribution of disease may be characterized as:

• Centrilobular
• Interlobular
• Perilobular
• Panlobular

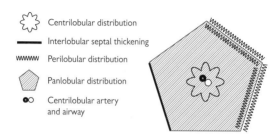

Centrilobular distribution

Interlobular septal thickening

Perilobular distribution

Panlobular distribution

Centrilobular artery and airway

Fig. 2.20 Distribution of pathology within the pulmonary lobule.

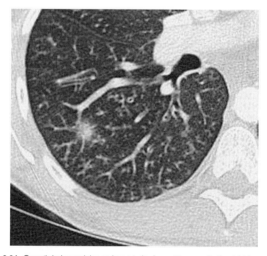

Fig. 2.21 Centrilobular nodules and tree-in-bud opacities seen in the right lower lobe in a patient with common variable immunodeficiency.

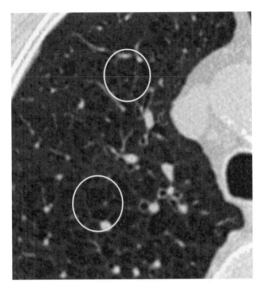

Fig. 2.22 Centrilobular emphysema seen on CT in which the areas of low attenuation are centred around the centrilobular core structures (rings).

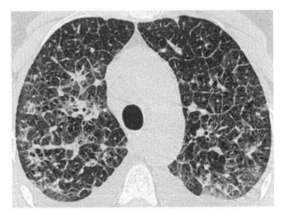

Fig. 2.23 Smooth interlobular septal thickening in a patient with pulmonary oedema.

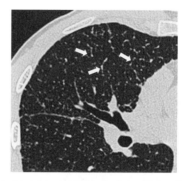

Fig. 2.24 Nodular interlobular septal thickening (arrows) in sarcoidosis.

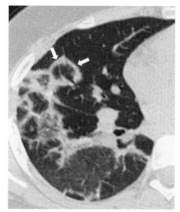

Fig. 2.25 Perilobular pattern in cryptogenic organizing pneumonia. The fuzzy perilobular opacity (arrows) affects both sides of the interlobular septa.

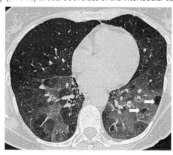

Fig. 2.26 Lobular air trapping (areas of low attenuation [arrows]) seen on CT obtained in end-expiration in subacute hypersensitivity pneumonitis.

Chapter 3

Common terms used in thoracic radiology reports

Consolidation

An homogeneous increase in lung parenchymal density which *obscures* vessels and airway walls (cf. ground-glass opacification) (Figs. 3.1–3.3). An air bronchogram/bronchiologram may be visible. At a pathological level, any process which occupies the air spaces with material can give rise to this pattern.

Causes of consolidation on CXR/CT

* Infection—bacterial, mycobacterial, protozoal, fungal, parasitic, or viral
* Organizing pneumonia—cryptogenic or otherwise
* Intra-alveolar haemorrhage—e.g. idiopathic pulmonary haemosiderosis, antiglomerular basement membrane disease, vasculitides, infarction
* Cancer—disseminated adenocarcinoma and lymphoma
* Eosinophilic lung disease
* Oedema—cardiogenic or non-cardiogenic
* Sarcoidosis—relatively uncommon pattern reflecting marked interstitial expansion by granulomas

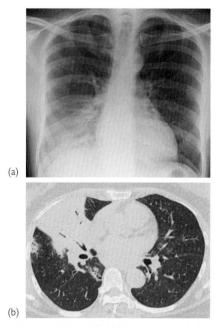

(a)

(b)

Fig. 3.1 Consolidation on CXR and CT. (a) PA projection showing increased opacification in the right lower zone which obscures vessel markings (contrast this with the visibility of vessels in other zones). (b) Consolidation in the middle lobe on CT in a different patient; vessel markings are not visible but air is easily seen in patent airways (giving rise to an 'air bronchogram').

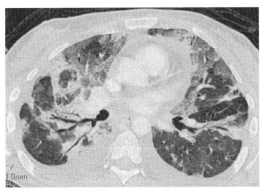

Fig. 3.2 Patchy bilateral consolidation (and ground-glass opacification) caused by Epstein–Barr virus infection following haematopoetic stem cell transplantation.

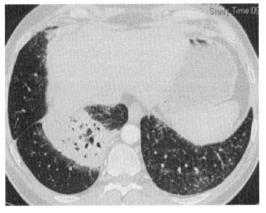

Fig. 3.3 Consolidation in a patient with sarcoidosis. There is dense opacification in the right lower lobe which obscures vessel markings. In sarcoidosis, this appearance is due to gross thickening of the interstitium.

Ground-glass opacification

On CXR, ground-glass opacification is a hazy increased density, through which the margins of the pulmonary vessels appear indistinct. The increased density may be localized or generalized (Fig. 3.4). In contrast, on CT, ground-glass density is defined as hazy increased attenuation of lung but with preservation of bronchial and vascular margins (Fig. 3.5) (as opposed to consolidation, in which these margins are obscured). At a microscopic level, ground-glass opacification is caused by partial filling of airspaces, interstitial thickening (due to fluid, cells, and/or fibrosis), partial collapse of alveoli, increased capillary blood volume, or a combination of these. The key factor in these different pathological processes is the partial displacement of air.

Causes of ground-glass opacification

- Pulmonary oedema
- Pulmonary haemorrhage
- Atypical infections (e.g. *Pneumocystis jiroveci*, cytomegalovirus)
- Drug toxicity
- Radiation pneumonitis
- Acute respiratory distress syndrome and acute interstitial pneumonia
- Adenocarcinoma
- Hypersensitivity pneumonitis
- Respiratory bronchiolitis-interstitial lung disease
- Non-specific interstitial pneumonia
- Desquamative interstitial pneumonia
- Sarcoidosis
- Lymphoid interstitial pneumonia
- Eosinophilic pneumonia

Ground-glass opacification not caused by disease

Because increased lung density can be caused by any process which partially displaces air from the lungs, ground-glass opacification is seen in some physiological (non-disease) states: the simplest example is the CT examination performed at or near residual volume (Fig. 3.6). A relative absence of air (due to the inability to expand the lungs fully) is the likely cause of ground-glass opacification in obese individuals (Fig. 3.7). Increased parenchymal density is also a feature of normal lungs in infants and young children by comparison with adults because there are fewer alveoli in the developing lung. Contrast administration can cause (unpredictably) a diffuse increase in lung density and, finally, inappropriate window settings will lead to a spurious appearance of ground-glass opacification on CT.

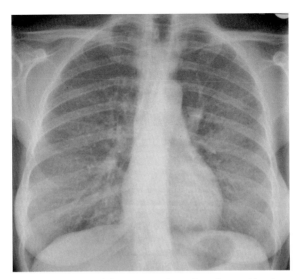

Fig. 3.4 Generalized ground-glass opacity on chest radiography caused by subacute hypersensitivity pneumonitis. Note the indistinct pulmonary vessels.

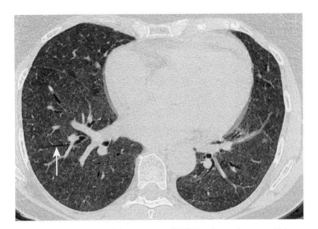

Fig. 3.5 Widespread ground glass opacity on HRCT in subacute hypersensitivity pneumonitis. There is increased conspicuity of the large airways because of the 'black' air (arrow) in the lumen contrasting with the ground-glass opacification in the surrounding lung. The bronchovascular margins are not obscured.

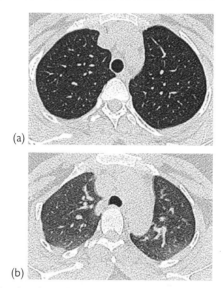

(a)

(b)

Fig. 3.6 Physiological ground-glass opacification. Images taken (a) at full inspiration and (b) end-expiration. There is increased density (ground-glass opacification) on expiration.

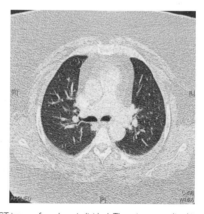

Fig. 3.7 HRCT image of an obese individual. There is a generalized increased lung density which may be (erroneously) interpreted as uniform diffuse lung disease.

Reticular pattern

On CXR, a reticular pattern is seen as innumerable interlacing linear opacities resembling a 'net' (Fig. 3.8). The finding usually represents established interstitial lung disease. The lines may be fine or coarse. CT more readily demonstrates the interlacing lines of a reticular pattern and this may be due to interlobular septal thickening, thickened intralobular lines, or the cyst walls of honeycombing (Fig. 3.9). NB Honeycombing and a reticular pattern may coexist but the terms are not synonymous.

Causes of a reticular pattern

Fibrotic lung diseases
Upper zone predominant:
- Sarcoidosis
- Post-tuberculosis
- Occupational lung diseases
- Post-fungal infection

Lower zone predominant:
- Idiopathic pulmonary fibrosis
- Asbestosis
- Connective tissue disease-related fibrosis
- Drug-induced fibrosis
- Hypersensitivity pneumonitis

Miscellaneous causes
- Langerhans' cell histiocytosis
- Lymphangioleiomyomatosis
- (Interstitial) oedema
- Lymphangitis carcinomatosis

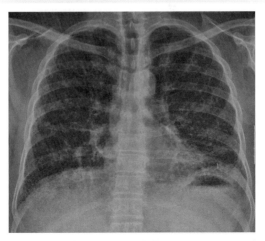

Fig. 3.8 A reticular pattern, most marked in the lower zones, in a patient with idiopathic pulmonary fibrosis.

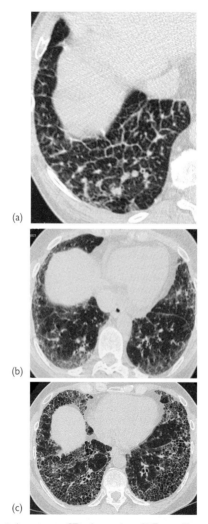

(a)

(b)

(c)

Fig. 3.9 A reticular pattern on CT in three patients. (a) Targeted image through the right lower lobe shows a reticular pattern caused by lymphangitis carcinomatosis: there are thickened interlobular septa in the right lower lobe. (b) CT through the lower zones in non-specific interstitial pneumonia; there is a fine reticular pattern and ground-glass opacification. (c) A coarse reticular pattern with honeycombing in a patient with usual interstitial pneumonia.

Honeycombing

Honeycombing refers to the cystic spaces seen in fibrotic and various lung diseases at an advanced stage. On CXR, honeycombing is seen as multiple cystic spaces (measuring 3–10mm in diameter) with thickened (1.0–3.0mm) walls (Fig. 3.10). On CT, honeycombing manifests as clustered cystic air spaces (usually subpleural) with a diameter of 3–10mm (Fig. 3.11). Honeycomb cysts may be difficult to distinguish from dilated airways in areas of fibrotic lung (see 📖 Radiological terms/ Traction bronchiectasis/bronchiolectasis, p75).

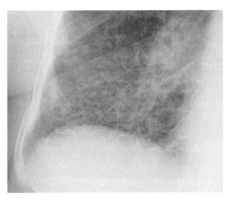

Fig. 3.10 Targeted CXR showing honeycomb cysts and reticulation in the right lower lobe in a patient with mixed connective tissue disease and UIP.

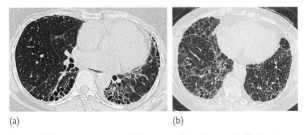

(a)   (b)

Fig. 3.11 CT in two patients with a UIP pattern of lung fibrosis. (a) CT through the lower lobes shows honeycomb destruction in a subpleural distribution. (b) Honeycombing is present in the lower lobes but some of the cystic spaces are probably dilated airways ('traction bronchiectasis') caused by fibrosis.

Nodules and nodular pattern

A nodule is a rounded opacity on CXR or CT, which may be well or poorly defined and measuring up to 3cm in diameter (Fig. 3.12). (NB lesions larger than 3cm in diameter are termed 'masses'.) Nodules can be sub-classified based largely on their appearance on CT:

- Micronodule—a rounded opacity measuring up to 3mm in diameter.
- Centrilobular nodule—a rounded opacity (of soft-tissue or ground-glass attenuation) which is usually ill-defined because of the localization; individual centrilobular nodules appear separated from adjacent nodules by normal intervening lung parenchyma.
- Non-solid nodule—an opacity composed, at least partially, of ground-glass attenuation.
- Solitary pulmonary nodule—(see also 📖 Lung tumours/Solitary pulmonary nodule or mass, p349). A single rounded opacity, usually of soft-tissue attenuation (± calcification).

A nodular pattern on CXR/CT is one in which there are *innumerable* small rounded opacities that are discrete and range in diameter from 2mm to 10mm. CT may allow distinction between a centrilobular, peri-lymphatic, or randomly-distributed nodular pattern.

Causes of pulmonary nodules

- Granulomatous—tuberculous, fungal
- Neoplastic—benign (e.g. hamartoma), malignant (e.g. lung cancer, metastases, carcinoid, lymphoma)
- Inflammatory—infection (e.g. abscess, hydatid), Wegener's granulomatosis, organizing pneumonia, amyloid, sarcoidosis, rheumatoid arthritis
- Miscellaneous—intrapulmonary lymph node, bronchogenic cyst

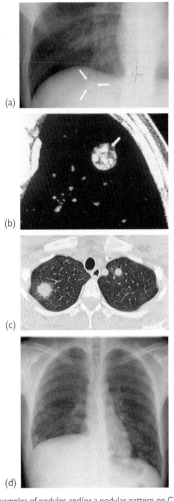

Fig. 3.12 Four examples of nodules and/or a nodular pattern on CXR and CT.
(a) Right lower lobe lung cancer. Targeted image of the right lower lobe shows
a well-defined 1.5cm diameter non-calcified nodule (arrows). (b) Targeted
prone CT through the right lower lobe showing a benign hamartoma; there are
amorphous foci of calcification and areas of low attenuation (arrow) indicating fat.
(c) Angioinvasive aspergillosis in a neutropenic patient following haematopoetic
stem cell transplantation; CT through the upper zones demonstrates two focal
nodules and (d) multiple soft-tissue density nodules in the lower zones bilaterally
caused by metastasis from a known hepatocellular carcinoma; the elevation of the
right hemidiaphragm was secondary to hepatomegaly.

Thickened interlobular septa and intralobular lines

Interlobular septal thickening

- The interlobular septa form the boundaries of the pulmonary lobule (see 📖 Key radiological anatomy/Pulmonary lobule, p45). These connective tissue septa are about 0.1mm thick and form part of the peripheral supporting structure of the lung.
- The pulmonary veins and lymphatics run in the interlobular septa.
- Normal interlobular septa are generally not visible on CXR but may be seen on HRCT.
- Pathological processes that lead to lymphatic or venous congestion or infiltration render the interlobular septa visible.
- On CXR, thickened septa appear as short (1–2cm in length), peripheral, horizontal thin lines perpendicular to and in contact with the lateral pleura (Fig 3.13), most easily seen at the lung bases (formerly called Kerley B lines) or as longer lines (2–6cm; Kerley A) in the upper zones radially-oriented from the hila. NB The terms septal thickening and septal lines are preferred to the eponymous Kerley lines.
- On CT, the boundaries of the individual pulmonary lobules are clearly demarcated by thickened interlobular septa, most often visible at the lung apices and bases (Fig. 3.14); thickening of the interlobular septa may be smooth or nodular (Fig. 3.15).

Causes of thickened interlobular septa

- Cardiogenic pulmonary oedema
- Lymphangitis carcinomatosis—typically causes nodular/irregular thickening of the interlobular septa
- Sarcoidosis—also nodular but often limited in extent
- Pulmonary veno-occlusive disease
- Septal amyloidosis
- Lipoid pneumonia
- Lymphoid interstitial pneumonia
- Leukaemic infiltration
- Amyloidosis
- Alveolar microlithiasis
- Diffuse pulmonary lymphangiomatosis
- Congential lymphangiectasia
- Rare storage diseases (e.g. Erdheim–Chester disease)

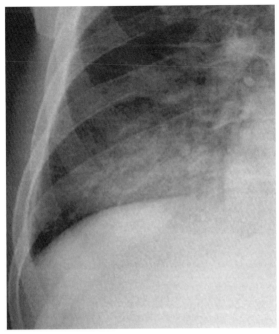

Fig. 3.13 Targeted image of the right lower zone in a patient with cardiogenic pulmonary oedema and septal thickening (short horizontal lines) demonstrated at the right base.

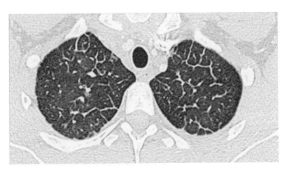

Fig. 3.14 Smooth bilateral interlobular septal thickening at the apices on HRCT in a patient with cardiogenic pulmonary oedema.

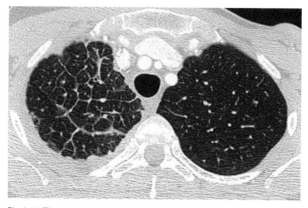

Fig. 3.15 Thickened interlobular septa in the right upper lobe caused by lymphangitis carcinomatosis, in a patient with known breast cancer.

Intralobular lines

- Intralobular lines are fine linear opacities in a lobule, rendered visible when interstitial tissue is abnormally thickened. Where this is extensive, they may appear as a very fine reticular pattern.
- Intralobular lines may be seen in various conditions, including any cause of interstitial fibrosis.
- Often thickened intralobular lines may be so fine that HRCT does not demonstrate discrete lines but a generalized increase in lung density (ground-glass opacification).

Tree-in-bud pattern

A descriptive term referring to the presence of centrilobular branching structures on HRCT; this appearance is likened to that of a 'budding tree'. The pattern most commonly (but not exclusively) reflects pathology in, and around, the peripheral airways; inflammatory exudate and inflammation in the walls of the small airways are responsible for this CT pattern. Depending on the orientation of the airways with respect to the plane of the CT section, there may be small nodules, 'V-shaped', 'Y-shaped' or branching linear opacities (Fig. 3.16). Because of the limited contrast resolution and summation, a tree-in-bud pattern is not seen on CXR.

Causes of a tree-in-bud pattern on CT

- Idiopathic—(Japanese) diffuse panbronchiolitis
- Infection (due to endobronchial spread)—bacterial, mycobacterial (tuberculous and non-tuberculous), fungal (e.g. airway-invasive aspergillosis), viral (e.g. cytomegalovirus or respiratory syncytial virus)
- Genetic/immunological—cystic fibrosis (± other causes of bronchiectasis), allergic bronchopulmonary aspergillosis, rheumatoid arthritis, Sjögren's syndrome
- Miscellaneous—recurrent aspiration, toxic fume inhalation

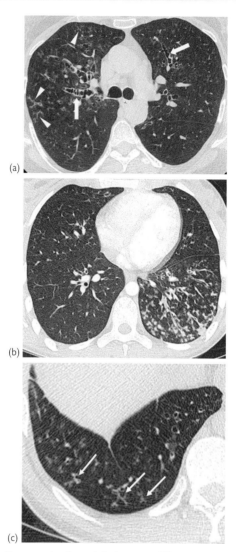

Fig. 3.16 Three examples of a tree-in-bud pattern on CT in patients with (a) allergic bronchopulmonary aspergillosis; there are peripheral branching 'V' and 'Y' shaped opacities (arrowheads). Central varicose bronchiectasis is also present (arrows) in the upper lobes; (b) localized left lower lobe bronchiectasis and (c) cystic fibrosis; targeted image through the right lower lobe shows a delicate tree-in-bud pattern (thin arrows).

Atelectasis and collapse

Atelectasis is defined as decreased inflation of all or part of the lung. Although often used interchangeably, the term collapse is ideally reserved for complete atelectasis but, common to both, is the reduced inflation of lung. Radiological collapse and atelectasis are distinguished from consolidation by the presence of *volume loss* and, where possible, the phrase 'collapse-consolidation' should be avoided. The severity of collapse or atelectasis ranges from:

- An entire lung, leading to a complete 'white-out' (Fig. 3.17).
- An entire lobe (Figs. 3.18–3.20).
- A segment or subsegment of lung (Fig. 3.21).

Miscellaneous causes of collapse and atelectasis may be subdivided according to whether or not there is an obstructive lesion:

Causes of atelectasis/collapse

- **Obstruction of a supplying bronchus**
  - Intrinsic (e.g. lung cancer, mucus plug or inhaled foreign body)
  - Extrinsic (e.g. hilar lymph node enlargement, mediastinal masses/fibrosis or cardiac enlargement).
- **Non-obstructive**
  - Passive (e.g. due to pneumothorax)
  - Compressive (e.g. due to mass or pleural effusion)
  - Adhesive (discoid or linear atelectasis, usually limited extent)
  - Replacement by tumour
  - Cicatrization due to contraction of fibrous tissue (local or generalized)

Broadly, the radiological features of atelectasis can be divided into direct and indirect signs:

Radiological features of atelectasis

- **Direct**
  - Displacement of fissures
  - Crowding of bronchi and vessels.
- **Indirect**
  - Increased opacity
  - Diaphragmatic elevation
  - Mediastinal displacement
  - Compensatory overinflation of remaining lung
  - Hilar displacement.

On CXR, increased density is seen with volume loss shown by displacement of fissures, diaphragm, or mediastinal or bronchovascular structures, depending on the extent of collapse. Similar signs of volume loss are seen on CT with increased attenuation of the affected lung.

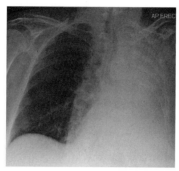

Fig. 3.17 Complete collapse of the left lung with a 'white-out' of the affected hemithorax and volume loss with mediastinal shift to the left. Volume loss is a useful sign for differentiating from other causes of a complete lung 'white-out' such as a large pleural effusion. The underlying cause in this patient was a mucus plug.

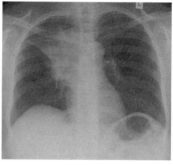

(a)

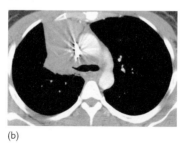

(b)

Fig. 3.18 Right upper lobe collapse caused by lung cancer. (a) CXR shows right upper lobe collapse with a convex bulge inferiorly due to an obstructing right hilar mass; the elevated horizontal fissure now has a roughly 'sigmoid' shape—called Golden S sign. (b) CT in the same patient shows narrowing of the right main bronchus and obliteration of the right upper lobe bronchus caused by a squamous cell carcinoma.

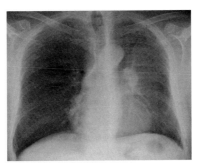

Fig. 3.19 CXR in a 71-year-old smoker shows left upper lobe collapse caused by squamous cell carcinoma. The typical veil-like increased density over the mid and upper left hemithorax and volume loss are seen.

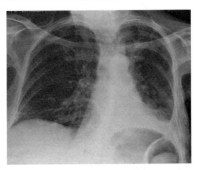

Fig. 3.20 Left lower lobe collapse with increased retrocardiac density and obscuration of the left hemidiaphragm caused by a mucus plug. Note the mediastinal shift to the left.

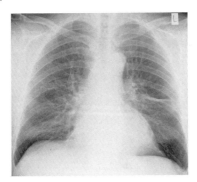

Fig. 3.21 Post-operative CXR showing an area of linear (or discoid) atelectasis in the left mid zone, a form of adhesive atelectasis secondary to hypoventilation.

Pulmonary air cysts

An air-containing space with a definable wall. The presence of a visible wall differentiates a cyst from other causes of focal decreased lung attenuation (e.g. centrilobular emphysema). Because of the two-dimensional nature of CXR, small cysts are more readily and confidently identified on HRCT. Miscellaneous causes of cysts are listed and illustrated (Figs. 3.22–3.25).

Causes of pulmonary air cysts

- Lymphangioleiomyomatosis (LAM)
- Langerhans' cell histiocytosis
- Post-infective pneumatocoeles
- Honeycomb lung
- Lymphoid interstitial pneumonia
- Tracheobronc hial papillomatosis
- Age-related

Miscellaneous rare causes:

Hydatid disease, sarcoidosis, hypersensitivity pneumonitis, desquamative interstitial pneumonia, Birt-Hogg-Dubé syndrome, cystic fibrohistiocytic tumour.

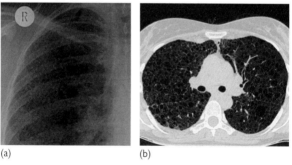

(a)   (b)

Fig. 3.22 Lymphangioleiomyomatosis on (a) targeted CXR and (b) CT showing numerous small, uniform cysts typical of LAM.

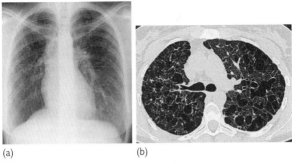

(a)   (b)

Fig. 3.23 Langerhans' cell histiocytosis. (a) CXR demonstrates fine reticulation (caused by multiple superimposed cysts) and (b) CT in which cysts are irregularly shaped. Both hilar points are raised on the CXR, reflecting upper lobe volume loss.

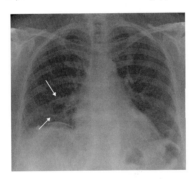

Fig. 3.24 CXR demonstrates a thin walled cystic structure (pneumatocele; arrows) in a patient with a past history of staphylococcal pneumonia.

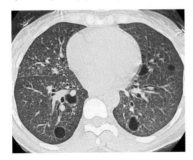

Fig. 3.25 Thin walled cysts and small nodules in a patient with lymphoid interstitial pneumonia.

Crazy-paving pattern

This CT pattern refers to the presence of relatively sharply-demarcated ('geographical') areas of ground-glass opacification within which there is interlobular septal thickening and intralobular lines (Fig. 3.26). The pattern was first reported in the context of pulmonary alveolar proteinosis and, in its classical form, is virtually pathognomonic of that diagnosis. Other conditions which, at least superficially, give rise to this CT appearance are recognized and listed in the box.

> **Causes of a crazy-paving pattern**
>
> - Pulmonary alveolar proteinosis
> - Lipoid pneumonia
> - Adenocarcinoma
> - Non-cardiogenic pulmonary oedema—diffuse alveolar damage (as seen in acute respiratory distress syndrome, acute interstitial pneumonia)
> - *Pneumocystis jiroveci* pneumonia
> - Pulmonary haemorrhage
> - Drug-induced toxicity
> - Non-specific interstitial pneumonia

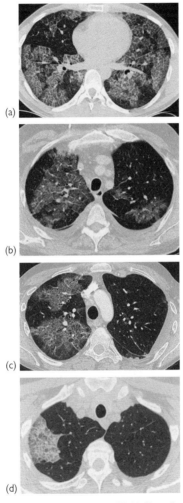

Fig. 3.26 Examples of a crazy-paving pattern on CT. (a) 'Classical' crazy-paving in a patient with pulmonary alveolar proteinosis. There are bilateral patchy ground-glass opacities in which there are thickened interlobular septa and intralobular lines. Areas of abnormal lung are sharply-demarcated from normal lung. (b) Pulmonary haemorrhage. (c) Unilateral pulmonary oedema in a known IV drug-abuser. The appearances largely resolved within 24 hrs. (d) Axial CT of a patient with bacterial pneumonia. There is a localized crazy-paving pattern in the right upper lobe which resolved with antibiotic treatment.

Mosaic attenuation pattern

This is a descriptive term that refers to a CT pattern comprising a 'patch-work' of regions of differing attenuation (put simply, areas of 'black and grey' lung).

Categories of causes of a mosaic attenuation pattern on CT

- Obliterative small-airways disease (e.g. obliterative bronchiolitis)
- Chronic occlusive vascular disease (e.g. chronic thromboembolic disease)
- Patchy infiltrative/interstitial disease (e.g. desquamative interstitial pneumonia, pulmonary haemorrhage)

Differentiating between causes of a mosaic attenuation pattern

Distinguishing between the different causes is not always straightforward on CT (Figs. 3.27–3.30), but features that may aid the interpretation of this pattern are listed below:

- A paucity in the number and/or a reduction in the calibre of vessels within the areas of black (low attenuation) lung indicates that the black lung is abnormal.
- The grey lung is abnormal if there is no disparity in the size of pulmonary vessels between the grey and black lung.
- In chronic occlusive vascular disease there may be dilation of the central (main and segmental) pulmonary arteries.
- In small airways disease, there is usually some dilatation (often minor) of the macroscopic bronchi in addition to the reduction in calibre of vessels within the abnormal black lung. Additionally, there is air-trapping on CT images performed at end-expiration.

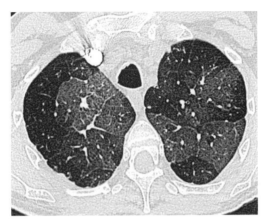

Fig. 3.27 CT through the upper lobes in a patient with primary ciliary dyskinesia shows a striking mosaic attenuation pattern. There was mild cylindrical bronchiectasis in areas of 'black lung' on other sections.

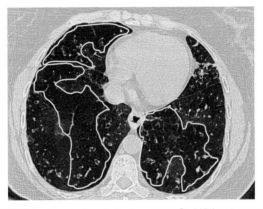

Fig. 3.28 CT in obliterative bronchiolitis. In contrast to Fig. 3.27 there is a more subtle mosaic attenuation pattern. The areas of 'black lung' (outlined in white) are abnormal. Note the reduction in pulmonary vasculature in these areas. There is evidence of mild cylindrical bronchiectasis suggesting that the areas of decreased attenuation are caused by small airways disease.

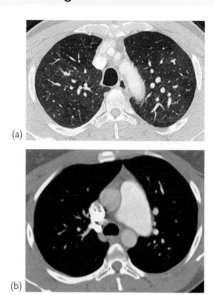

(a)

(b)

Fig. 3.29 CT in two patients with chronic thromboembolism. (a) Image through the upper lobes shows a mosaic attenuation pattern; there is a marked difference in the calibre and number of vessels between regions of black and grey lung. (b) Post-contrast CT showing dilatation of the main pulmonary artery by comparison with the transverse diameter of the ascending aorta.

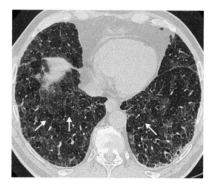

Fig. 3.30 Patchy areas of ground glass opacification are present in conjunction with lobular areas of low attenuation (arrows) in this patient with hypersensitivity pneumonitis. The areas of low attenuation are a result of small airways disease.

Traction bronchiectasis/ bronchiolectasis

Traction bronchiectasis/bronchiolectasis is defined as irreversible bronchial/bronchiolar dilatation caused by surrounding retractile fibrosis. This CT sign is an important ancillary finding in many fibrosing lung diseases (Fig. 3.31). Depending on the orientation of the airway relative to the plane of scanning, differentiation from surrounding honeycomb cysts may be difficult particularly if the typical branching structure of the airways cannot be identified (Fig. 3.32). Traction bronchiectasis/bronchiolectasis is seen on a background of abnormal lung (usually a reticular pattern or ground-glass opacification).

Conditions in which traction bronchiectasis/ bronchiolectasis occurs

- Usual interstitial pneumonia
- Non-specific interstitial pneumonia
- Chronic hypersensitivity pneumonitis
- Asbestosis
- Sarcoidosis
- Drug-induced fibrosis
- Post-infectious fibrosis (e.g. following tuberculosis)
- Organizing pneumonia (fibrosing variant)

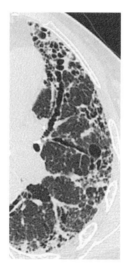

Fig. 3.31 Severe traction bronchiectasis in the left upper lobe anteriorly on HRCT in a patient with idiopathic pulmonary fibrosis. Note the irregular airway dilatation.

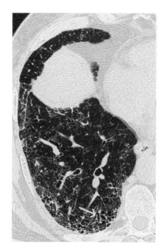

Fig. 3.32 A patient with idiopathic pulmonary fibrosis shows traction bronchiolectasis (arrow) amongst honeycombing. The branching nature of the airway allows the distinction from adjacent honeycomb cysts.

Emphysema

Emphysema is defined histopathologically as the abnormal permanent enlargement of airspaces distal to the terminal bronchiole with destruction of alveolar walls usually in the absence of 'obvious' fibrosis. On CT emphysema is seen as focal areas or regions of decreased density usually without visible walls. (Figs. 3.33–3.36). The main morphological subtypes of emphysema are:

● Centrilobular (sometimes called centriacinar)
● Paraseptal
● Panlobular (panacinar)

Recognized causes of emphysema

● Cigarette smoking (centrilobular and paraseptal)
● Marijuana smoking
● α_1-antitrypsin deficiency (panlobular or panacinar)
● HIV infection
● Dust inhalation (e.g. silicosis, rare association with hypersensitivity pneumonitis)

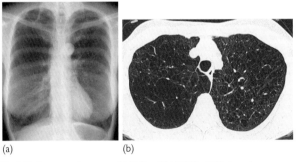

(a)   (b)

Fig. 3.33 Severe emphysema on (a) CXR and (b) CT. The CXR shows large volume lungs with flattening of the hemidiaphragms and a paucity of vessels in the upper zones (particularly on the right). The corresponding CT through the upper lobes shows extensive emphysema. There are widespread focal areas of decreased density mostly without visible walls.

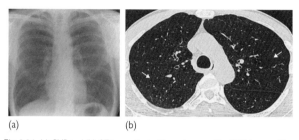

Fig. 3.34 (a) CXR and (b) CT in a patient with emphysema. The CXR is normal but on CT there are patchy ill-defined low attenuation foci in the upper zones (arrows) indicating centrilobular emphysema.

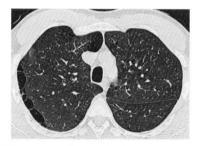

Fig. 3.35 HRCT in a 65-year-old heavy smoker showing paraseptal emphysema in the right upper lobe.

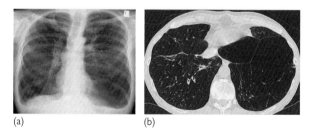

Fig. 3.36 Panacinar emphysema in a patient with homozygous α_1-antitrypsin deficiency. (a) CXR shows large volume lungs with lower zone predominant emphysema. (b) On HRCT, there is diffusely decreased attenuation in the left lower lobe and there are thin long lines indicating 'remnant' interlobular septa. Mild cylindrical bronchiectasis is present in the right lower lobe.

Bullae

A bulla is an airspace greater than 1cm in diameter, demarcated by a thin wall, no greater than 1mm thick. On CXR and CT bullae are thin-walled (<1mm thickness) focal areas of decreased attenuation (identical to air), and measuring more than 1cm in diameter (Figs. 3.37 and 3.38). Bullae are occasionally very large and distinction from a loculated pneumothorax may be almost impossible.

Principal causes of bullae

- Cigarette smoking (coexistent centrilobular and paraseptal emphysema)
- Idiopathic giant bullous disease ('vanishing lung syndrome') or destructive lung disease (e.g. pulmonary sarcoidosis or Langerhans' cell histiocytosis)
- Marijuana smoking

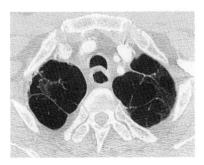

Fig. 3.37 CT through the apices in an adult smoker showing large bullae at both apices.

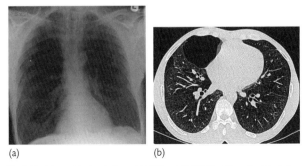

(a)   (b)

Fig. 3.38 A large right lung bulla on (a) CXR and (b) CT. The thin wall of the bulla are difficult to define on CXR but CT of the same individual clearly demonstrates a large bulla in the right middle lobe.

Air space diseases

A radiological approach to air space diseases

Diseases that principally involve the air spaces are common. Any pathological process which displaces air from the alveoli can cause a pattern of air space opacification.

A guide to reviewing the CXR in air space disease

The CXR is usually the first investigation in patients with suspected lung disease. With experience, it is usually possible to offer a short list of differential diagnoses (Table 4.1) for the cause of air space opacification on CXR. For this, the observer should pay particular attention to the following:

- Associated clinical features
- Distribution of abnormalities on CXR
- Changes on serial CXRs

Table 4.1 Causes of air space opacification on CXR

Common causes
- Infection/inflammatory diseases
- Oedema (hydrostatic or increased permeability)

Miscellaneous (less common) causes
- Eosinophilic lung disease
- Organizing pneumonia
- Adenocarcinoma
- Primary pulmonary lymphoma (MALToma)
- Sarcoidosis
- Alveolar proteinosis
- Aspiration pneumonia
- Pulmonary haemorrhage

The importance of associated clinical features

A review of the radiology together with knowledge of the clinical features may be diagnostic in some instances (Fig. 4.1):

- In a patient with pyrexia, a productive cough, and an elevated white cell count, air space opacification on a CXR is most likely to be caused by infection.
- In the context of known left ventricular dysfunction, bilateral air-space opacification is likely to represent pulmonary oedema.
- The appearance of air space opacities in a patient reporting haemoptysis is likely to reflect intra-alveolar blood.

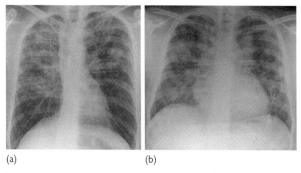

(a)   (b)

Fig. 4.1 Two patients with air space opacification on CXR. (a) Bilateral air space opacification in a patient complaining of fever, weight loss, and night sweats. The main radiological diagnosis is that of infection. Microbiological tests in this patient confirmed a diagnosis of tuberculosis. (b) Bilateral patchy air space opacities, representing blood, in a patient with haemoptysis.

The importance of the identifying the predominant distribution of disease

Recognition of the distribution of air space opacities on CXR can be also helpful (Fig. 4.2):

- In cryptogenic organizing pneumonia, the classical finding is of multifocal areas of consolidation in the peripheral and lower zones of the lung.
- In chronic eosinophilic pneumonia, the airspace opacification is typically in the upper zones and parallels the chest wall.

The importance of reviewing serial CXRs

A review of *serial* radiographs, to ascertain disease progression or regression, can be invaluable.

- Relatively rapid improvement on follow-up CXRs (sometimes occurring over a period of hours or, at most, a few days) suggests pulmonary oedema or intra-alveolar blood as the cause.
- Air space opacities that are transient and migratory may suggest the diagnosis of an eosinophilic pneumonia or cryptogenic organizing pneumonia.
- Persistent opacification in a patient who has had treatment (perhaps empiric) of the more common causes of air space opacification (e.g. infection, oedema) should start to raise the possibility of malignancy (see Table 4.1).

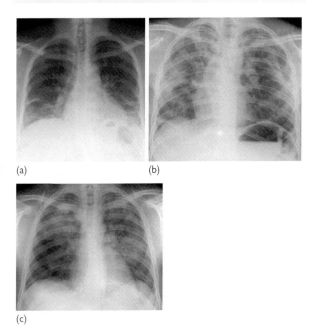

(a) (b)

(c)

Fig. 4.2 CXRs in three patients with multifocal air space opacification in whom the distribution of disease is of diagnostic value. (a) Predominant lower zone air space opacities in cryptogenic organizing pneumonia. (b) Characteristic upper zone peripheral air space opacities (which roughly parallel the chest wall) in chronic eosinophilic pneumonia. (c) Air space opacities are centrally disposed (sometimes called a 'bat's wing' distribution); this is uncommonly found in cardiogenic pulmonary oedema.

Computed tomography (CT) in air space diseases

CT may be requested in patients with a pattern of air space disease on CXR and no clear diagnosis. In some patients, CT together with the clinical information will permit a reasonably confident diagnosis to be made. However, in general, the real advantage of CT over plain CXR in the diagnosis of air space diseases is debatable.

Infectious pneumonia: general principles

Patients with a suspected lower respiratory tract infection will generally have a CXR. In addition to defining the zonal/lobar location of infection, the CXR is also useful in establishing the extent of lung involvement. Furthermore, because of the relatively low radiation burden, another important role—in contrast to CT—is that the progress of an infection can justifiably be followed on serial CXRs. In the following pages, the imaging findings of some infectious pneumonias which illustrate the general principles are considered.

Radiological signs of infection

- Consolidation (± cavitation)—this may be focal, lobar, upper zone, or lower zone; involving one whole lung or both lungs
- Ground-glass opacification
- Nodules/nodular pattern ± cavitation
- Tree-in-bud pattern
- Reticular or reticulonodular pattern
- Lymph node enlargement—hilar and/or mediastinal
- Parapneumonic effusions/empyema

CXR features of diagnostic value include

Distribution
- Upper zone opacification (e.g. *Mycobacterium tuberculosis* or fungal infection) vs lower zone (e.g. aspiration pneumonia).
- Lobar—a feature of bacterial pneumonia (e.g. Streptococcal).

Pattern of opacification and ancillary findings
- Consolidation with cavitation—Staphylococcal, *Klebsiella*, *Pseudomonas* pneumonias or mycobacterial infections.
- Consolidation with bulging of fissures—*Klebsiella, Staphylococcus*.
- Consolidation with reticulonodular opacities—viral pneumonias or mycoplasma infection.
- Large pleural effusion—usually with bacterial infections.
- Nodal enlargement.

Streptococcal (pneumococcal) pneumonia

- The commonest cause of community acquired pneumonia due to *S. pneumonia*.
- Predisposing factors: smoking, age (very young and elderly), immunosuppression, 'institutionalized' living, alcoholism, chronic cardiopulmonary disease.
- Infection is most common in children (aged <5yrs) and the elderly (aged >65yrs).

Imaging of streptococcal pneumonia

CXR findings (Fig. 4.3)

The CXR is the first investigation in patients with suspected pneumonia and is of value in follow-up. The typical CXR features include:

- Consolidation—generally non-segmental or involving entire lobe but may be multilobar and bilateral.
- Pleural effusion—ipsilateral to the consolidation.
- Cavitation —more readily appreciated on CT.
- Lymph node enlargement—ipsilateral to consolidation.

CT findings (Fig. 4.4)

- CT rarely adds to management in routine clinical practice. However, in specific scenarios, CT may be vital for:
  - Detecting complications
  - Evaluating patients responding slowly, or not at all, to treatment.
- CT features of clinical importance that may be masked on CXR include:
  - Cavitation or abscess formation.
  - Parapneumonic effusion or empyema.
  - Lymph node enlargement.
  - Causative endobronchial lesion.
  - Bronchopleural fistula.
  - Malpositioned chest drain.

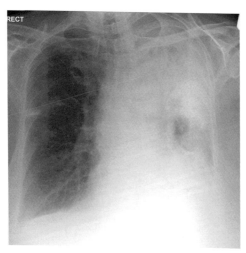

Fig. 4.3 CXR in a patient with pneumococcal pneumonia. There is consolidation in the left upper lobe and lucencies suggesting cavitation. Air bronchograms are just visible and there is evidence of volume loss.

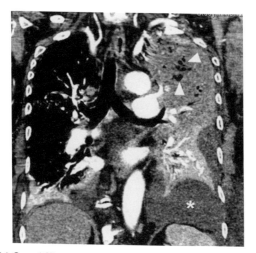

Fig. 4.4 Coronal CT reconstruction (on mediastinal window settings) in the same patient as above. There are multiple gaseous densities (indicating cavitation [arrowheads]) and a large pleural effusion (asterisk) but other than this no additional diagnostic information has been provided by CT when compared with the CXR.

Staphylococcal pneumonia

- Infection is usually via the tracheobronchial tree but may be due to haematogenous dissemination. Recent emergence of methicillin-resistant *Staphylococcus aureus* (MRSA) is a worldwide concern.
- Hospital-acquired (nosocomial) infection: most common—typically in intensive care units or following solid-organ transplantation.
- Community-acquired MRSA: predisposing factors include age <2 years or >60 years, alcoholism, IV drug-use, COPD, recent influenza, malnutrition, ethnicity (higher incidence in Afro-Caribbeans), institutionalization.

Imaging of staphylococcal pneumonia

CXR findings (Fig. 4.5)

- Lobar or multilobar consolidation—most commonly in one lobe (~60% of patients). Consolidation is usually homogeneous and more often seen in the lower lobes.
- Cavitation—associated with abscess formation.
- Pneumatocoeles (± air-fluid levels)—thin-walled cystic spaces. More common in children.
- Ancillary CXR features: bulging of fissures, pneumothorax (mostly children), parapneumonic pleural effusion/empyema, lobar or segmental collapse.

CT findings (Fig. 4.6)

- Consolidation may be in one lobe or multiple lobes, segmental or subsegmental ± cavitation.
- Other features include centrilobular nodules and tree-in-bud pattern, pleural effusion, pneumatocoeles, and abscesses.

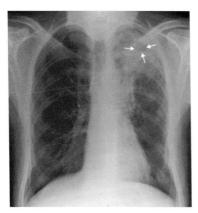

Fig. 4.5 CXR in a patient with staphylococcal pneumonia. There is consolidation in the left upper lobe with evidence of cavitation (arrows).

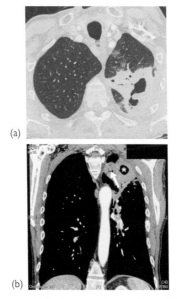

(a)

(b)

Fig. 4.6 Axial and coronal CT in the same patient as in Fig. 4.5. (a) There is consolidation in the left upper lobe with obvious cavitation. (b) The coronal reconstruction, imaged on soft-tissue settings, also demonstrates the cavity (asterisk) and an obvious air-bronchiolram (arrow); apart from the clearer depiction of the cavity, the CT does not add significantly to the findings on CXR.

Pulmonary tuberculosis

- An airborne infectious disease caused by *Mycobacterium tuberculosis*—an aerobic, non-motile, non-spore forming rod.
- 9 million new cases are diagnosed annually worldwide; highest rates per capita are in Africa and strongly linked to HIV/AIDS.
- The primary site of infection is called the Ghon focus. In the early stages, organisms spread to regional hilar and mediastinal nodes but the initial infection is usually clinically silent.
- In 5% of infected individuals, immunity is inadequate and clinically active disease develops within a year of infection (called 'progressive primary infection') and, in another 5%, endogenous reactivation of latent infection develops (termed 'post-primary' or 'reactivation' TB).

Imaging of tuberculosis

The CXR is the imaging test of choice in suspected TB and the radiological diagnosis is frequently suggested if key imaging features are present in the appropriate clinical setting. Serial CXRs are particularly useful for monitoring response to treatment; the indications for CT in TB are summarized in Table 4.2. The principal CT features of tuberculosis vary depending on the 'stage' at which imaging is undertaken.

Table 4.2 Indications for CT in tuberculosis

- Detection of intrathoracic disease in patients with a high clinical suspicion of TB but a normal CXR.
- Identification of features that may suggest 'active' disease (e.g. consolidation, cavitation, tree-in-bud pattern, necrotic lymph nodes).
- Demonstration of complications (see Table 4.3).

Primary tuberculosis

CXR and CT findings (Figs. 4.7 and 4.8)

- Lymph node enlargement—usually unilateral hilar and/or mediastinal. On CT, there may be central low attenuation (because of caseous necrosis) and peripheral rim enhancement (representing the vascular rim of the granulomatous inflammatory tissue).
- Consolidation—typically dense and homogeneous but may also be patchy, nodular, or mass-like; segmental or lobar.
- Pleural effusion—with or without evidence of parenchymal disease.

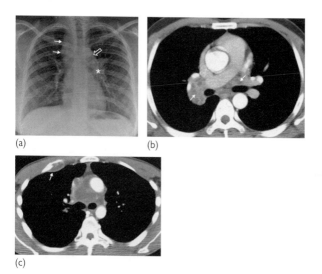

Fig. 4.7 Primary tuberculosis on CXR and CT manifest as hilar and mediastinal lymph node enlargement. (a) CXR shows extensive lymph node enlargement in the right paratracheal region (line arrows), AP window (block arrow) and at the left hilum (asterisk). (b) CT on mediastinal window setting shows central low attenuation (arrows) indicating necrosis in enlarged lymph nodes, (c) mediastinal lymph node enlargement with rim enhancement and a chest wall abscess (arrow).

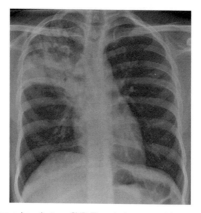

Fig. 4.8 Primary tuberculosis on CXR. There is dense consolidation in the right upper lobe.

Post-primary (reactivation) tuberculosis

CXR and CT findings (Figs. 4.9–4.11)

- Consolidation—focal or patchy usually in the upper lobes or apical segments of the lower lobes.
- Poorly-defined nodules—caused by bronchogenic spread of necrotic and granulomatous inflammation filling and surrounding terminal and respiratory bronchioles and alveolar ducts. On CT these are manifest as a tree-in-bud pattern.
- Cavitation—the CXR and CT hallmark of reactivation TB.
- Hilar/mediastinal lymph node enlargement—uncommon, seen in 5–10% (compare with primary TB).
- Pleural effusion ± thickening—may be the sole manifestation. New subpleural lung nodules may develop during treatment of a tuberculous effusion and should not be regarded as treatment failure; subpleural nodules eventually resolve.

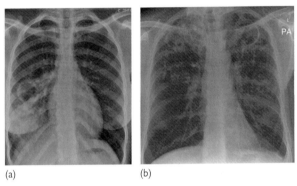

(a)   (b)

Fig. 4.9 Reactivation TB on CXR in two patients. (a) There is a well-defined cavity and consolidation in the right lower lobe. (b) Multiple cavities and ill-defined nodules in the mid and upper zones.

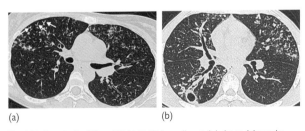

(a)   (b)

Fig. 4.10 Reactivation TB on CT. (a) Multiple small centrilobular nodules and a tree-in-bud pattern (arrows) caused by bronchogenic spread. (b) Right lower lobe cavity with multiple small nodules and also some larger nodules in the lingula.

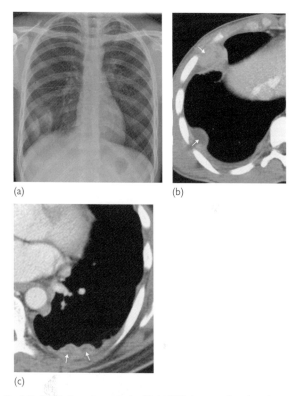

Fig. 4.11 Pleural disease in reactivation TB. (a) CXR shows two lens-shaped opacities in the right lower zone. There is also ill-defined nodularity in the left upper zone. (b) CT in the same patient as in (a) confirms the presence of two pleurally-based lesions (arrows) and pleural thickening. The diagnosis of TB was confirmed from bronchial washings from the left upper lobe. (c) CT in a different patient with proven TB, showing focal pleural thickening with low attenuation areas (arrows) indicating necrosis.

Miliary tuberculosis

The term 'miliary' refers to a CXR and CT pattern caused by haematogenous dissemination (not necessarily confined to the lungs) of TB. This pattern of disease occurs in ~2–6% of patients with primary disease and is also seen in reactivation TB.

CXR and CT findings (Fig. 4.12)

- Multiple 1–3mm nodules—distributed *randomly* throughout the lungs.
- Thickening of interlobular septa and intralobular structures.
- Ground-glass opacity—diffuse or localized; may indicate the onset of acute lung injury/acute respiratory distress syndrome.
- Pneumothorax—rare but recognized feature in children, possibly because small areas of confluent subpleural miliary nodules undergo caseation/necrosis and rupture into the pleural space.

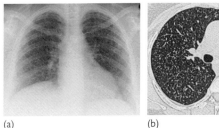
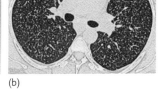

(a)   (b)

Fig. 4.12 Miliary tuberculosis. (a) CXR with widespread micronodular opacities. A CXR performed 5 months earlier was normal. (b) CT in another patient demonstrates innumerable randomly-distributed small nodules.

Imaging of TB in different clinical situations

Multi-drug resistant TB (MDR-TB)

The imaging features of MDR-TB do not differ substantially from those of drug-sensitive disease. However, a number of potentially important differences are highlighted below:

- Multiple cavities and features of chronicity such as bronchiectasis and calcified granulomata are more common in patients with MDR-TB.
- Patients who develop MDR-TB without a history of anti-TB chemotherapy or those who have been treated for less than 1 month tend to present with non-cavitary consolidation, pleural effusions and a pattern of disease that is similar to that in patients with primary TB.
- Patients with MDR-TB and a treatment history of over 1 month often show cavitary consolidation and a pattern of disease mirroring that seen in reactivation TB.

Extensively-drug resistant TB

- Extensively-drug resistant disease manifests as an advanced pattern of primary TB. Consolidation (± lymph node enlargement) may be particularly widespread.
- In non-AIDS patients, disease manifests as an advanced pattern of MDR TB (i.e. multiple cavitary lesions and consolidative or nodular lesions).

TB in immunocompromised hosts

Risk factors for the development of active TB include HIV infection, malnutrition, drug and alcohol abuse, malignancy, diabetes mellitus, immunosuppressive therapy and other drugs (e.g. infliximab and etanercept).

- TB is a major cause of death in patients with HIV infection or AIDS.
- The radiographic manifestations of pulmonary TB are dependent on the level of immunosuppression; HIV-seropositive patients with a CD4 T-lymphocyte count <200/mm^3 have a higher prevalence of mediastinal or hilar lymph node enlargement, a lower prevalence of cavitation, and often extrapulmonary involvement as compared with HIV-seropositive patients with a CD4 T-lymphocyte count >200/mm^3.
- Miliary or disseminated disease has also been reported to be associated with severe immunosuppression.

Complications of pulmonary tuberculosis

There are myriad complications of TB, some of which are listed in Table 4.3. The CXR and CT features of many of the entities listed are covered in other sections.

Table 4.3 Complications and sequelae of pulmonary tuberculosis

- **Parenchymal complications**
  - Acute lung injury/acute respiratory distress syndrome
  - Aspergilloma (in pre-existing post-TB fibro-cavities)
- **Airway complications**
  - Bronchiectasis
  - Tracheobronchial stenosis
  - Broncholithiasis
  - Laryngeal TB secondary to active pulmonary disease
- **Vascular complications**
  - Pulmonary and bronchial arteritis
  - Pulmonary artery pseudoaneurysm (Rasmussen aneurysm)
- **Mediastinal complications**
  - Fibrosing mediastinitis
  - Constrictive pericarditis
  - Oesophageal TB secondary to active pulmonary disease causing ulceration, fistulas, and strictures
- **Pleural and chest wall complications**
  - Empyema
  - Pneumothorax
  - Bronchopleural fistula
  - Osteitis of vertebral bodies/ribs caused by haematogenous or direct spread

Non-tuberculous mycobacterial infections

- The non-tuberculous mycobacteria are a group of ubiquitous low-grade pathogens (Table 4.4) that typically infect cervical lymph nodes, skin, soft tissues and the lung.

Table 4.4 Clinically important non-tuberculous mycobacterial species

- *M. avium-intracellulare* complex (MAC)
- *M. kansasii*
- *M. malmoense*
- *M. xenopi*
- *M. fortuitum*
- *M. chelonae*

- Non-tuberculous mycobcterial infections account for approximately half of all mycobacterial infections.
- Infection in immunocompetent hosts occurs in two groups: males aged >50 years with pre-existing chronic lung disease (e.g. COPD, cystic fibrosis) and elderly females with otherwise normal lungs. Other predisposing factors include alcoholism, diabetes mellitus, AIDS and corticosteroid treatment.
- Infection is caused by inhalation or ingestion of aerosolized organisms from environmental reservoirs such as soil and dusts; human-to-human transmission of non-tuberculous mycobacterial infection has not been reported.
- The diagnosis of pulmonary non-tuberculous mycobacterial infections is difficult and often delayed. The clinical course of non-tuberculous mycobacterial infections is generally more indolent than in tuberculosis.

CXR and CT findings

The features on CXR and/or CT (Figs. 4.13–4.15) which should suggest the diagnosis of non-tuberculous mycobacterial infection are described below:

- Bronchiectasis—in the upper or lower lobes (NB localization to the right middle lobe and lingula [termed the Lady Windemere syndrome] is a feature of MAC infection); bronchiectasis may progress.
- Nodules/tree-in-bud pattern—small (<2cm diameter). In contrast to other non-tuberculous mycobacterial infections, nodules are common in MAC infection.
- Cavitation—thin- or thick-walled and may be in the upper zones (especially in *M. kansasii* infection); NB Cavities are less common in MAC infection.
- Consolidation—seen to a greater or lesser degree in all non-tuberculous mycobacterial infections.
- Other features include lymph node enlargement, pleural effusions and fibrosis.

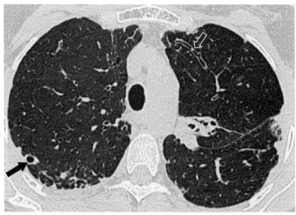

(a)

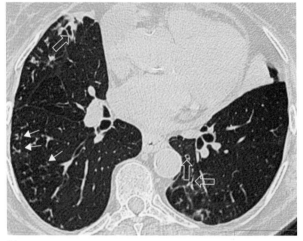

(b)

Fig. 4.13 CT through the (a) upper lobes and (b) mid zone in a patient with proven MAC infection. There is mild cylindrical bronchiectasis (open arrows) in multiple lobes. Centrilobular nodules/tree-in-bud pattern (line arrows) and a cavitating nodule (black arrow) are seen. There is also consolidation in the inferior lingular segment.

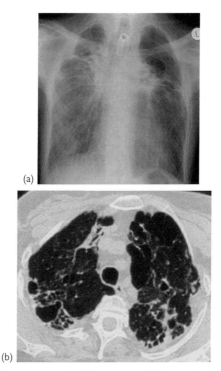

Fig. 4.14 *M. kansasii* infection. (a) CXR in a patient with *M. kansasii* infection. There is extensive cavitation in the upper lobes with coexisting fibrosis. (b) CT in a different patient showing upper lobe cavitation and emphysema.

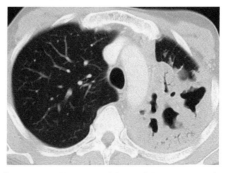

Fig. 4.15 Cavitating consolidation in the left upper lobe in a patient with confirmed *M. malmoense* infection.

Viral pneumonias

- The predisposing factors for the development of viral respiratory infection are listed in Table 4.5.
- In children, the common viruses which cause lower respiratory tract infection are respiratory syncytial virus (RSV), adenovirus, influenza, and parainfluenza virus. In immunocompetent adults, the commonest pathogens are influenza and adenovirus.
- In recent years, emerging pathogens causing epidemics of severe pneumonia in immunocompetent hosts have also been described (e.g. a corona virus causing severe acute respiratory syndrome and influenza pandemics (e.g. H1N1). Cytomegalovirus (CMV) is the commonest viral pathogen in immunosuppressed individuals.

Table 4.5 Risk factors associated with increased incidence of viral pneumonia

- Extremes of age (very young or elderly)
- Malnutrition
- Immunosuppression
- Overcrowding

Imaging of viral pneumonias

The radiological features of viral pneumonias are often non-specific. Thus, the primary role of imaging (particularly CT) is a) to exclude superadded bacterial or fungal infection and b) to guide bronchoalveolar lavage in order to isolate an organism.

CXR findings

- Widespread ill-defined small nodules which may coalesce (common) (Fig. 4.16).
- Peribronchial opacities and bronchial wall thickening may be prominent.
- Cavitation and pleural effusions are very unusual.

CT findings

- Bilateral consolidation and ground glass opacity (Fig. 4.17).
- Not typically seen in a lobar distribution (by contrast to bacterial pneumonia).

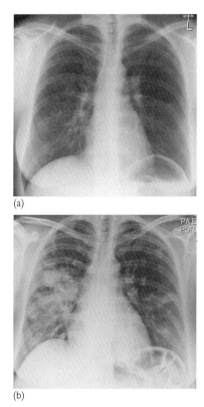

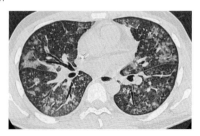

Fig. 4.16 Two CXRs in a patient with chronic lymphocytic leukaemia and H1N1 (swine flu) infection. (a) subtle ill-defined nodules in the right midzone on the initial CXR and, (b) subsequent coalescence to cause confluent bilateral consolidation 72 hours later.

Fig. 4.17 CT in a patient with acute myeloid leukaemia and pneumonia due to respiratory syncytial virus. There is patchy bilateral ground-glass opacification and multiple nodules.

Specific viral respiratory tract infections

Respiratory syncytial virus (RSV)

- A major cause of bronchiolitis and bronchopneumonia in infants and young children.
- In adults, RSV causes pneumonia in the immunosuppressed.

CXR findings (Fig. 4.18)

- 'Streaky' peribronchial opacities (sometimes with hyperinflation).
- Hilar lymph node enlargement—variably present.
- Lobar collapse—relatively common.
- Lobar consolidation—infrequently seen.

CT findings

- Generally non-specific and similar to findings on CXR.
- Air-trapping, bronchial dilatation, and wall thickening are recognized sequelae.

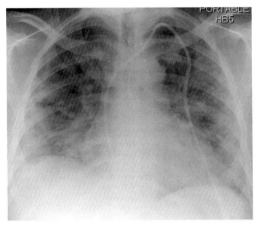

Fig. 4.18 CXR in a patient with acute myeloid leukaemia and viral pneumonia caused by RSV infection. There is patchy bilateral consolidation.

Adenovirus

- A frequent cause of mild upper respiratory tract infection.
- Causes pneumonia in infants, young children and young adults (e.g. military recruits).
- Long term sequelae of adenovirus infection include bronchiectasis or obliterative bronchiolitis and are common in children.

CXR findings
- Consolidation—patchy or widespread and confluent; lobar consolidation is unusual.
- Peribronchiolar opacities and bronchial wall thickening.
- Air-trapping and lobar collapse—common.
- Small pleural effusions—relatively common.

Influenza virus
- Sporadic, epidemic, or pandemic infections.
- Superadded bacterial pneumonia (*S. pneumoniae*, *S. aureus*, or *H. influenzae*) is common in contrast to infections caused by other viruses.

CXR findings
- Consolidation—multifocal and rapidly progressing to bilateral basal opacification; lobar/segmental consolidation is unusual. Appearance may resemble pulmonary oedema.
- Cavitation—very rare.
- Pleural effusions—an occasional feature.

Parainfluenza virus
- Mainly affects children during winter outbreaks.
- Bronchiolitis and croup are common; pneumonia is rare but superadded bacterial pneumonia is a problem.

CXR findings
- Consolidation—patchy, basal and peribronchiolar.

Severe acute respiratory syndrome (SARS)
- Severe pneumonia due to coronavirus; epidemics reported in Southern China in 2003 (with spread to Hong Kong, Singapore) and Toronto; fatal in approximately 10% of cases.
- Lymphopenia and raised liver transaminases are common.

CXR findings
- Ground-glass opacities progressing to consolidation—usually bilateral; ± cavitation.
- Lymph node enlargement and pleural effusions—uncommon.

CT findings
- Focal ground-glass opacities—may occur in the context of a normal CXR in early disease. Initial peripheral basal distribution of ground-glass opacities and progressing to admixed ground-glass and consolidation (resembling ARDS (see 🕮 Air space diseases/Miscellaneous causes of pulmonary oedema, p130)).
- Ancillary features: mild bronchial dilatation within areas of ground-glass opacification and thickening of intralobular structures and interlobular septa (the 'crazy-paving' pattern).
- Complete resolution over time.

Cytomegalovirus (CMV)

- Commonest viral pathogen in immunocompromised hosts (e.g. AIDS, haematological malignancy, and following solid-organ transplantation); predisposes to and/or coexists with *Pneumocystis jiroveci* pneumonia.

CXR findings

- Nodules—basal and bilateral; small nodules ('miliary' pattern) are sometimes seen.
- Consolidation—resembling bacterial pneumonia.
- Pleural effusions—a recognized finding.
- Spontaneous pneumothorax and pneumomediastinum may occur.

CT findings (Fig. 4.19)

- Ground-glass opacities.
- Small nodules (<5mm in diameter).
- Consolidation.
- Reticular pattern.

Herpes simplex and Varicella-zoster viruses

- May cause pneumonia in immunocompromised adults (especially in patients with lymphoma). Not common in children.

CXR and CT findings (Fig. 4.20)

- Nodules—Multiple, bilateral nodules with a tendency to become confluent. Usually resolve but can persist. In small proportion, nodules may calcify.
- Hilar lymph node enlargement—uncommon.
- Pleural effusion—uncommon

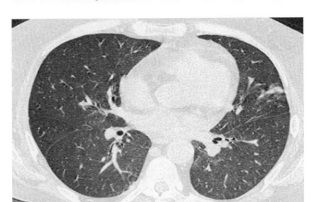

Fig. 4.19 CT in a patient with CMV pneumonitis showing subtle ground-glass opacity and consolidation in the lingula.

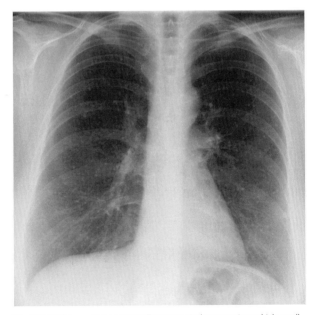

Fig. 4.20 CXR in a patient post varicella pneumonia demonstrating multiple, small, bilateral calcified nodules.

Fungal infections

- Fungal infections occur in immunocompetent hosts and immuno-compromised patients.
- In immunocompetent hosts, endemic fungal pathogens e.g. *Histoplasma capsulatum, Coccidioides immitis, Paracoccidioides brasiliensis,* and *Blastomyces dermatitidis* are the important causative organisms.
- Opportunistic fungal organisms e.g. *Aspergillus, Candida, Mucor* species, *Cryptococcus*, and *Pneumocystis jiroveci* tend to cause pneumonia in patients with congenital or acquired defects in their host defences.

Risk factors associated with the development of pulmonary fungal infection

- **Endemic fungal infections**
  - Workers or farmers with heavy exposure to bird, bat, or rodent droppings and other animal excreta in endemic areas.
- **Opportunistic fungal infections**
  - Haematopoetic stem cell transplantation
  - Solid-organ transplantation
  - Myeloablative chemotherapy in acute leukaemia or lymphoma
  - AIDS and congenital immunodeficiency syndromes
  - Prolonged corticosteroid therapy
  - Neutropenia.

Imaging in fungal infections

As with the viral pneumonias, the imaging features of fungal infections are non-specific and there are overlapping radiological appearances.

Opportunistic fungal infections

Pneumocystis jiroveci **pneumonia**

- Formerly called *Pneumocystis carinii* and now re-termed *Pneumocystis jiroveci* pneumonia (although the acronym PCP remains in common use).
- *Pneumocystis jiroveci* is a unicellular fungus which classically causes infection in patients with AIDS but also in patients undergoing transplantation.
- In patients with AIDS, CD4 levels are generally <100 cells/μL at the time of diagnosis of the first episode of PCP.

CXR findings (Fig. 4.21)

- Normal appearances.
- Ground-glass opacification—typically bilateral and predominantly in the peri-hilar regions; may be diffuse or involve the lower or upper lung zones.
- Reticulonodular pattern.
- Consolidation—perihilar or diffuse bilateral may be seen in progressive disease.
- Pleural effusions and lymph node enlargement—uncommon findings (the presence of these on CXR should prompt consideration of alternative diagnoses).

CT findings (Fig. 4.22)

- Ground-glass opacification—patchy or diffuse intermingled with areas of normally aerated lung. Sparing of the peripheral (sub-pleural) lung may be seen.
- Fine reticular/linear pattern—may be superimposed on ground-glass opacification creating a 'crazy-paving' pattern.
- Consolidation.
- Cysts—usually multiple and associated with an increased risk of spontaneous pneumothorax. More prevalent in AIDS patients receiving prophylactic aerosolized pentamidine and trimethoprim.
- Mass lesions/pulmonary nodules—multiple.
- Pleural effusions and lymph node enlargement—uncommon.

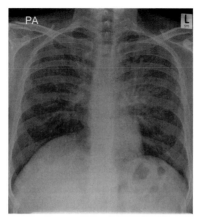

Fig. 4.21 *Pneumocystis jiroveci* pneumonia. CXR shows typical perihilar ground-glass opacification and a fine reticular pattern.

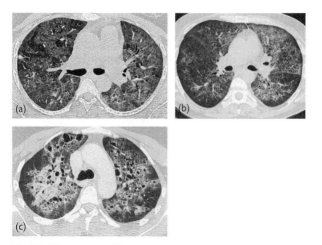

Fig. 4.22 CT appearances of *Pneumocystis jiroveci* pneumonia in three patients with AIDS. (a) CT at the level of the carina shows patchy ground-glass opacities admixed with regions of normal lung and (b) extensive ground-glass opacification with superimposed fine reticulation resulting in a 'crazy-paving' pattern. (c) CT in a third patient showing multiple cysts on a background of consolidation and ground-glass opacification.

Aspergillus infection

- *Aspergillus* is a genus with a large number of species (~250–300) found ubiquitously. The common species causing disease in man is *Aspergillus fumigatus*. In the following section, only those infections which manifest predominantly as patterns of air-space disease will be discussed.
- The risk of developing *Aspergillus*-related disease depends on the interplay between virulence, the presence/absence of pre-existing lung 'damage', host hypersensitivity and the ability of the host to resist infection.
- Disease patterns known to be caused by *Aspergillus* species in man are summarized in Table 4.6. However, it must be stressed despite these apparently discrete entities, there is considerable overlap. It is also known that, in any patient, one form may evolve into another with changes in virulence and immunity.

Table 4.6 Spectrum of *Aspergillus*-related pulmonary disease

- **Aspergilloma**
- **Indolent through to invasive pulmonary aspergillosis**
  - Chronic necrotizing/semi-invasive pulmonary aspergillosis ('chronic aspergillosis')
  - Angioinvasive aspergillosis
  - Acute airway invasive aspergillosis—acute tracheobronchitis, exudative bronchiolitis ± bronchopneumonia
- **Allergic disease**
  - Allergic bronchopulmonary aspergillosis (ABPA)
  - Bronchocentric granulomatosis
  - Acute hypersensitivity pneumonitis

Adapted from Buckingham SJ and Hansell DM. Aspergillus in the lung: diverse and coincident forms. *Eur Radiol* 2003;**13**:1786–1800)

Chronic aspergillosis

- An indolent, granulomatous, cavitary infection which occurs because of local invasion by *Aspergillus fumigatus*; the infection runs a progressive course (typically over months to years). The two main subtypes are chronic cavitary pulmonary aspergillosis and chronic necrotizing pulmonary aspergillosis—the former having no invasive features whereas the latter is locally invasive.
- This form of *Aspergillus* infection commonly occurs in patients with pre-existing abnormal lung (e.g. COPD or lung fibrosis caused by tuberculosis/sarcoidosis) and some underlying immune defect (e.g. caused by corticosteroid therapy, diabetes, or AIDS) and may coexist with non-tuberculous mycobacterial infection.
- A robust diagnosis of truly invasive aspergillosis requires the histopathological demonstration of invasion by fungal hyphae through the basement membrane of bronchial walls. In practice, diagnosis is usually achieved via a combination of clinical, radiological ± serological tests for *Aspergillus fumigatus*, or the isolation of the same from respiratory samples.

CXR findings (Fig. 4.23)

- Consolidation—typically in the upper zones and progressing to cavitation.
- Nodules.
- Pleural thickening—adjacent to areas of consolidation/cavitation.

CT findings (Fig. 4.24)

- Consolidation—predominantly in the upper lobes; may be extensive. Cavitation in foci of consolidation may be seen and mycetomas may develop within cavities.
- Nodules.
- Pleural thickening—adjacent to areas of consolidation/cavitation.
- Cavitary lesions.
- Features of coexistent non-tuberculous mycobacterial infection (☐ see Air space diseases/Non-tuberculous mycobacterial infections, p96).

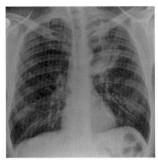

Fig. 4.23 CXR in a diabetic patient with chronic necrotizing pulmonary aspergillosis. There is left upper lobe consolidation.

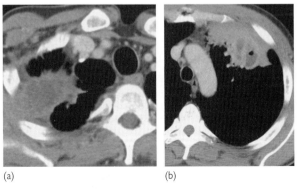

(a)   (b)

Fig. 4.24 Chronic necrotizing pulmonary aspergillosis in two patients. (a) CT through the right apex demonstrates consolidation in the right upper lobe with foci of low attenuation suggesting necrosis and pleural thickening. (b) Left upper lobe consolidation with associated necrosis and cavitation; *Aspergillus* hyphae were seen on biopsy.

Invasive aspergillosis

The two main patterns of aggressive and invasive disease are i) angioinvasive (due to invasion of the pulmonary artery branches) and ii) airway-invasive (related to the invasion of bronchi and bronchioles) aspergillosis.

Risk factors for the development of invasive aspergillosis

- Profound neutropenia <1000 cells/mm^3 for >3 weeks is the most significant risk factor
- Haematopoietic stem cell or solid-organ transplantation
- Immunosuppressive therapy
- Prolonged corticosteroid use
- AIDS
- Marijuana smoking (in immunocompetent hosts)

Angioinvasive aspergillosis

- There are two classical pathological features of angioinvasive pulmonary aspergillosis in which involvement of vessels appears to be central to pathogenesis:
  - Invasion of major proximal pulmonary arteries with resultant thrombosis and infarction of lung distally leading to a roughly wedge-shaped lesion with its base abutting the visceral pleura.
  - A well-circumscribed spherical nodule with a vessel in the centre of the lesion, infiltrated by *Aspergillus* hyphae. The nodule has a pale centre which consists of an area of coagulative necrosis. This central necrotic core is surrounded by a rim comprised of congested and haemorrhagic lung. This pathological nodule is termed the 'target' lesion or mycotic 'sequestrum'.

CXR findings

- Nodules—single or multiple.
- Consolidation—segmental or subsegmental.
- Ground-glass opacification.

CT findings (Figs. 4.25–4.28)

- Nodules—multiple and of variable size ± surrounding halo of ground-glass attenuation (the 'halo' sign) corresponding to a rim of alveolar haemorrhage. NB the halo sign is not specific for angioinvasive aspergillosis.
- Areas of segmental/subsegmental consolidation.
- Cavitation—in nodules/consolidation. Cavitation may appear as a peripheral crescent of low density (called the 'air crescent' sign). Seen in up to ~50% of patients and occurs during the recovery of neutrophil levels.

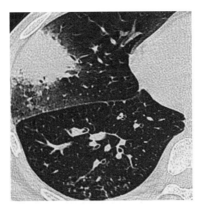

Fig. 4.25 CT through the right mid zone in a patient with angioinvasive aspergillosis. There is a focal, peripheral wedge-shaped lesion caused by an area of infarction.

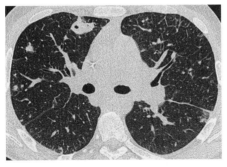

Fig. 4.26 CT section below the level of the carina in a patient being treated for haematological malignancy. There are multiple focal lesions of varying size, one of which, in the right upper lobe, is cavitating.

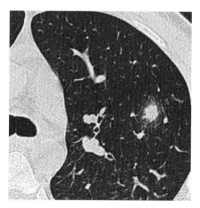

Fig. 4.27 The CT 'halo sign' in angioinvasive aspergillosis. There is a ground-glass margin around the nodule in the left upper lobe.

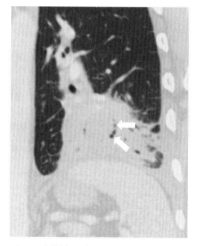

Fig. 4.28 Targeted coronal CT through the left lower lobe in a patient with Hodgkin's lymphoma. There is a large area of consolidation, with an 'air crescent' (arrows) seen during the phase of neutrophil recovery.

Pulmonary candidiasis

- *Candida* species are increasingly problematic in patients with haematological malignancies (i.e. in those undergoing chemotherapeutic conditioning or following haematopoietic stem cell transplantation), in IV drug abusers, and in AIDS.
- A definitive diagnosis of *Candida* pneumonia is difficult to establish since 'colonization' is common in immunocompromised hosts.
- There is no reliable test for the diagnosis of a *Candida* infection and a definitive diagnosis of invasive candidiasis is often only made on the histopathological demonstration of yeasts in lung tissue, the presence of fungus in normally sterile tissues or the demonstration of invasion in other organs.

CXR and CT findings (Fig. 4.29)

- Nodules—multiple and varying in size (3–30mm diameter); mainly in the lower zones.
- Ground-glass opacification.
- Consolidation ± cavitation.
- Tree-in-bud opacities.
- Nodules may be surrounded by discrete areas of ground-glass opacity (CT halo sign).

The CT manifestations of pulmonary candidiasis are similar to those described in other pulmonary infections and may be indistinguishable from those caused by other opportunistic infections, particularly invasive aspergillosis and mucormycosis.

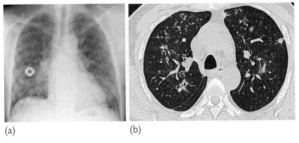

(a)   (b)

Fig. 4.29 CXR and CT in pulmonary candidiasis. (a) CXR demonstrates multiple nodules predominantly in the mid and lower zones in an immunosuppressed patient. (b) CT through the upper zones shows multiple irregular nodules and ill-defined opacities (some with surrounding ground-glass halos) in the same patient with proven pulmonary candidiasis.

Pulmonary cryptococcosis

- Caused by infection with *Cryptococcus neoformans*, an organism normally found in soil (especially that containing pigeon or avian excrement).
- Infection occurs predominantly (but not exclusively) in immunocompromised patients; ~50–60% of symptomatic infections occur in the context of AIDS.
- In immunocompetent subjects, cryptococcal infections are commonly localized to the lung and patients may be asymptomatic; in immunocompromised patients, cryptococcal infections often cause symptomatic pulmonary infections and disseminate to the central nervous system, skin, and bones.

CXR and CT findings (Fig. 4.30)

- Nodules—solitary or multiple nodules, usually small and well-defined with a middle/upper zone and subpleural distribution.
- Consolidation—patchy, segmental or lobar.
- Reticular/reticulonodular pattern.
- Cavitation within nodules and areas of consolidation are common in immunosuppressed individuals.
- Hilar/mediastinal lymph node enlargement and pleural effusions—not common but more prevalent in AIDS-related cryptococcosis.

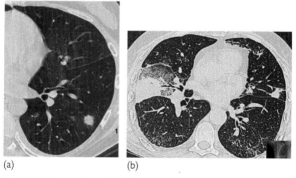

(a) (b)

Fig. 4.30 CT in two patients with pulmonary cryptococcosis. (a) Targeted CT shows a solitary left lower lobe nodule in a patient with biopsy-proven *Cryptococcus* infection. (b) CT at the level of the pulmonary venous confluence with patchy, multifocal consolidation.

Endemic fungal infections

Pulmonary histoplasmosis

- Caused by the dimorphic fungus *Histoplasma capsulatum*, endemic in Mississippi, Ohio, and the St. Lawrence river valleys.
- The different manifestations of pulmonary infection with *Histoplasma* are summarized in Table 4.7.

Table 4.7 Patterns of *Histoplasma* infection and imaging findings

- **Fleeting focal pneumonitis** (usually asymptomatic and self-limiting)
  - Usually not seen on CXR.
  - Occasionally, enlargement or coalescence of several inflammatory foci results in single or multiple poorly-defined areas of air space opacification.
- **Histoplasmoma(s)**
  - Solitary or multiple nodules (Fig. 4.31) corresponding to a focus or foci of necrotizing granulomatous inflammation.
  - Central or diffuse calcification (caused by dystrophic calcification of necrotic material).
- **Disseminated disease** (generally in immunocompromised hosts)
  - Miliary or diffuse reticulonodular pattern.
  - Focal/patchy areas of consolidation.
- **Mediastinal histoplasmosis**
  - Enlarged lymph nodes.
  - Inflammation may extend into the adjacent pericardium (pericarditis) or mediastinum (fibrosing mediastinitis—leading to obstruction of the SVC, major bronchi or central vessels).
- **Chronic histoplasmosis** (rare manifestation occurring in ~1 in 2000 exposed patients and almost exclusively in those with COPD).
  - Patchy consolidation (± cavitation), typically in the apical and posterior segments of the upper lobes.
  - Calcification of hilar and mediastinal nodes is commonly seen; nodes may erode into the lumen of adjacent bronchi (i.e. broncholithiasis).

Adapted from JW Gurney, DJ Conces Jr. Pulmonary histoplasmosis. *Radiology*. 1996;**199**:297–306.

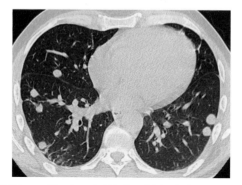

Fig. 4.31 Pulmonary histoplasmosis. Multiple well defined soft tissue nodules (resembling pulmonary metastases). Histopathological examination of a biopsied nodule confirmed the diagnosis of benign histoplasmomas.

Pulmonary coccidioidomycosis

- Caused by inhalation of the spores of the fungus *Coccidioides immitis*; endemic in the south western United States of America and Mexico.
- Infection may be acute or chronic: acute coccidioidomycosis is usually a mild illness and may be asymptomatic in ~40%. Chronic (persistent) disease is seen in some patients whose symptoms persist beyond 1–2 months.

Acute coccidioidomycosis
CXR and CT findings
- Normal CXR—in many patients, particularly if asymptomatic.
- Nodules—small (± calcification).
- Consolidation—solitary focus or multifocal.
- Thin-walled cavities—uncommon.
- Lymph node enlargement—uncommon.

Chronic coccidioidomycosis
CXR and CT findings
- Nodules—usually small; may cavitate (thin- or thick-walled, usually with homogeneous attenuation on CT); ranging in size from 0.5–3.0cm diameter. Subpleural and predominantly in the lower lobes.
- Consolidation—sometimes with cavitation.
- Volume loss.
- Disseminated ('miliary') nodules.

Pulmonary blastomycosis

- Caused by the dimorphic fungus *Blastomyces dermatitidis*.
- Infection is most common in the central and south eastern United States of America, central/southern America, and southern Canada.

CXR and CT findings
- Consolidation—most common radiological finding; usually patchy or confluent and may be segmental, subsegmental, or non-segmental. Cavitation in ~50%.
- 'Masses'—mass-like areas of consolidation: seen in ~30%. Usually well-circumscribed, measuring 3–10cm in diameter. Masses have a tendency to be paramediastinal or perihilar. Some reports have found a correlation between masses and more chronic manifestations of blastomycosis.
- Nodules—(0.5–3cm in diameter) occur infrequently. Nodules can be numerous but patients may also have only one or two nodules. Identification of intermediate-sized nodules in combination with other manifestations such as consolidation should raise suspicion for fungal disease and may help make the diagnosis. Miliary dissemination accompanies clinically overwhelming infection.
- Pleural effusion—in 10–15% of patients.
- Hilar or mediastinal lymph node enlargement—occasionally seen.
- Calcification—uncommon.

Lung abscess

- An inflammatory mass containing central purulent necrosis.
- Any infectious pneumonia may be complicated by a lung abscess, although abscess formation is not generally a feature of uncomplicated viral pneumonias.
- An abscess usually occurs as a consequence of lung necrosis.
- Multiple abscesses usually occurs when there is haematogeneous spread from a source of sepsis (e.g. infective endocarditis).
- The differentiation between a lung abscess and empyema is not always straightforward; the CT features which may favour the diagnosis of one over the other are listed on page 121).

Pathogens commonly associated with pulmonary abscess formation

- *Mycobacterium tuberculosis*
- *Staphylococcus aureus*
- Gram negative bacteria (*Klebsiella pneumoniae, Pseudomonas aeruginosa and Proteus*)
- Anaerobic bacteria e.g. *Bacteroides* spp. (from aspiration of oropharyngeal secretions)

Imaging of lung abscess

The CXR is the standard investigation in patients with a pulmonary abscess, not only for the diagnosis (NB relatively low sensitivity in early stages) but also for the identification of complications and follow-up after treatment.

CXR findings (Fig. 4.32)

- Single or multiple masses—typically >2cm in diameter. Commonest sites: posterior segments of the upper lobes and superior segments of the lower lobes.
- Cavitation—an air-fluid level may be apparent, but in practice, is often difficult to detect when there is extensive consolidation.

CT findings (Figs. 4.33–4.36)

- Consolidation—with central (necrotic) low attenuation which may progress to cavitation, sometimes with an air-fluid level.
- Fluid density—helps to distinguish an abscess from other cavitating lesions.
- Thickened wall—differentiates an abscess from other cystic lesions.
- Rim enhancement of the wall post-IV contrast injection.

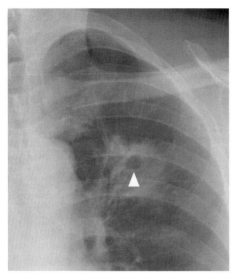

Fig. 4.32 Targeted CXR in a young non-smoker with cough and fever. There is a cavitating abscess in the left upper zone with an air-fluid level (arrowhead).

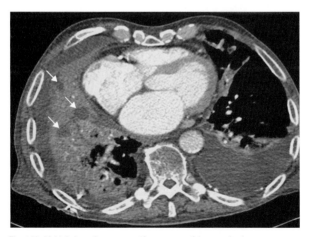

Fig. 4.33 Multiple lung abscesses manifest as areas of decreased enhancement (arrows) post IV contrast in consolidated right lung. There are bilateral pleural effusions.

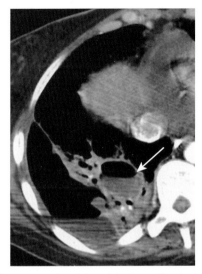

Fig. 4.34 CT in a patient with a right lower lobe abscess. There is an air-fluid level and rim enhancement (arrow). Note the adjacent hydropneumothorax due to a complicating bronchopleural fistula.

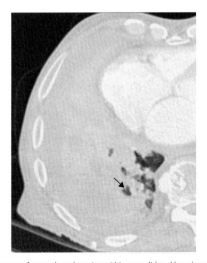

Fig. 4.35 An area of parenchymal sparing within consolidated lung (arrow) which mimics an area of cavitation. However, the density of this area of spared lung is identical to that of normally aerated lung rather than (black) air surrounding the patient.

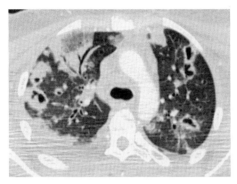

Fig. 4.36 CT showing multiple pulmonary abscesses in both lungs in a patient with infective endocarditis.

CT features which may differentiate between lung abscess and empyema

Empyema
- Lens-shaped (unless very large)
- Obtuse or tapering angle with chest wall
- A change in shape with altered patient position
- Smooth wall with two layers of enhancing pleura separated by fluid (the so called 'split-pleura' sign)
- Compressed underlying lung with displacement of bronchovascular structures

Lung abscess
- Spherical shape
- Acute angles with chest wall
- Fixed shape regardless of patient position
- Irregular/nodular wall, containing locules of air or air-bronchograms
- Uncompressed surrounding lung with the bronchovascular structures undisplaced or drawn toward abscess

Pulmonary infections in the immunocompromised host

The population of potentially immunocompromised hosts is large and partly reflects the widespread use of immunosuppressive agents in clinical medicine. Pulmonary infections are common and linked with high morbidity and mortality. The CXR is usually the first radiological test requested but the appearances on CXR and CT are seldom specific. The diagnostic approach must therefore integrate the radiological findings with knowledge of which pathogens are likely to cause disease. This in turn will depend on the:

- Specific epidemiological or environmental exposure.
- Nature of the underlying immune defect (e.g. neutropenia, immunoglobulin deficiency).
- Duration and severity of immunocompromise.

The following section highlights the infections in different groups of immunocompromised patients. The imaging features are described in other sections.

Infections in specific groups of immunocompromised patients

Human immunodeficiency virus infection (HIV)/acquired immunodeficiency syndrome (AIDS)

The list of causative agents is dependent on the circulating levels of CD4 positive cells:

CD4 count >200 cells/μL
- Bacterial pneumonias:
  - *Streptococcus pneumoniae*
  - *Haemophilus influenzae*
  - *Pseudomonas aeruginosa*
  - *Streptococcus viridans*
  - *Staphylococcus aureus*
- *Mycobacterium tuberculosis*

CD4 count <200 cells/μL
- *Pneumocystis jiroveci* (PCP)
- *Mycobacterium tuberculosis* (usually disseminated)
- *Cryptococcus neoformans*
- *Coccidioides immitis*
- *Histoplasma capsulatum*
- *Blastomyces dermatitidis*

CD4 count <50 cells/μL
- Non-tuberculous mycobacteria (typically *M. avium intracellulare* or *M. kansasii*)
- *Candida albicans*
- *Aspergillus* (rare in HIV patients: incidence <1%). Most common presentation is chronic necrotizing aspergillosis manifesting as cavitary pneumonia. Airway invasive aspergillosis, manifesting as acute tracheobronchitis, bronchiolitis, or bronchopneumonia also occurs.
- Cytomegalovirus

Solid-organ transplant recipients

In this group of patients there are three important time-points to consider following transplantation:
- **1 month following transplantation**
  - Bacterial pneumonias dominate (usually caused by oral flora or gram negative bacilli and septic emboli related to the use of indwelling IV catheters).
- **From 1 month to 6 months following transplantation**
  - Cytomegalovirus
  - Epstein–Barr virus
  - Herpes simplex virus
  - *Pneumocystis jiroveci*
  - *Aspergillus* species
- **Beyond 6 months**
  - Opportunistic infections (in those who have impaired graft function and require high levels of immunosuppression).

Haematopoetic stem cell transplantation (HSCT)

In HSCT recipients, pulmonary infections occur in up to 50% of patients and are a major cause of morbidity and mortality.

* Fungi are the most common cause of pulmonary infection during the neutropaenic phase following HSCT (up to three weeks after transplantation). *Aspergillus*, *Candida* and *Histoplasma* are the usual pathogens.
* CMV pneumonia is the most significant viral infection in HSCT patients occurring 3 weeks to 100 days after transplantation (early phase).
* Respiratory syncytial virus pneumonia.

Mild immunosuppression

Patients with chronic debilitating illnesses (e.g. diabetes mellitus, malnutrition, alcoholism, advanced age and those on prolonged corticosteroid treatment) often have mild immunosuppression and are prone to infection. In these patients, a form of *Aspergillus* infection (termed chronic aspergillosis) may occur.

Utility of CT in immunocompromised patients

Thoracic CT is not infrequently requested in immunocompromised patients with suspected infection. However, the added benefit of CT over and above a review of serial CXR and the clinical data is often questionable.

Specific situations in which CT may aid management

* Confirmation of pulmonary infection in the face of an apparently normal CXR.
* More detailed evaluation of sometimes complex CXR abnormalities.
* Identification of concurrent pleural effusions/empyema.
* Detection of other complications.
* Guiding diagnostic procedures (e.g. biopsy, diagnostic aspiration, or drainage of pleural fluid).

CT findings of diagnostic value in immunocompromised patients

Highlighted below are some CT findings, which in the appropriate clinical context, may point to a particular infectious agent (Table 4.8).

* Tuberculous infection—a tree-in-bud pattern, foci of consolidation/ nodules (± cavitation) with intrathoracic lymph node enlargement.
* Invasive aspergillosis—nodule or mass surrounded by ground-glass halo in a neutropaenic patient.
* *Pneumocystis jiroveci*—diffuse ground-glass opacification and a superimposed fine reticular pattern in a perihilar or geographical distribution.
* Bacterial infection—segmental or lobar consolidation.

Table 4.8 Combinations of CT and clinical features which suggest a specific infection in immunosuppressed hosts

CT findings	Clinical setting	Organism
Lobar consolidation	Community-acquired AIDS (CD4 >200)	S. pneumoniae
	Mild immunosuppression	Chronic aspergillosis
	Solid-organ transplantation	Gram negative bacilli Staphylococcus
Ground-glass opacity	AIDS (CD4 <200)	P. jiroveci
	Haematopoetic stem cell transplantation	CMV
Bronchopneumonia	Neutropenia	Airway invasive aspergillosis
Interstitial pneumonia	Haematopoetic stem cell transplantation	CMV
	AIDS	P. jiroveci
Multiple small nodules	Haematopoetic stem cell transplantation	CMV
	AIDS	Cryptococcosis
		Varicella
		Herpes
	Neutropenia	Angioinvasive aspergillosis
		Candida
Tree-in-bud pattern	Transplantation	Endobronchial TB
		Airway invasive aspergillosis

Adapted from Franquet T. Imaging of pneumonia: trends and algorithms. *Eur Resp J* 2001;**18**:196–208.

Pulmonary oedema

- Pulmonary oedema is an excess of extravascular lung water.
- The causes of pulmonary oedema can be divided into those related to an increase in hydrostatic pressure and those caused by increased vascular permeability (Table 4.9). This dichotomous classification has the advantage of simplicity but in practice the cause of pulmonary oedema, in individual patients, may be multifactorial and the clinical distinction between hydrostatic and increased permeability oedema is not always clear.
- The terms cardiogenic and non-cardiogenic oedema are sometimes applied but, in the following discussion, the more mechanistic division into hydrostatic and increased permeability oedema is used.

Table 4.9 Causes of pulmonary oedema

- **Hydrostatic**
  - Left ventricular dysfunction
  - Mitral valve stenosis
  - Chronic liver disease
  - Renal disease
  - Fluid overload
  - Pulmonary veno-occlusive disease
- **Increased permeability**
  - Acute respiratory distress syndrome and acute lung injury
- **Uncertain mechanism**
  - Re-expansion oedema
  - Re-perfusion oedema
  - Neurogenic (e.g. intracranial tumours, haemorrhage, head injury)
  - High-altitude oedema

Pathophysiology of pulmonary oedema

- Knowledge of the pathophysiology of oedema is of relevance to the interpretation of radiological tests.
- Hydrostatic pulmonary oedema occurs in situations where there is an increase in pulmonary venous pressure or a decrease in plasma oncotic pressure.
- As the term implies, in increased permeability oedema, the key pathological event is 'injury' to the alveolar–capillary cellular barrier.

- Regardless of mechanism, there is a more or less predictable sequence: as the normal capacity of the pulmonary lymphatics to remove extravascular fluid is exceeded, the volume of fluid in the central (bronchovascular) and peripheral interstitium increases. If the inciting event is not corrected, oedema fluid then leaks into the air spaces, leading to alveolar oedema.

Imaging of pulmonary oedema

CXR findings (Figs. 4.37 and 4.38)

For clarity, the CXR signs of interstitial and alveolar oedema are considered separately. In most cases, there is a recognizable CXR sequence (mirroring the pathophysiological changes) from normal, through appearances indicating interstitial oedema, and finally air space opacification.

Interstitial oedema

- Septal lines—indicating thickening of interlobular septa. Two morphological types of septal lines may be seen: a) short (~1cm), parallel, thin lines seen in the periphery of the mid/lower zones which contact the visceral pleural (also called Kerley B lines) and b) longer (up to 4cm), thin lines radiating from the hila in the mid/upper zones (called Kerley A lines). Septal lines are not synonymous with oedema since any cause of infiltration of the interlobular septa may render these lines visible (e.g. lymphangitis carcinomatosis).
- Peribronchial 'cuffing' and peri-hilar haziness—due to oedema fluid in the central interstitium surrounding the bronchovascular structures.
- Lamellar effusion—fluid collecting between the lung and visceral pleura (NB *not* in the pleural space).

Intra-alveolar oedema

- Ground-glass opacification ± consolidation—indicating oedema fluid in the air spaces; typically bilateral and symmetrical but may be asymmetric and, rarely, unilateral. Unlike other causes (e.g. infection) air space opacification due to oedema may alter in severity relatively rapidly (over a period of hours sometimes). Thus, review of serial chest radiographs is of diagnostic value.

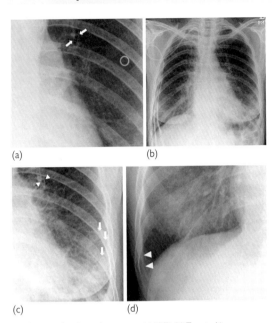

(a)

(b)

(c)

(d)

Fig. 4.37 Interstitial oedema shown on serial CXR. (a) Targeted image demonstrating a normal segmental airway seen 'end-on' in the left lung (arrows); the wall of the airway is uniform and thin. (b) CXR in the same patient on another day shows increased linear markings, particularly in the mid and lower zones but there is no evidence of air space opacification to indicate intra-alveolar fluid. (c) Targeted image of the same examination as (b) showing a lack of clarity of the wall of the segmental airway (arrowheads; termed 'peri-bronchial cuffing') and multiple linear septal (Kerley B) lines (arrows). (d) Targeted CXR in another patient showing a lamellar effusion (arrowheads) at the right base.

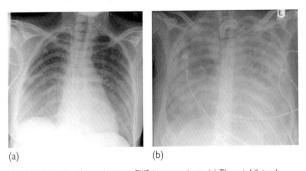

(a)

(b)

Fig. 4.38 Intra-alveolar oedema on CXR in two patients. (a) There is bilateral mid- and lower zone ground-glass opacification due to intra-alveolar oedema. (b) Bilateral patchy consolidation reflecting severe oedema.

CT findings (Fig. 4.39)

As with CXR, the CT appearances of pulmonary oedema reflect the pathophysiological sequence. The CT features that indicate pulmonary oedema are as follows:

- **Interstitial oedema**
  - Ground-glass opacification—may be subtle but typically bilateral and widespread. There may be sparing of the sub-pleural lung.
  - Thickened interlobular septa—smooth thickening is the usual finding; may be associated with the thickening of intralobular structures. When the thickening of septa is associated with ground-glass opacification, a crazy-paving pattern may be seen.
- **Intra-alveolar oedema**
  - Ground-glass opacification.
  - Consolidation.
- **Ancillary features**
  - The following features may be present: bilateral pleural effusions, pericardial effusion, cardiac enlargement (± left ventricular enlargement), increased density of mediastinal fat, enlarged mediastinal lymph nodes.

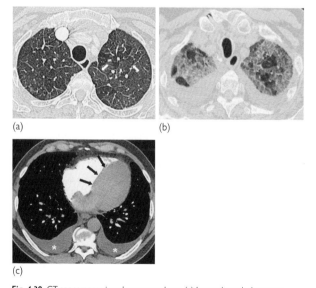

(a) (b)

(c)

Fig. 4.39 CT appearances in pulmonary oedema. (a) Image through the upper zones demonstrating smooth interlobular septal thickening (arrows) and subtle ground-glass opacification. (b) CT in another patient with more obvious ground-glass opacities and thickening of interlobular septa and intralobular structures (giving a crazy-paving appearance). (c) Ancillary CT findings in a patient with pulmonary oedema. There are bilateral pleural effusions (asterisks) and convex bowing of the interventricular septum towards the right (arrows).

Miscellaneous causes of pulmonary oedema

Acute respiratory distress syndrome (ARDS)

- ARDS is a non-specific but stereotypical and potentially life-threatening response of the lung to direct (pulmonary) or indirect (extra-pulmonary) injury.

- **Direct injury (pulmonary ARDS)**
    - Aspiration
    - Severe pneumonia
    - Toxic fume inhalation
    - Near-drowning
    - Trauma with lung contusion
- **Indirect injury (extrapulmonary ARDS)**
    - Severe systemic (non-pulmonary) sepsis
    - Non-thoracic trauma
    - Hypertransfusion response/transfusion-related acute lung injury (TRALI)

- Regardless of cause, the catastrophic cascade in ARDS begins with the exudative phase (0–24hrs after injury) in which there is capillary congestion and endothelial swelling followed by sloughing of cells from the alveolar epithelium and capillary endothelium. There is widespread exudation of proteinaceous fluid and inflammatory cells (first into the interstitium and then into air spaces); characteristic hyaline membranes subsequently form.
- In the next, proliferative phase (24–36hrs), there is proliferation of fibroblasts and type II pneumocytes.
- Finally, there is a chronic phase (36hrs onwards) when 'repair' occurs but there may be considerable residual lung fibrosis.

Diagnosis of ARDS

The diagnosis of ARDS is based on physiological criteria and *not* imaging tests; radiology plays a supporting role in diagnosis (Table 4.10). The key physiological parameter is the ratio of the arterial oxygenation (PaO_2) to the fraction of inspired oxygen (FiO_2). A PaO_2/FiO_2 ratio < 300mmHg in a patient with acute onset of respiratory symptoms, no evidence of cardiac dysfunction, and infiltrates on CXR indicates acute lung injury whereas a PaO_2/FiO_2<200mmHg defines patients with acute respiratory distress syndrome.

Table 4.10 Indications for imaging in ARDS

Indication	Role of imaging test	
	CXR	**CT**
Supporting a diagnosis of ARDS	++	+/−
Detection of complications ('silent' or otherwise)	++	++
Monitoring progression/resolution	++	+/−
Determining the cause of ARDS	−	+/−
Quantifying for 'staging' severity	−	++
In follow-up of survivors	+/−	+/−

++ definite role; +/− possible role in specific circumstances; − no defined role

Imaging in ARDS
CXR findings (Fig. 4.40)
The CXR features of ARDS broadly reflect the sequence of histopathological changes:

- 0–24hrs—the CXR is usually normal.
- 24–36hrs—increasingly extensive homogeneous air space opacities with ground-glass opacification ± consolidation, diffusely and symmetrically distributed in all lung zones.
- 36hrs onwards: severity/distribution of air space opacities persist for a variable period after 36hrs and followed by radiographic resolution; signs of fibrosis (parenchymal distortion, reticulation, volume loss) of variable severity, may be seen.
- In addition to the CXR signs of ARDS, it is important to review CXRs for features indicating complications or iatrogenic injury:
  • Pneumothoraces (due to barotrauma)
  • Nosocomial/ventilator-associated pneumonia
  • Pleural effusions
  • Fluid overload/left ventricular dysfunction

The radiological signs which indicate complications may be modified considerably because of the (sometimes unavoidable) suboptimal radiographic technique in critically-ill patients and, not infrequently, coexistent pathology (e.g. left ventricular dysfunction/fluid overload or emphysema on a background of ARDS).

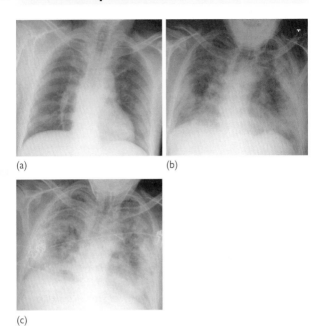

(a)

(b)

(c)

Fig. 4.40 CXR series in ARDS following major trauma. (a) Normal CXR taken at admission. (b) and (c) show progressive air space opacification caused by filling of the interstitium and then the air spaces with oedema and haemorrhagic fluid.

CT findings (during the 'acute' period) (Fig. 4.41)

In contrast to CXR, the appearances on CT may be markedly inhomogeneous. Two broad groups of appearances are recognized:

- Typical—symmetrical abnormalities with a gradient of increasing parenchymal density from the ventral (non-dependent) to dorsal (dependent) regions; in dependent lung there is dense opacification (representing atelectatic lung units) whereas in the non-dependent lung there is ground-glass opacification (representing oedematous but non-atelectatic parenchyma) admixed with more normally aerated lung. This distribution is more commonly associated with extrapulmonary ARDS.
- Atypical—greater inhomogeneity with a less obvious gradient. Foci of consolidation in non-dependent lung. Atypical CT appearances are more commonly associated with pulmonary ARDS.

CT findings (in survivors)

With improved ICU support and management of the critically-ill, an increasing proportion now survive the acute period. CT demonstrates:

- Reticulation in the anterior (non-dependent) lung—probably representing fibrosis and disruption related to the relatively greater effects of barotrauma on the non-atelectatic ('unprotected') ventral lung in the acute stages.
- Ground-glass opacities ± traction bronchiectasis/bronchiolectasis—also concentrated in the anterior lung and denoting finer fibrosis but below the limits of CT resolution.
- Normal or near-normal posterior (dependent) lung.

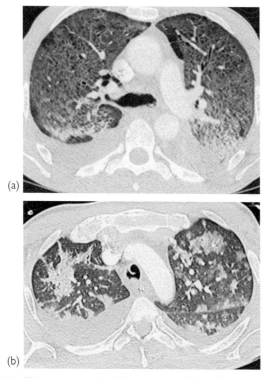

(a)

(b)

Fig. 4.41 CT in two patients with ARDS demonstrating (a) 'Typical' appearance with a symmetrical gradient of increasing density from the ventral (non-dependent) to dorsal (dependent) lung and (b) 'Atypical' appearances with widespread ground-glass opacification but also non-dependent foci of consolidation. There are small-volume bilateral pleural effusions in both patients.

Re-expansion pulmonary oedema
- Pulmonary oedema which follows drainage of large pleural collections, pneumothoraces, or after thoracoscopic intervention.
- Probably related to a combination of mechanical vascular injury during rapid re-expansion and reperfusion injury, both leading to increased permeability oedema.
- Usually occurs in 1–2hrs after re-expansion but can be up to 24hrs later; resolves within one week.
- CXR shows ground-glass opacities/consolidation, typically in the ipsilateral lower lobe but may be bilateral and, rarely, in the contralateral lung (Fig. 4.42).

Neurogenic pulmonary oedema
- Pulmonary oedema related to many and varied intracranial pathologies (e.g. severe head or spinal cord injury, CNS tumours, subarachnoid or spinal haemorrhage, extradural haematoma, and severe grand mal seizures).
- Onset of neurogenic pulmonary oedema may be very rapid and resolving in 24–48hrs.

High-altitude pulmonary oedema
- Pulmonary oedema related to rapid ascent to heights over 2500m.
- Generally occurs 36–72hrs after ascent to altitude.

Transfusion-related acute lung injury (TRALI)
- Acute lung injury which occurs following transfusion of blood/blood products; possibly related to transfusion of anti-HLA, class I or II antigens or anti-granulocyte antibodies leading to activation of complement-mediated sequestration and activation of neutrophils in the lung.
- Commonest cause of transfusion-related death in UK and USA; mortality = 5–25%.
- Pulmonary oedema occurring either during transfusion or within 1–2hrs in the majority; most patients recover within 72hrs.
- The CXR appearances are indistinguishable from those of ALI/ARDS.

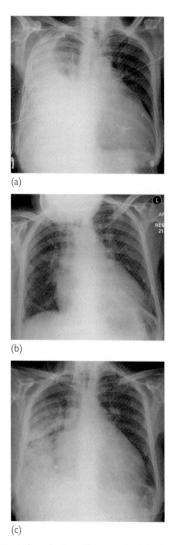

(a)

(b)

(c)

Fig. 4.42 Pulmonary oedema due to rapid re-expansion following drainage of pleural fluid. (a) Large right pleural effusion associated with mediastinal shift to the left. (b) CXR taken 2 hrs following chest drain insertion. There is no residual pleural fluid on the right. (c) CXR taken the following day shows unilateral air space opacification caused by pulmonary oedema.

Diffuse pulmonary haemorrhage

Diffuse haemorrhage into the lungs is a relatively rare occurrence; the common causes of diffuse pulmonary haemorrhage are listed in Table 4.11. Most patients present with haemoptysis and anaemia. However, widespread pulmonary haemorrhage may not be accompanied by any haemoptysis. Regardless of the underlying cause the imaging features of diffuse pulmonary haemorrhage are non-specfic.

The CXR and CT features of specific causes of diffuse pulmonary haemorrhage are discussed elsewhere. A useful diagnostic feature, particularly on serial CXRs, is that (in the absence of on-going haemorrhage), opacities caused by intra-alveolar blood, resolve relatively quickly. This contrasts with other possible causes of air space opacification (e.g. infection, malignancy) which tend to resolve/progress more slowly.

Table 4.11 Common causes of diffuse pulmonary haemorrhage

- Idiopathic pulmonary haemosiderosis
- Anti-glomerular basement membrane disease (Goodpasture's syndrome)
- Wegener's granulomatosis
- Microscopic polyangiitis
- Churg–Strauss syndrome
- Drug-induced (e.g. cyclophosphamide, anticoagulants, cocaine)
- Systemic lupus erythematosus
- Other connective tissue diseases (e.g. rheumatoid arthritis)
- Henoch-Schönlein disease
- Antiphospholipid syndrome
- Behçet's disease
- Diffuse alveolar damage

Air space opacification caused by malignant disease

A few malignant lung diseases can manifest with a pattern of air space opacification (i.e. consolidation and/or ground-glass opacity). The diagnosis of these disorders is potentially difficult and may be delayed, particularly if the clinical features are non-specific. At first presentation, findings are not infrequently interpreted as being representative of more benign pathology (e.g. infection); in this regard, CT often offers no diagnostic advantage over CXR. Indeed, more often than not, a review of serial CXRs (as opposed to CT), in a patient with 'non-resolving' air space opacities raises the possibility of a malignant (or potentially pre-malignant) cause.

Premalignant and malignant causes of air space opacification (consolodation and/or ground-glass opacity)

- Atypical adenomatous hyperplasia
- Adenocarcinoma—primary or secondary
- Adenocarcinoma in situ
- Primary pulmonary lymphoma (MALToma)*

* see 📖 Lung tumours/Other primary lung tumours, p348.

Atypical adenomatous hyperplasia

- Focal proliferation of atypical cuboidal or columnar epithelial cells along the alveoli and respiratory bronchioles.
- Atypical adenomatous hyperplasia (AAH) is believed to be a precursor lesion to adenocarcinoma. Foci of AAH are incidentally discovered in up to 16% of patients with lung cancer.
- The number of detected AAH lesions has been increasing due to the widespread use of CT and because of screening in some countries.

Imaging of AAH

The lesions of AAH are seldom, if ever, detectable on CXR.

CT findings (Fig. 4.43)

- Nodule—ground-glass attenuation, spherical or oval nodular area of pure ground-glass opacification with smooth margins. Typically <5mm in diameter.
- The interface between AAH lesions and surrounding normal lung is usually well-defined.
- Although AAH is usually smaller than adenocarcinoma, lesion size cannot be used as a reliable discriminating feature.

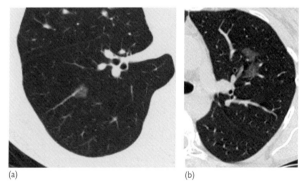

(a)   (b)

Fig. 4.43 Atypical adenomatous hyperplasia in two patients. (a) single, and (b) multiple lesions of AAH demonstrating the typical appearance of 'pure' ground glass nodules.

Adenocarcinoma

- Adenocarcinoma is the most common histological subtype of lung cancer.
- The classification of lung adenocarcinoma has proven difficult and has been subject to change over many years. The latest IASLC/ATS/ERS International Multidisciplinary Lung Adenocarcinoma Classification proposes the following
  - Preinvasive lesions:
    - Atypical adenomatous hyperplasia.
    - Adenocarcinoma in situ (previously called bronchioloalveolar cell carcinoma)—mucinous, non-mucinous or mixed non-mucinous/mucinous.
  - Minimally invasive adenocarcinoma.
  - Invasive adenocarcinoma (subdivided into the following patterns: lepidic predominant, acinar predominant, papillary predominant, micropapillary predominant and solid predominant).
  - Variants of invasive adenocarcinoma.

Imaging of adenocarcinoma

Small foci of adenocarcinoma are unlikely to be identified on CXR. The CXR findings of larger peripheral adenocarcinomas is covered elsewhere (see 📖 Lung tumours/Lung cancer p328). The CT appearances of small adenocarcinomas vary.

CT findings (Fig. 4.44)

- Nodule(s)—single or multiple. Lobulated or spiculated (sometimes with a pleural 'tag'). Nodules may be of pure ground-glass attenuation, pure 'solid' density or with mixed ground-glass and solid elements. Focal bubble-like lucencies (termed pseudocavitation) and air bronchograms/bronchiolograms may be present. Nodules may be small (i.e. < 2 cm diameter).
- Consolidation—In a single or multiple lobes (with or without nodules); pseudocavitation and bulging of fissures may be present. On contrast-enhanced CT, vessels may seen coursing through consolidated lung (the CT angiogram sign). In some patients there is predominant ground-glass opacification with thickening of inter and intralobular septa (the crazy-paving pattern).

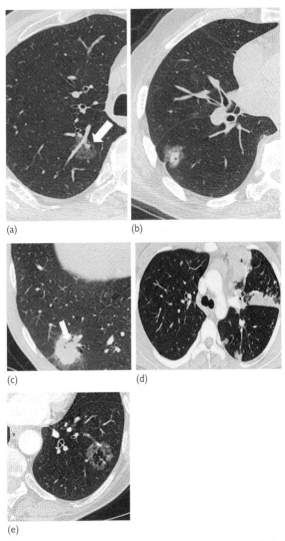

(a)   (b)

(c)   (d)

(e)

Fig. 4.44 Variable CT appearances of adenocarcinoma in different patients. (a) Focal non-solid nodule (arrow) in the right upper lobe. (b) Part-solid nodule in the right lower lobe. There are ground-glass and more dense (solid) elements. (c) Rounded area of consolidation in the right lower lobe; an air bronchiologram is visible (arrow). (d) Multifocal consolidation and multiple small nodules in the left upper and lower lobes. (e) Focal ground-glass nodule in the left lobe with central bubble-like lucencies (pseudocavitation) in another patient with proven adenocarcinoma.

Chapter 5

141

Airways diseases

Imaging in airways disease

Diseases of the airways are common and comprise those which affect the large (i.e. trachea, main, lobar, segmental, and subsegmental bronchi) and/or the small airways (Table 5.1).

Table 5.1 Causes/categories of airways disease

- **Large airways (tracheal/bronchial):**
  - Tracheomalacia and tracheobronchomalacia
  - Tracheobronchomegaly (Mournier–Kuhn syndrome)
  - Tracheal stenosis (e.g. infections, tumours, Wegener's granulomatosis, Saber-sheath trachea, Tracheobronchopathia osteochondroplastica, sarcoidosis)
  - Relapsing polychondritis
  - Bronchiectasis
  - Broncholithiasis
- **Small airways**:
  - Obliterative bronchiolitis
  - Exudative bronchiolitis
- **Miscellaneous disorders**:
  - Follicular bronchiolitis
  - Hypersensitivity pneumonitis
  - Sarcoidosis
  - Respiratory bronchiolitis

Imaging tests for airways disease

The radiological tests most commonly used in the investigation of patients with suspected airways disease are:
- CXR
- CT

CXR in airways disease

The signs of airways disease will vary according to the principal site of abnormality. However, the signs on CXR that suggest airways disease are:

- Direct signs
    - Airway wall thickening (trachea, main, segmental, or subsegmental bronchi).
    - Focal narrowing (trachea, main airways—easily overlooked).
    - Airway dilatation.
    - Non-tapering segmental/subsegmental airways or ring shadows.
    - Large branching opacities (mucus-filled dilated bronchi).
    - Nodular opacities.
- Indirect signs
    - Hyperinflation.
      Hyperlucency (focal or diffuse).
    - Paucity of vascular markings/vessel 'pruning'.

CT in airways disease

CT (and specifically, HRCT) more readily demonstrates the features of airways disease. The advent of multi-detector row CT acquisitions now allows sophisticated reconstructions (e.g. volume-rendering or minimum intensity projections) and analysis of the airways. This may be of particular value in the evaluation of tracheal disorders. The HRCT signs of airways disease include:

- Direct signs
    - Abnormal dilatation of airways.
    - Abnormal narrowing of airways.
    - Greater than expected collapse of central airways on expiration.
    - Tracheal/bronchial wall thickening.
    - Abnormal dilatation or narrowing—either focal or diffuse.
    - Plugging/branching opacities in large airways (bronchocoeles) or the peripheral airways (tree-in-bud pattern).
- Indirect signs
    - Mosaic attenuation pattern.
    - Volume loss.

Tracheomalacia/tracheobronchomalacia

- Weakness of the trachea and main bronchi due to hypoplasia/atrophy of the longitudinal elastic fibres or a weakness of cartilage rendering the airways excessively susceptible to collapse during expiration (NB a small reduction in the cross-sectional area (typically up to 35% but sometimes exceeding 50%) is a normal phenomenon during expiration).
- Tracheomalacia (TM) and tracheobronchomalacia (TBM) occur at any age; congenital and acquired forms are recognized (Table 5.2). Both are common and underdiagnosed.

Table 5.2 Causes and associations of TM/TBM

- **Congenital**
  - Prematurity
  - Cartilage abnormalities (Ehlers–Danlos syndrome, dyschondroplasia, chondromalacia)
  - Mucopolysaccharidoses (Hurler's syndrome, Hunter's syndrome)
  - Chromosomal/genetic disorders (trisomy 9, trisomy 21, 11p13 and 22q11 deletion)
  - Associations with tracheo-oesophageal fistula and bronchopulmonary dysplasia
- **Acquired**
  - Prolonged intubation/tracheostomy
  - Relapsing polychondritis
  - Severe tracheobronchitis
  - Chronic extrinsic compression (vascular anomalies (e.g. right-sided aortic arch, aberrant right subclavian artery), left atrial enlargement, scoliosis, tumours)
  - Post-infectious
  - Post-traumatic

Adapted from Carden KA et al. *Chest* 2005; **127**:984–1005.

Imaging of tracheomalacia/tracheobronchomalacia

CXR findings
In the era of multidetector CT, the CXR probably has a limited or no role in the accurate diagnosis of TM/TBM.

CT findings (Fig. 5.1)
MDCT is the radiological investigation of choice for the diagnosis of TM/TBM. The key findings of TM/TBM are:
- Reduction of airway cross-sectional area; a reduction of >50% has been the traditional threshold for diagnosis, although it is recognized that more severe collapsibility (e.g. >70%) may be present in normal volunteers.
  - At suspended end-expiration—CT performed at end-inspiration and followed by images through the airways at full end-expiration.
  - During dynamic expiration—the CT acquisition occurs during a forced expiratory manoeuvre; a more sensitive method than (non-dynamic) paired inspiratory-expiratory CT.
- 'Frown' sign—tracheal lumen becomes crescentic on expiratory CT due to marked anterior bowing of the posterior membrane and near apposition with the anterior wall. Normal outline on inspiratory CT in majority.

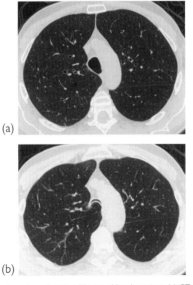

Fig. 5.1 Tracheobronchomalacia in a 79-year-old male patient. (a) CT image at full suspended inspiration shows the normal configuration of the posterior tracheal membrane (bowing convex posteriorly); there is cylindrical bronchiectasis in both lungs. (b) CT at residual volume demonstrates marked reduction in the cross-sectional area of the tracheal lumen. Note the anterior bowing of the posterior tracheal membrane leading to a crescentic lumen (the 'frown sign').

Tracheal stenosis

- Abnormal reduction in the cross-sectional area of the tracheal lumen; stenosis may be focal (e.g. in the subglottic region) or diffuse.
- The trachea may be narrowed because of extrinsic compression or there may be intrinsic tracheal disease (Table 5.3).

Table 5.3 Cause of tracheal stenosis

- **Extrinsic compression**
  - Vascular anomalies (aberrant right subclavian artery, pulmonary artery sling, thoracic aortic aneurysm)
  - Non-tracheal tumours
  - (Iatrogenic) haematoma
- **Intrinsic**
  - Congenital tracheal stenosis
  - Idiopathic laryngotracheal stenosis
  - Iatrogenic (post-endotracheal intubation)
  - Post-lung transplantation/other surgery (at airway anastomotic site)
  - Inflammatory/immunological (Wegener's granulomatosis, relapsing poly-chondritis, amyloidosis, sarcoidosis)
  - Infections (tuberculosis, fungal, viral (e.g. laryngotracheal papillomatosis))
  - Tracheal tumours (benign or malignant)
  - Miscellaneous (mucopolysaccharidoses, tracheobronchopathia osteochon-droplastica, multifocal fibrosclerosis)

Imaging of tracheal stenosis

CXR findings

CXR plays a minor role in the accurate diagnosis and evaluation of the severity of tracheal stenosis. However, there may be signs suggesting tracheal narrowing (e.g. due to thyroid enlargement) on CXR.

CT findings (Fig. 5.2)

CT is the non-invasive investigation of choice for suspected tracheal stenosis. With MDCT machines different image reconstruction formats are available. Depending on the cause of tracheal stenosis there may be:
- Focal/diffuse narrowing of the tracheal wall ± wall thickening.
- External compression (e.g. an anomalous vessel, a thyroid goitre).

The following image reconstruction formats, of varying complexity, are now routinely available on CT machines:

- Axial CT—the standard method for reviewing CT images.
- Multiplanar reconstruction (MPR)—with the thin-section contiguous ('volume') image acquisition from MDCT, the trachea may be viewed in the coronal and/or sagittal planes in conjunction with the axial images; curved MPRs may also be used.
- Minimum intensity projection—these reconstructions 'enhance' the lowest attenuation elements in an image. Thus, the air-containing airways are optimally visualized.
- Three-dimensional (3D) surface-shaded display—a reconstruction technique which creates the impression of a 3D image with depth due to (computer-generated) 'shading'.
- Volume rendering—another 3D image reconstruction technique in which a 3D external impression of the trachea is generated.
- Virtual CT bronchoscopy—a 3D reconstruction of the internal appearance of the trachea. This technique has one potential advantage over bronchoscopy in that the airway lumen beyond a significant obstruction (not accessible to the bronchoscope) may be examined.

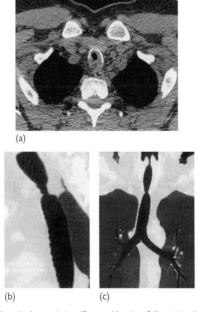

(a)

(b)   (c)

Fig. 5.2 Focal tracheal stenosis in a 47-year-old patient following intubation. (a) Axial CT showing narrowing of the tracheal lumen and concentric wall thickening. (b) Sagittal and (c) coronal minimum intensity projections more accurately demonstrate the site and extent of focal tracheal narrowing which gives rise to an 'hour-glass' configuration.

Miscellaneous large airway diseases

Tracheobronchopathia osteochondroplastica (or tracheopathia osteoplastica)

- Rare condition of unknown aetiology, characterized by the presence of multiple osteocartilagenous nodules in the trachea and sometimes the central bronchi.
- Most cases occur in males and typically present in the 5th or 6th decades (NB the condition is recognized in childhood and old age).

CXR findings

- Usually normal; nodularity ± calcification may be rarely discernible along the anterior tracheal wall on a lateral CXR, particularly in advanced disease.
- Narrowing of the trachea may be seen on a frontal CXR.

CT findings (Fig. 5.3)

- Multiple nodular submucosal lesions ± calcification projecting into the tracheal lumen—by definition, lesions spare the posterior tracheal membrane (because of the absence of cartilaginous elements.
- Tracheal (± main bronchi) narrowing—if severe, the trachea may narrow in its coronal dimension.

Saber-sheath trachea

- The term refers to the morphology of the intrathoracic trachea in which the sagittal diameter is increased and the coronal diameter decreased (ratio of sagittal:coronal diameter >2).
- Related to COPD in >90% and almost exclusively in males.

CXR findings

- Diffuse narrowing of the trachea on a frontal CXR, below the level of the thoracic inlet.
- Smooth luminal surface (cf. tracheobronchopathia osteochondroplastica).

CT findings (Fig. 5.4)

- Diffuse narrowing of the tracheal lumen in the coronal plane. NB The trachea returns to normal calibre or configuration at the thoracic inlet and just above the carina.
- Important 'negative' findings include the smooth luminal surface and the absence of tracheal wall thickening.

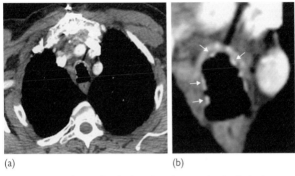

(a)   (b)

Fig. 5.3 Incidental finding of tracheobronchopathia osteochondroplastica in an adult male patient. (a) Axial CT on soft-tissue window settings demonstrates irregularity of the tracheal lumen caused by multiple nodules. (b) Magnified image of the same section clearly shows multiple calcified nodules around the inner tracheal wall (arrows).

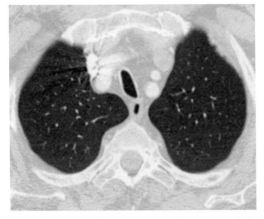

Fig. 5.4 Saber-sheath trachea. CT through the apices demonstrates marked reduction in the coronal diameter of the trachea (compared to the antero-posterior diameter).

Relapsing polychondritis

- A multisystem disorder characterized by chondral inflammation that affects any cartilage-containing structure (e.g. the pinna, nose, joints, and airways).
- Equal sex incidence but respiratory involvement is more common in females; typically presenting in the 5th to 6th decades. Airway involvement occurs in up to 50% of patients at some time during the course of the illness.

CXR findings

- Usually normal—tracheal calcification may occasionally be identified.

CT findings (Fig. 5.5)

- Tracheal and bronchial wall thickening with sparing of the posterior tracheal membrane; bronchial wall thickening without tracheal involvement is recognized but less common. Wall thickening is usually smooth and diffuse but is occasionally focal and nodular.
- Increased density of anterior and lateral walls of the trachea and bronchial walls (NB the posterior tracheal membrane is spared); overt calcification may be present.
- Airway stenosis: usually diffuse, rarely focal and subglottic.
- There may be excessive collapse of the trachea and bronchi (tracheomalacia/tracheobronchomalacia) on end-expiratory or dynamic expiratory CT.

Tracheobronchial papillomatosis

- A rare disorder caused by human papilloma virus infection: typically localized to the larynx but tracheal and bronchial involvement with multiple sessile or polypoidal papillomas can occur. Pulmonary parenchymal involvement is less common but recognized.

CXR findings (Fig. 5.6)

- Polypoidal mass(es) in the trachea and large airways may be seen if the lesions are large.
- Multiple pulmonary nodules ± cavitation.
- Secondary effects of obstructing tracheal and bronchial mass(es) include atelectasis and distal obstructive pneumonia.

CT findings (Fig. 5.6)

- Single or multiple tracheal or bronchial nodules.
- Multiple intrapulmonary nodules ± cavitation.

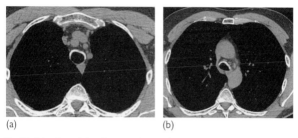

Fig. 5.5 Relapsing polychondritis in a 49-year-old male. Axial CT images (a) at the level of the great vessels and (b) below the level of the aortic arch. Both images show thickening and calcification of the anterior and lateral walls of the trachea but with sparing of the (non-cartilaginous) posterior tracheal membrane.

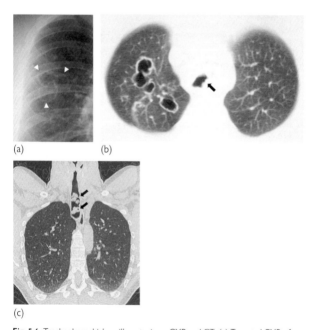

Fig. 5.6 Tracheobronchial papillomatosis on CXR and CT. (a) Targeted CXR of the right lung demonstrating a cluster of thin-walled cavities (arrowheads). (b) CT through the upper zones in the same patient as in (a) shows the same cavities in the right lung. There is nodularity along the left lateral wall of the trachea (black arrow). (c) Coronal CT in another patient with multiple polypoid lesions in the tracheal lumen (black arrows).

Bronchiectasis

- Bronchiectasis is irreversible (localized or diffuse) bronchial dilatation typically caused by inflammation.
- The relative frequency with which the recognized causes (Table 5.4) of bronchiectasis are encountered has changed over the years: most notably, post-infectious bronchiectasis is less commonly a cause in Western countries but remains frequent in the developing world.
- Despite appropriate investigations, a cause for bronchiectasis is not found in up to 50% of patients.

Table 5.4 Causes of bronchiectasis

- **Idiopathic**
- **Immunodeficiency** including panhypogammaglobulinaemia, post-chemotherapy or immunoglobulin-related disorders (IgG4-disease).
- **Cystic fibrosis**
- **Post-infective**
  - McLeod's/Swyer–James syndrome
  - Viral/mycoplasma/pertussis pneumonia
  - Mycobacterial—TB and non-tuberculous
- **Other congenital disorders**
  - Williams–Campbell syndrome
  - Mounier–Kuhn syndrome
  - α_1-antitrypsin deficiency
- **Chronic mechanical airway obstruction**
- **Impaired mucus transport**
  - Primary and secondary ciliary dyskinesia
  - Young's syndrome
- **Immunological**
  - Allergic bronchopulmonary aspergillosis
  - Following solid-organ or haematopoetic stem cell transplantation
- **Miscellaneous**
  - Ulcerative colitis
  - HIV infection
  - Rheumatoid arthritis
  - Coeliac disease

Imaging in bronchiectasis
CXR findings (Fig. 5.7)
The low sensitivity and specificity means that the CXR can not be relied on to make a confident diagnosis in anything but advanced disease. The CXR features of bronchiectasis include:
- Prominent ring-shaped opacities—for airways that are seen 'end-on'; cystic opacities (± air-fluid levels) in more severe disease.
- Tramline opacities—for airways that are seen longitudinally.
- Ancillary CXR features—hyperexpansion (caused by airflow obstruction), volume loss/crowding of airways.

CT findings
HRCT is the gold-standard for a diagnosis of bronchiectasis; however, it should be noted that for one of the key diagnostic signs (i.e. the absence of bronchial tapering) high-resolution CT reconstructions from a *volume*

acquisition (as opposed to interspaced HRCT images) may be superior. The CT features of bronchiectasis can be divided into the cardinal signs (i.e. without which a CT diagnosis *cannot* be made) and ancillary signs. Except for a minority of conditions (e.g. in *some* patients with cystic fibrosis, allergic bronchopulmonary aspergillosis, or α_1-antitrypsin deficiency) CT provides no clue as to the underlying cause of bronchiectasis.

- **Cardinal CT findings (Fig. 5.8)**
  - Non-tapering airways—most reliable sign and best appreciated on axial CT images in the mid-zone (typically the middle lobe and lingular airways). NB The morphological appearance of bronchiectatic airways may be:
    - cylindrical—parallel-walled.
    - varicose—dilated bronchi with a 'beaded' appearance.
    - cystic—cystic dilatation ± air-fluid levels.
  - Signet ring sign—the luminal (internal) diameter of the airway exceeds the transverse diameter of the homologous pulmonary artery. This sign should be looked for in airways in the upper and lower lobes, which are oriented perpendicular to the usual axial imaging plane.
  - Airways visible within 2cm of the pleural surface.
- **Ancillary CT signs (Fig. 5.9)**
  - Bronchial wall thickening.
  - Bronchial crowding/volume loss.
  - Mucus filling of large (central) and smaller (peripheral) airways manifests as bronchocoeles and tree-in-bud opacities respectively.
  - Mosaic attenuation pattern reflecting constrictive obliterative bronchiolitis (see 📖 Airway diseases/Constrictive obliterative bronchiolitis, p166) (present to a greater or lesser degree in virtually all patients with bronchiectasis); NB may be present in lobes without overt evidence of bronchiectasis.
  - Smooth thickening of interlobular septa.
  - Segmental/subsegmental atelectasis.

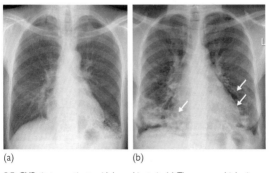

(a) (b)

Fig. 5.7 CXRs in two patients with bronchiectasis. (a) There are multiple ring-shaped opacities in the left lower zone. CT in this patient showed that bronchiectasis was most severe in, but not restricted to, the left lower lobe. (b) Cystic bronchiectasis in both lungs. There are multiple 'cysts' (arrows) with variable wall thickness. Air-fluid levels are also clearly shown in the lumen of many airways.

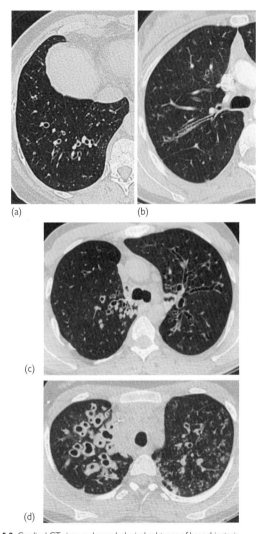

Fig. 5.8 Cardinal CT signs and morphological subtypes of bronchiectasis. (a) Targeted image through the right lower lobe showing mild cylindrical dilatation of subsegmental airways (by comparison with homologous pulmonary arterial branch (the signet ring sign). (b) Targeted image shows a non-tapering airway in the right upper lobe. (c) Varicose bronchiectasis in the left upper lobe and (d) severe cystic bronchietasis in the right upper lobe in a patient with cystic fibrosis. There are tree-in-bud opacities in the left upper lobe.

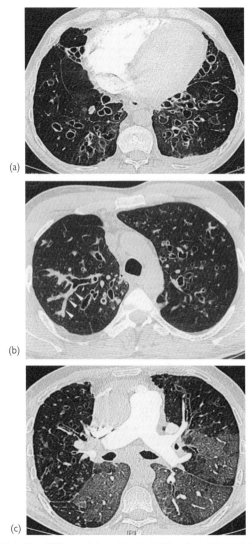

Fig. 5.9 Ancillary CT features in bronchiectasis. (a) 'Crowding' of thick-walled subsegmental airways in the lower lobes and also in the lingula and middle lobe, (b) mucus plugging of a bronchiectatic airway in the periphery of the right upper lobe (arrowheads) and (c) bilateral mosaic attenuation pattern (caused by obliterative bronchiolitis) in a patient with widespread bronchiectasis.

Specific causes of bronchiectasis

A detailed discussion of all causes of bronchiectasis is not the purpose of the following section. However, a brief description of some of the potentially recognizable conditions, in imaging terms, are discussed.

Cystic fibrosis (CF)

Autosomal recessive disease due to genetic mutation on chromosome 7; most commonly affecting the lungs and pancreas.

CXR and CT findings (Figs. 5.10 and 5.11)

- Bronchiectasis—most severe in upper lobes on CXR but can be seen to affect all lobes on CT.
- Bronchial wall thickening.
- Bronchocoeles—caused by mucoid impaction in large airways ('finger-in-glove' sign).
- Consolidation—related to infection but usually not extensive. Transient, migratory areas of consolidation (± bronchocoeles) should suggest the diagnosis of allergic bronchopulmonary aspergillosis.
- Hilar prominence—this may be related to lymph node enlargement and/or pulmonary hypertension.
- Mosaic attenuation pattern—due to obliterative bronchiolitis which is invariably present.
- Nodules—multiple nodules ± cavitation (± focal areas of consolidation) may indicate infection with non-tuberculous mycobacterial infection.

Allergic bronchopulmonary aspergillosis (ABPA)

Allergic disorder related to type I and III hypersensitivity reaction to *Aspergillus* species (most commonly *A. fumigatus*) colonizing the airways. Patients with ABPA exhibit a peripheral blood eosinophilia and the disorder occurs almost exclusively in atopic subjects with asthma or cystic fibrosis.

CXR and CT findings (Fig. 5.12)

- Bronchiectasis—central, usually varicose.
- Tubular, branching ('gloved-finger') or clustered and rounded ('bunch of grapes') opacities, due to mucoid impaction in the large airways; typically in the upper zones, although all lobes may be affected. Opacities may be transient and related to clearing of mucoid plugs from airways.
- Tree-in-bud opacities—caused by plugging of peripheral airways.
- Consolidation (± cavitation)—usually multifocal, segmental, and generally transient.
- Upper lobe scarring and contraction.

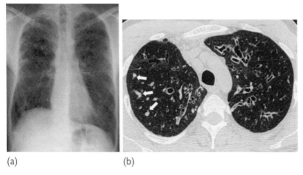

(a)   (b)

Fig. 5.10 CXR and CT in a patient with cystic fibrosis. (a) CXR shows predominantly upper lobe ring-shadows and tramline opacities. (b) On CT through the upper lobes there is varicose bronchiectasis (best seen on the left) and plugging of large airways on the right (arrows).

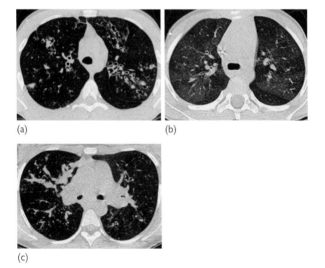

(a)   (b)

(c)

Fig. 5.11 CT appearances in three patients with cystic fibrosis. (a) CT at the level of the aortic arch in a patient with *Mycobacterium abscessus* infection. In addition to bronchiectasis there are multiple nodules in both lungs. (b) CT at the level of the carina demonstrating striking mosaicism caused by obliterative bronchiolitis and (c) mucous plugging of large airways in the right lung.

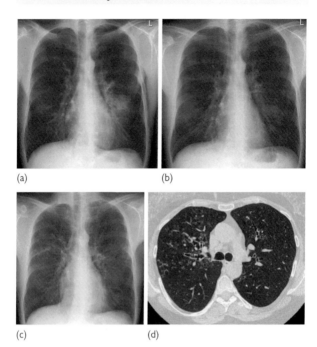

(a) (b)

(c) (d)

Fig. 5.12 CXRs and CT in allergic bronchopulmonary aspergillosis. Serial CXRs in the same patient: (a) initial CXR, (b) 5 months later and (c) 15 months after (b) showing 'flitting' consolidation. There is consolidation in the lingula on the initial CXR which has largely cleared 5 months later but there is now ill-defined opacification in the right upper zone. 15 months later, there are ill-defined opacities in both mid zones together with thick-walled dilated airways. (d) CT at the level of the carina in another patient shows characteristic 'central' varicose bronchiectasis in both upper lobes. There are multiple peripheral tree-in-bud opacities on the right.

Tracheobronchomegaly (Mounier–Kuhn syndrome)

A congenital defect characterized by atrophy/absence of the longitudinal elastic and muscular layers of the trachea. The muscular defect leads to marked dilatation of the trachea and main bronchi. Tracheobronchomegaly is significantly more common in males and in black populations.

CXR and CT findings (Fig. 5.13):

- Tracheal dilatation—transverse diameter >25mm in men and >21mm in women; sagittal diameter >27mm in men and >23mm in women. The thin mucosa prolapses between the cartilage causing a corrugated or sacculated outline.
- Main bronchial dilatation—right main bronchus: >21mm in men and >19.8mm in women; left main bronchus: >18mm in men and >17.4mm in women.
- Localized cystic bronchiectasis with exquisitely thin-walls.

Kartagener's syndrome

This autosomal recessive syndrome, a specific type of ciliary dyskinesia, is characterized by bronchiectasis, situs inversus, and chronic rhino-sinusitis. Kartagener's (or Siewert–Kartagener's) syndrome is found in up to 50% of patients with ciliary dysmotility.

CXR and CT findings (Fig. 5.14):

- Widespread bronchiectasis—tends to be most severe in the middle lobe and lingula.
- Situs inversus totalis—dextrocardia, gastric air-bubble under the right hemidiaphragm, liver in left upper quadrant, spleen in right upper quadrant.
- Sinusitis/nasal polyps.

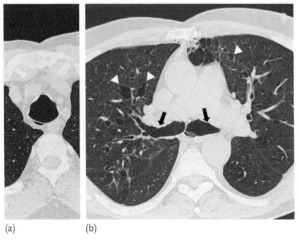

(a)   (b)

Fig. 5.13 CT in Mounier–Kuhn syndrome. (a) Targeted image demonstrating gross dilatation of the trachea and (b) the left and right main bronchi (black arrows). There is varicose bronchiectasis in both lungs; note that dilated airways have very thin walls (arrowheads).

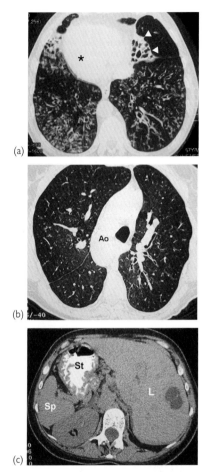

Fig. 5.14 CT in a patient with Kartagener's syndrome. (a) CT through the lower zones demonstrates florid bronchiectasis with a widespread tree-in-bud pattern. There is dextrocardia with the left ventricle on the right (asterisk). The morphological right middle lobe (seen on the left) is atelectatic (arrowheads) (b) Image through the upper zones shows that the aortic arch (Ao) is right sided. (c) CT through the upper abdomen demonstrates total visceral situs (L = liver; Sp = spleen and St = stomach).

Broncholithiasis

- A rare bronchial disorder caused by calcified/ossified material in the lumen of bronchi or the distortion of the tracheobronchial tree by calcified peribronchial nodes.
- In most patients, broncholithiasis is caused by the extrusion (and subsequent erosion) of calcific material ('broncholiths') into the adjacent airway from adjacent lymph nodes and lymph node calcification is typically caused by chronic granulomatous infection (e.g. tuberculosis, histoplasmosis and actinomycosis).

Imaging in broncholithiasis

CXR findings
The CXR signs of broncholithiasis are either due to the presence of calcification in or adjacent to central bronchi or as a consequence of erosion into or obstruction of airways. The key CXR signs are:
- Central calcification—a useful diagnostic sign on serial CXRs is the change in the position of the calcification relative to the airway.
- Segmental or lobar collapse.
- Consolidation—in the segment/lobe subtended by the partially obstructed airway.

CT findings (Fig. 5.15)
The findings on CT mirror those seen on CXR except that the relationship of calcified material to the lumen/wall of the airway is more readily evident:
- Calcification—endobronchial or peri-bronchial but with no associated soft-tissue mass.
- Segmental atelectasis.
- Lobar collapse.
- Consolidation—due to 'obstructive' pneumonia.
- Bronchiectasis.

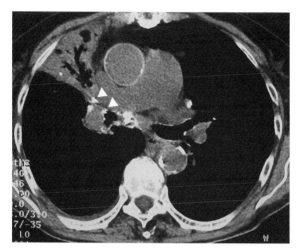

Fig. 5.15 CT just below the level of the carina. There are multiple calcified mediastinal nodes, a number of which (arrowheads) are impinging on the middle lobe bronchus (the lobe is partially collapsed).

Bronchial diverticula

- Small air-filled outpouchings related to the bronchial wall.
- The key pathogenetic process is that of hypertrophy and obstruction of bronchial mucosal glands together with weakness in the airway wall. When intra-airway pressure is raised (e.g. during coughing), mucosa and enlarged glands herniate through the smooth muscle layer and coalesce to form diverticula.

Principal causes and associations of bronchial diverticula

- COPD
- Smoking
- Tracheobronchomegaly (Mournier–Kuhn syndrome)

Imaging of bronchial diverticula

CXR findings

Because diverticula are generally small, CXR has little or no role in detection.

CT findings (Fig. 5.16)

Diverticula are typically seen along the walls of central airways. The CT features are:

- Rounded or tubular blind-ending outpouchings.
- Common ancillary features: bronchial wall thickening, emphysema.

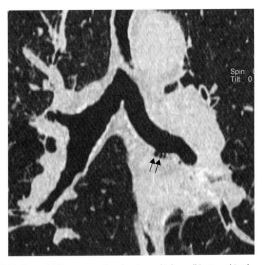

Fig. 5.16 Coronal CT reconstruction showing multiple small 'outpouchings' (diverticula) arising from the inferior wall of the left main bronchus (arrows).

Small airways disease

Terminological considerations

The small airways are defined as those with an internal diameter of <2mm. The terminology of small airways disease has been plagued by confusion: one of the main problems is that clinicians, pathologists, and radiologists have used the apparently simple term 'small airways disease' to describe a range of disparate entities. Pathologists have categorized small airways diseases into many different subtypes which have no clear radiological/clinical correlates.

Although not a comprehensive classification, a more practical approach has been suggested (Table 5.5) which divides the small airway diseases into two broad subgroups. This categorization has the attraction that it accounts for the majority of cases of small airways disease encountered in clinical practice and, perhaps more importantly, has recognizable clinico-radiological manifestations. NB The term bronchiolitis obliterans organizing pneumonia (BOOP) has now been abandoned (see 📖 Diffuse parenchymal lung diseases/Organizing pneumonia, p240).

Table 5.5 Subtypes of the two commonest categories of small airways disease in clinical practice

- **Constrictive obliterative bronchiolitis** Characterized by narrowing of the small airways by peribronchiolar inflammation and, subsequently, fibrosis which progresses to complete obliteration.
- **Exudative bronchiolitis** Characterized by inflammatory exudate in and around the small airways.

Adapted from Hansell DM. Small airways disease: detection and insights with computed tomography *Eur Respir J* 2001; **17**:1294–1313.

Constrictive obliterative bronchiolitis

- A pathological lesion affecting the small airways characterized by peribronchiolar inflammation and fibrosis.
- Constrictive obliterative bronchiolitis (OB) is a surprisingly common finding on histopathological examination. The recognized causes of constrictive OB are shown in Table 5.6.

Table 5.6 Causes of constrictive obliterative bronchiolitis

- **Post infective**
  - Viral (e.g. adenovirus, influenza, parainfluenza, respiratory syncytial virus)
  - Mycoplasma
- **Connective tissue diseases**
  - Rheumatoid arthritis
  - Sjögren's syndrome
- **Allograft recipients**
  - Solid-organ and haematopoietic stem cell transplantation.
- **Drugs** (e.g. penicillamine)
- **Toxic fumes or gas inhalation**
  - Nitrogen dioxide, sulphur dioxide, ammonia, chlorine, phosgene
- **Idiopathic**
- **Miscellaneous**
  - Bronchiectasis
  - Hypersensitivity pneumonitis
  - Sarcoidosis
  - Diffuse idiopathic pulmonary neuroendocrine hyperplasia
  - *Sauropus androgynus* (sweet leaf) ingestion

Imaging of constrictive obliterative bronchiolitis

CXR findings (Fig 5.17)

CXR is relatively insensitive to even severe OB. Moreover, the CXR signs are non-specific and include:
- Hyperinflation—probably the commonest CXR sign of constrictive OB.
- Bronchial wall thickening.
- Paucity/pruning of vessels.

CT findings (Fig. 5.18)

CT is very sensitive and may demonstrate abnormalities even when disease is asymptomatic.

- Mosaic attenuation pattern—the cardinal CT sign of constrictive OB. The areas of decreased attenuation are due to hypoxic vasoconstriction and subsequent vascular remodelling with shunting of blood to normally-ventilated lung (which appears of increased density). Vessels in regions of decreased attenuation are reduced in number and/or calibre; NB in extensive disease, differentiation of mosaicism from panacinar emphysema may be difficult.
- Air-trapping—accentuation of the areas of decreased attenuation (i.e. there is increased conspicuity of 'black' lung because of an increase in the density of adjacent unaffected parenchyma) while maintaining the relative area on end-expiratory CT.
- Dilatation of segmental/subsegmental airways—the severity/extent of large airway dilatation is variable.

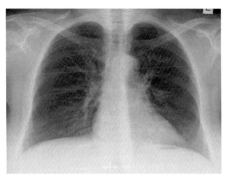

Fig. 5.17 Near normal CXR of a patient with disabling OB caused by previous viral infection.

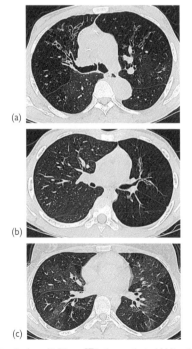

(a)

(b)

(c)

Fig. 5.18 Obliterative bronchiolitis on CT in three patients. (a) Idiopathic bronchiectasis, (b) Swyer-James (McLeod) syndrome and (c) following haematopoetic stem cell transplantation. In all three cases there are regions of decreased lung density in which there is a reduction in the number and calibre of vessels.

Exudative bronchiolitis

- A pattern of small airways disease characterized by inflammatory exudate in the lumen of airways, and in the immediately adjacent lung parenchyma.
- The important categories of causes of this pathological and radiological pattern are given in Table 5.7.

Table 5.7 Miscellaneous causes of an exudative bronchiolitis

- **Idiopathic**—typified by (Japanese) diffuse panbronchiolitis
- **Bronchiectasis**
- **Infectious**
  - Mycobacterial infection—tuberculous and non-tuberculous
  - Mycoplasma pneumonia
- **Chronic/recurrent aspiration**
- **Allergic bronchopulmonary aspergillosis**

Imaging of exudative bronchiolitis

By contrast with OB, in which the imaging features are an *indirect* manifestation of the underlying pathological process, in the exudative bronchiolitides, it is the abnormal airways that are seen. NB a mosaic attenuation pattern is not usually a feature, but can coexist.

CXR findings

As with OB, it is difficult to make a confident diagnosis of an exudative bronchiolitis on CXR. Features that may be seen include:

- Nodules—the branching nature of which cannot be appreciated on CXR.
- Bronchial wall thickening.
- Bronchiectasis.

CT findings (Figs. 5.19 and 5.20)

- Tree-in-bud pattern—the characteristic CT manifestation of exudative bronchiolitides. Depending on the orientation of the abnormal airways, in relation to the plane of imaging, there may be branching linear, 'v-' or 'y-shaped' opacities.
- Ancillary features: bronchial wall thickening, bronchiectasis, nodules and consolidation.

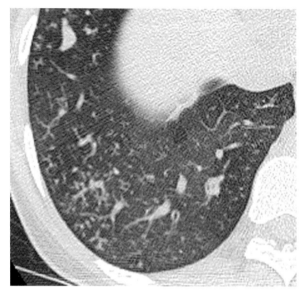

Fig. 5.19 Targeted CT through the right lower lobe in a patient with cystic fibrosis. There is a tree-in-bud pattern with branching opacitites and nodules in the right costophrenic recess.

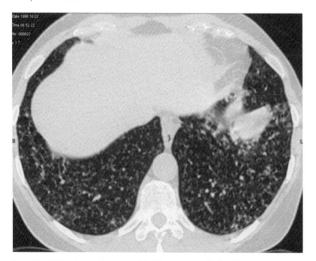

Fig. 5.20 CT in a Japanese patient with diffuse panbronchiolitis showing widespread tree-in-bud opacities and mild large airway dilatation.

Chronic obstructive pulmonary disease

Chronic obstructive pulmonary disease (COPD) encompasses a group of diseases characterized by chronic or recurrent obstruction to airflow. Traditionally, four disorders have been considered to be encompassed by the term COPD. (NB Bronchiectasis is discussed separately (see Airways diseases/Bronchiectasis, p152)).

- Emphysema
- Asthma
- Chronic bronchitis
- Bronchiectasis.

Emphysema

- Emphysema is defined as the abnormal, permanent enlargement of airspaces distal to the terminal bronchiole accompanied by destruction of alveolar walls, but without obvious fibrosis.
- Cigarette smoking is by far the most important cause of emphysema worldwide. However, up to 10% of patients with emphysema have never smoked or are infrequent smokers.
- Two pathophysiological mechanisms are considered important:
  - Structural weakness caused by elastolysis (secondary to a constitutional disorder or to increased proteolysis).
  - Airway obstruction caused either by loss of support or inflammation in the walls of small airways.
- The recognizable morphological subtypes (broadly characterized by their distribution with respect to the pulmonary lobule) include centrilobular, paraseptal, and panlobular emphysema.

Causes of emphysema

- **Cigarette smoking**—commonest and most important cause.
- **α_1-antitrypsin deficiency**—associated with panacinar emphysema.
- **Connective tissue diseases**—cutis laxa, Marfan syndrome, Ehlers–Danlos syndrome.
- **IV drug abuse**—2% of IV drug abusers develop emphysema, related to pulmonary vascular damage from injecting insoluble filler (cornstarch, cotton fibres, cellulose, talc) contained in methadone or methylphenidate. In addition, people who inject cocaine or heroin may develop upper zone bullous disease.
- **HIV infection**—emphysema with bullae occurs in 12% of HIV-seropositive patients, regardless of *Pneumocystis jiroveci* infection.
- **Hypocomplementaemic urticarial vasculitis syndrome.**
- **Malnutrition and rare metabolic disorders.**

Adapted from Lee P et al. Emphysema in nonsmokers: alpha-1-antitrypsin deficiency and other causes. *Cleveland Clinic Journal of Medicine* 2002; **69**:928–946.

Imaging in emphysema

The CXR is the most frequently requested radiological test for patients with emphysema. However, in specific circumstances, CT will provide information about the morphological characteristics, extent, and distribution of emphysema. In patients with complex CXR appearances, CT will also be of value in the identification of complications of emphysema (e.g. pneumothorax, infection) and those related to smoking (i.e. lung cancer).

CXR findings (Fig. 5.21)

The CXR signs of relatively advanced emphysema are overinflation and parenchymal destruction. However, the limitations of a CXR in the diagnosis of emphysema include low specificity, low sensitivity in the context of mild disease, and the inability to quantify the severity of emphysema.

CXR findings (Fig. 5.21):

- Signs indicating hyperinflation
  - Diaphragmatic depression—right hemidiaphragm in the mid clavicular line at or below the anterior end of the seventh rib.
  - Diaphragmatic flattening—loss of the normal curvature of the hemidiaphragms.
  - Increased retrosternal lucency—on a lateral CXR.
  - Obtuse costophrenic angle—on a PA or lateral CXR.
  - Reduced transverse cardiac diameter measuring <11.5cm.
- Signs indicating parenchymal destruction
  - Increased transradiancy.
  - Reduced number/size of pulmonary vessels and their branches.
  - Distorted vessels.
  - Bullae—transradiant, avascular areas with fine curvilinear margins.

CT findings (Figs. 5.22–5.24)

CT should not be considered as a 'routine' investigation in the management of patients with emphysema.

Indications for CT in emphysema

- To determine the distribution of emphysema—'heterogeneous' (i.e. upper zones > lower) versus 'homogeneous' (i.e. no zonal predominance) in patients being considered for lung volume reduction surgery.
- 'Objective' quantification of extent of emphysema—e.g. patient stratification for clinical trials/research studies.
- For the detection of ancillary findings or alternative diagnoses (e.g. bronchiectasis but no emphysema).
- To detect complications (e.g. pneumothorax versus bullae formation).

On CT, emphysema is characterized by the presence of foci or regions of low attenuation with or without well-defined walls. The CT features of the different morphological subtypes of emphysema are as follows:

- Centrilobular emphysema
  - Characterized on CT by ill-defined focal low attenuation areas. Foci of lucency are distributed at the centre of the pulmonary lobule.
  - Most prevalent in the upper lobes and apical segment of the lower lobe.

- Paraseptal emphysema
  - Characterized by subpleural and peribronchovascular areas of decreased attenuation which are separated by distinct hairline walls; this pattern of emphysema can be likened to a 'saw tooth'. Frequently coexists with a pattern of centrilobular emphysema.
- Panacinar emphysema
  - Uniform decrease of the lung parenchyma with a reduction in the calibre of vessels in the abnormal lung (this may be indistinguishable from constrictive OB (see 📖 Airways diseases/Constrictive obliterative bronchiolitis, p166) affecting the lower lobes.
  - Long lines—thin intersecting lines in the lower zones (representing 'remnant', adjoining interlobular septa).
  - Bronchiectasis—mild cylindrical bronchiectasis is a recognized accompaniment of α_1-antitrypsin related emphysema.
  - Bronchial wall thickening.

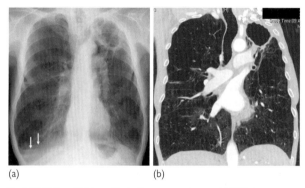

(a)   (b)

Fig. 5.21 CXR and CT in a patient with severe emphysema. (a) CXR shows a paucity of vessel markings and hyperinflation. There is flattening of the hemidiaphragms; the diaphragmatic attachments to the ribs are clearly seen on the right (arrows). Note the left apical cavity caused by tuberculosis. (b) Coronal CT shows severe emphysema especially in the upper zones.

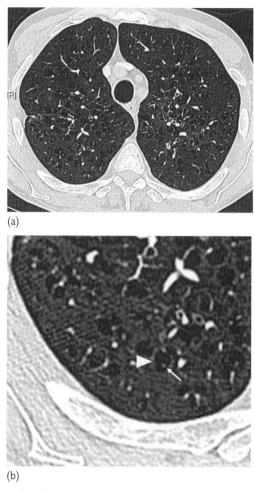

(a)

(b)

Fig. 5.22 Centrilobular emphysema on CT. (a) Image through the upper lobes shows multiple foci of decreased attenuation without obvious walls. (b) Targeted image of the same section shows the typical appearance: there is a focal area of low density (arrowhead) in the centre of which the centrilobular artery (arrow) is seen.

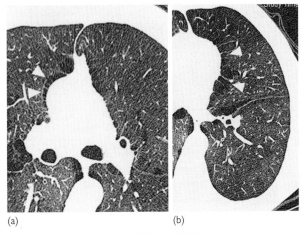

(a) (b)

Fig. 5.23 Paraseptal emphysema on CT. Targeted CT images in the same patient (a) just below the carina and (b) at the level of the left pulmonary venous confluence. There is emphysema with a 'saw tooth' appearance (arrowheads) which highlights the interlobular septa.

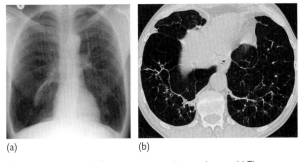

(a) (b)

Fig. 5.24 α_1-antitrypsin deficiency causing panacinar emphysema. (a) There is a marked paucity of vessels in the lower lobes in association with increased transradiancy on CXR. (b) CT demonstrates decreased attenuation of the lung parenchyma in the lower lobes with loss of the normal pulmonary vasculature and long thin intersecting lines.

Asthma

- Asthma is defined in functional terms as a disorder characterized by reversible episodes of airway obstruction.
- Airway inflammation, hyper-reactivity and, in the long-term, remodelling are the histopathological hallmarks of asthma.
- The diagnosis of asthma is made on *clinical* grounds and based on 'probabilities' rather than fixed criteria; clinical features that increase the probability of a diagnosis including episodic wheezing, cough, chest tightness, and 'difficulty in breathing'.

Imaging in asthma

Radiological tests have no routine role in the evaluation of patients with suspected or established asthma. The CXR (and even more so, CT) should be reserved only for those with severe disease, those in whom an alternative underlying diagnosis (e.g. cystic fibrosis, allergic bronchopulmonary aspergillosis) is a possibility or in patients who have developed a complication (e.g. intercurrent infection, pneumothorax/pneumomediastinum).

CXR findings

- Bronchial wall thickening—most common finding and more pronounced in children.
- Diaphragmatic depression—indicating hyperinflation; may be transient, during acute episodes (especially in children) but also during apparently 'quiescent' phases when disease is chronic and associated with airway remodelling.

CT findings (Fig. 5.25)

- Bronchial wall thickening—the most consistent CT abnormality.
- Bronchiectasis ± mucoid impaction. Usually mild (cylindrical) dilatation. May be reversible in some patients.
- Mosaic attenuation pattern—reflecting obstruction at the level of the small airways.

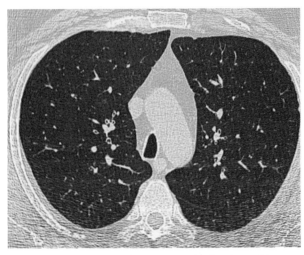

Fig. 5.25 CT through the upper lobes in a patient with asthma shows mild bronchial wall thickening only.

Chronic bronchitis

- Chronic bronchitis is defined clinically as a chronic or recurrent increase in the volume of bronchial secretions sufficient to cause sputum expectoration that occurs on most days for 3 months in 2 or more successive years.
- Strongly linked to smoking cigarettes.
- On histopathological examination, there is mucus gland hypertrophy and hyperplasia. Squamous metaplasia of the epithelium is also present and there is frequently a mild, chronic inflammatory cell infiltrate.

Imaging in chronic bronchitis

As with emphysema and asthma, radiological tests are not indicated for the routine management of patients with chronic bronchitis. Indeed, in a majority of patients with a diagnosis of chronic bronchitis, imaging tests (and particularly CXR) will show no abnormality.

CXR findings (Fig. 5.26)
- Bronchial wall thickening.
- Increased lung markings (so-called 'dirty lungs')—the exact pathological correlate of this non-specific sign is not clear but may reflect perivenous oedema, inflammation, and fibrosis.
- Cardiomegaly with enlarged central pulmonary vessels—features suggesting cor pulmonale.

CT findings
- Bronchial wall thickening.
- Focal areas of air trapping.
- Emphysema—often coexisting and of variable severity.

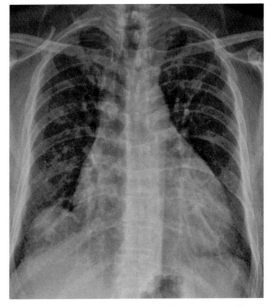

Fig. 5.26 CXR in a patient with chronic bronchitis. There are increased lung markings bilaterally.

Diffuse parenchymal lung diseases

Diffuse parenchymal lung diseases (DPLDs)

Diffuse parenchymal lung diseases (DPLDs; synonymous with interstitial lung diseases) are a diverse group of pulmonary disorders (Table 6.1). The term DPLD is generic and encompasses four broad categories of diseases which are summarized below.

Table 6.1 Categories and causes of DPLD

Category of DPLD	Key examples
Granulomatous DPLD	Sarcoidosis
DPLD of known cause	Connective tissue disease-related
	Hypersensitivity pneumonitis
	Drug-induced
	Radiation-induced
	Pneumoconioses
Idiopathic interstitial pneumonia	Usual interstitial pneumonia
	Non-specific interstitial pneumonia
	Cryptogenic organizing pneumonia
	Acute interstitial pneumonia
	Respiratory bronchiolitis associated interstitial lung disease
	Desquamative interstitial pneumonia
	Lymphoid interstitial pneumonia
Miscellaneous DPLDs	Langerhans' cell histiocytosis
	Lymphangioleiomyomatosis
	Tuberous sclerosis
	Neurofibromatosis
	Pulmonary vasculitides
	Eosinophilic lung diseases
	Alveolar microlithiasis
	Diffuse pulmonary ossification
	Pulmonary amyloidosis
	Pulmonary alveolar proteinosis
	Erdheim–Chester disease

An approach to the HRCT diagnosis of DPLDs

Introduction

Although the CXR is a cornerstone of pulmonary imaging, HRCT is the investigation of choice in patients with suspected DPLD. However, it must be remembered that HRCT interpretation is not straightforward: there are well over 200 known DPLDs manifesting in a surprisingly small number of histopathological patterns (e.g. fibrosis, consolidation, diffuse alveolar damage) which, in turn, are reflected by a relatively small group of HRCT features. Thus, a systematic approach to HRCT interpretation is recommended. A proposed schema of questions that the observer should ask (in roughly the order given) is as follows:

Key questions in HRCT interpretation

Is there a 'real' abnormality?

This is an important first question and not as simple to answer as it might first appear! HRCT features attributable to technical factors/normal variation (e.g. a poor inspiratory effort, inadequate mAs, regions of physiological dependent atelectasis) may be over interpreted and reported as 'disease'. Making the distinction between normality and abnormality can also be difficult when there is apparently minimal disease or, conversely, when there is diffuse abnormality (e.g. widespread decreased attenuation or uniform ground-glass opacity) (Fig. 6.1).

If there is an abnormality, what is/are the predominant HRCT pattern(s)?

The observer should always make an attempt to identify the dominant pattern(s) using standard terms (see 📖 Common terms used in thoracic radiology reports, p49). The use of non-standard terminology (e.g. patchy opacification, parenchymal opacities) or descriptive terms in which there is an implied pathology (e.g. interstitial pattern or alveolitis) is misleading and may lead to erroneous diagnoses.

What is the distribution of disease?

Because many DPLDs have a predilection for certain zones, an evaluation of dominant distribution is of diagnostic value (Fig. 6.2).

- Upper zone versus lower zones—in the majority of patients with idiopathic pulmonary fibrosis (IPF), disease is most prevalent in the mid to lower zones. This contrasts with fibrosis in patients with sarcoidosis which typically has a predilection for the upper lobes.
- Central versus peripheral—In addition to the cranio-caudal distribution (and in contrast to CXR), an assessment of the axial distribution can be made on CT. Using the examples of IPF and sarcoidosis again, the former is commonly peripheral (subpleural) whereas in the latter, disease tends to be central and bronchocentric.
- Perilobular distribution—this distinctive distribution of opacification is seen in patients with organizing pneumonia.

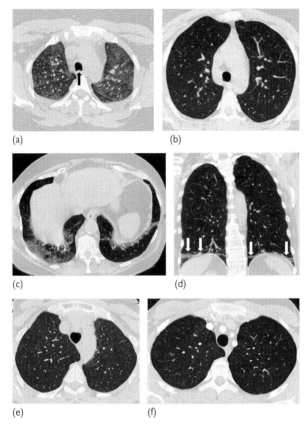

Fig. 6.1 Some pitfalls in HRCT interpretation. (a) Expiratory versus (b) inspiratory HRCT image pair at the level of the aortic arch. The generalized increase in lung density on the expiratory image should not be interpreted as an 'infiltrative' process; the expiratory nature of the study is betrayed by the anterior bowing of the posterior tracheal membrane (black arrow; compare this with the more ovoid tracheal configuration on the inspiratory image). (c) Axial and (d) coronal image of basal atelectasis; there is ground-glass attenuation in both costophrenic recesses which, on the axial image, could be interpreted as infiltrative disease. The coronal reconstruction confirms that the increased densities are caused by focal areas of linear atelectasis (arrows). (e) Diffuse increased attenuation (in subacute hypersensitivity pneumonitis) and (f) diffusely decreased lung density (caused by constrictive OB following haematopoietic stem cell transplantation); in both cases, such a uniform abnormality may be overlooked.

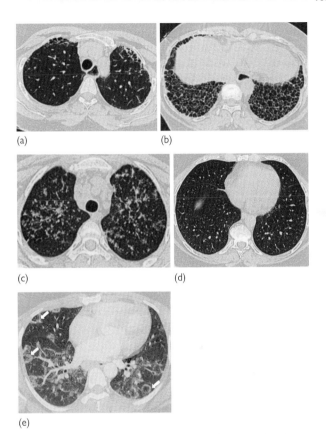

(a)

(b)

(c)

(d)

(e)

Fig. 6.2 Diagnostic importance of disease distribution. HRCT images through (a) the upper and (b) the lower lobes in a patient with fibrosis secondary to systemic sclerosis; there is reticulation with honeycombing (consistent with a pattern of UIP) more pronounced at the lung bases. (c) HRCT through the upper and (d) lower zones in sarcoidosis. Disease is clearly most marked in the upper zones; there are multiple nodules with a striking peribronchovascular predilection. (e) HRCT showing characteristic perilobular distribution of consolidation (arrows) in organizing pneumonia.

Are there any ancillary findings?

The presence or absence of additional HRCT features may be important in suggesting or, indeed, excluding certain diagnoses (Fig. 6.3):

- Pleural thickening/effusions/plaques (± calcification)—suggests asbestos-related lung disease as opposed to IPF as a possible cause of lung fibrosis.
- Lymph node enlargement (hilar/mediastinal)—reactive intrathoracic nodal enlargement is recognized in fibrotic DPLDs. However, symmetrical hilar nodal enlargement may suggest a diagnosis of sarcoidosis or occupational lung disease. Intrathoracic nodal enlargement is uncommon in pulmonary vasculitides (e.g. Wegener's granulomatosis).
- Bronchiectasis—coexistent suppurative airways disease in a patient with established pulmonary fibrosis may point to a diagnosis of an underlying connective tissue disease such as rheumatoid arthritis.
- Intrapulmonary cysts—in the appropriate clinical context, suggests a range of diagnoses including Langerhans' cell histiocytosis, lymphangioleiomyomatosis and lymphoid interstitial pneumonia.
- Consolidation—organizing pneumonia may coexist with signs of fibrosis and parenchymal distortion particularly in patients with connective tissue disease-related lung disease.

What is the likely pathology?

Knowledge of the relationship between HRCT patterns and their his-topathological correlates is vital. Thus, at a basic level, in a patient with predominant consolidation it is reasonable to conclude that the dominant pathology involves the air spaces whereas with reticulation, the likely pathological process affects the interstitium.

What is the clinical background?

Clinical data should be considered *after* formulating a radiological differ-ential diagnosis (Fig. 6.3). Specific clinical features that may be important include:

- Basic demographic data—age, gender, ethnicity.
- Smoking history—is the patient a current or ex-smoker, or a life-long non-smoker?
- Time course of the illness—have the respiratory symptoms developed over hours and days or weeks and months?
- Relevant medical history—drugs, background connective tissue disease, or travel.

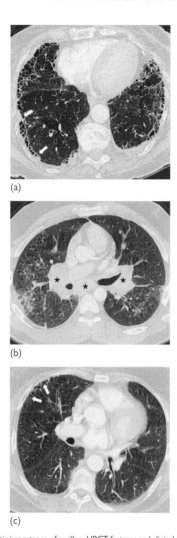

(a)

(b)

(c)

Fig. 6.3 Diagnostic importance of ancillary HRCT features and clinical data. CT images through (a) the lower zones in a patient with coarse reticulation and honeycombing. There are multiple discrete pleural plaques (arrows) indicating previous asbestos exposure; (b) the mid zone in a patient with a curious pattern of peripheral nodules; the symmetrical hilar and subcarinal lymph node enlargement (asterisks) was suggestive of sarcoidosis, a diagnosis that was confirmed at biopsy and (c) localized reticulation seen anterolaterally on the right (arrows) in a patient with a known history of treated breast carcinoma. These CT appearances are typical of previous tangential beam radiotherapy.

The clinical utility of HRCT in DPLDs

HRCT has contributed significantly to the understanding of DPLDs and is an integral part of investigation in clinical practice. However, all tests have limitations and the following section examines some of the issues surrounding the utility of HRCT in the diagnosis of DPLD.

Diagnostic accuracy

Diagnostic accuracy, expressed as the sensitivity and specificity for specific diagnoses, compared to a reference ('gold') standard is an important measure of clinical utility. Most studies show that HRCT is superior to CXR in the evaluation of DPLDs: radiologists' confidence is almost doubled when reviewing HRCT images and, when a confident diagnosis is given, it is almost always correct (particularly for certain diagnoses (Table 6.2)). The imaging features of the individual disorders listed below are covered in relevant sections of this book.

Table 6.2 Diagnoses of DPLD that can often be made with confidence on HRCT

Usual interstitial pneumonia
Sarcoidosis
Langerhans' cell histiocytosis
Lymphangioleiomyomatosis
Lymphangitis carcinomatosis
(Subacute) hypersensitivity pneumonitis
Pulmonary alveolar proteinosis

From Wells AU and Hirani N. Interstitial lung disease guideline: the British Thoracic Society in collaboration with the Thoracic Society of Australia and New Zealand and the Irish Thoracic Society. *Thorax* 2008; **63**:Suppl.v1–v58 (with permission from BMJ Publishing Group Ltd).

Observer agreement for HRCT diagnoses

Observer agreement is an important aspect of radiological interpretation and is usually expressed as the kappa coefficient (reflecting the strength of agreement). Values for kappa coefficient range from 0 to 1: where 1 indicates perfect agreement; values below 0.4 are considered below the limits of clinical acceptability and values above 0.8 represent excellent agreement. Observer agreement for the most commonly diagnosed DPLDs is, for the most part, well within clinically-acceptable limits (Table 6.3).

Table 6.3 Weighted kappa (κ_ω) for common DPLDs

Diagnostic category	Median κ_ω
Idiopathic pulmonary fibrosis/UIP	0.63
Non-specific interstitial pneumonia	0.51
Sarcoidosis	0.70
Hypersensitivity pneumonitis	0.60
Cryptogenic organizing pneumonia	0.49
Smoking-related interstitial lung disease	0.51

From Aziz A et al. HRCT diagnosis of diffuse parenchymal lung disease: interobserver variation. *Thorax* 2004; **59**:506–511 (with permission from BMJ Publishing Group Ltd).

Impact of HRCT on clinical practice

One of the true measures of the utility of a test is its impact on the clinical act of diagnosis. In the initial assessment of the patient with suspected DPLD, there is a dynamic process requiring the integration of clinical data (including laboratory results), CXR features, and where available, histopathological findings; HRCT may refine or radically change a presumptive diagnosis. Thus, the diagnostic process proceeds with a series of consecutive estimations of the probability of a particular disease and evolves with the accumulation of further test results. Thus, the real usefulness of a diagnostic test is the degree to which it alters clinical perception. In some cases of sarcoidosis, for example, the combination of erythema nodosum, a history of cough, and a CXR showing the typical features of bilateral hilar lymph node enlargement is more than sufficient for a confident diagnosis to be made because the pre-test probability is high. The addition of HRCT in this scenario does little to change the clinician's pre-test assumptions. However, in many situations, a change in the diagnosis often occurs once HRCT findings are integrated with the clinical details.

Granulomatous DPLD: sarcoidosis

- A granulomatous disease, of unknown aetiology, which can affect multiple organ systems but most commonly involves the lungs and lymphatic system.
- Variable worldwide prevalence (ranging from <1 to 40 per 100,000 population); higher in Danish, Swedish, and African-American populations. Overall there is a slight female predominance particularly in black populations. Occurs across all age groups (except the very young) but most common in young adults (<40 years of age).
- Well-formed caseating epithelioid cell granulomata, the archetypal lesions of sarcoidosis, have a predilection for lymphatic structures (i.e. lymph nodes, along the bronchovascular bundles, in the subpleural lung and along fissures), tend to resolve over time but can lead to extensive fibrosis in a minority of patients.

Imaging in pulmonary sarcoidosis

The typical radiological findings in sarcoidosis reflect its propensity for lymph nodes and lung parenchyma.

CXR findings

The overwhelming majority (>90%) of patients with sarcoidosis have an abnormal CXR at some time during the course of the disease.

Lymph node enlargement

Seen in 70–80% of patients and generally decrease in size over time, resolving completely by 2-years; as a rule, sarcoid nodes do not enlarge following complete resolution. Lymph node calcification may be present in up to 20% on CXR (higher on CT); 'egg-shell' calcification may be seen in some patients. Different distributions of intrathoracic nodal enlargement may be seen:

- Bilateral and symmetrical hilar ± right paratracheal or bilateral paratracheal—the commonest distribution(s).
- Bilateral and asymmetrical hilar (less common than symmetrical and should suggests alternative diagnoses (e.g. lymphoma, tuberculosis)).
- Unilateral hilar lymph node enlargement—an uncommon pattern.
- Anterior/posterior mediastinal or subcarinal—may be enlarged but rarely seen without hilar nodal disease; if nodes are isolated to these regions, alternative diagnoses should be considered.

Parenchymal disease

Parenchymal infiltration occurs in about 50% of patients and usually begins as nodal disease regresses. The common CXR patterns of disease include:

- Nodular or reticulonodular pattern—nodules are of soft tissue density with irregular margins, measuring 2–4mm in diameter. Most prevalent in the mid/upper zones bilaterally.
- Coarse linear opacities—indicating fibrosis. Typically bilateral, symmetrical, and most pronounced in the mid/upper zones. Upper zone fibrosis may be associated with 'tenting' of the hemi-diaphragms.

Rare CXR manifestations

Parenchymal calcification, cavitation, multifocal consolidation, pleural effusion/thickening, a solitary pulmonary nodule and multiple large nodules.

Chest radiographic 'staging' in sarcoidosis

Based on the presence or absence of nodal enlargement and lung disease, the CXR appearances are used to 'stage' sarcoidosis (Table 6.4; Fig. 6.4). There is a broad relationship between functional impairment and CXR stage (20% in stage I versus 40–70% in stages II–IV). However, CXR staging does not 'capture' disease activity accurately: thus, sarcoid granulomata, for example, are almost always present, even if not evident radiographically, in patients with stage I disease. Furthermore, patients do not, as a rule, progress from one stage to the next: 2/3 of patients with stage I disease at presentation resolve completely. Thus, the exact clinical and prognostic significance of CXR staging has not been established.

Table 6.4 CXR staging of sarcoidosis

Stage	CXR appearance	% patients at presentation
0	Normal	5–10%
I	Bilateral hilar nodes (BHL) alone	40–60%
II	BHL + parenchymal disease	25–30%
III	Parenchymal disease alone	10–20%
IV	Lung fibrosis/end-stage lung	~20%

Adapted from Hunninghake GW et al. Statement on Sarcoidosis. *Am J Respir Crit Care Med* 1999; **160**:736–755).

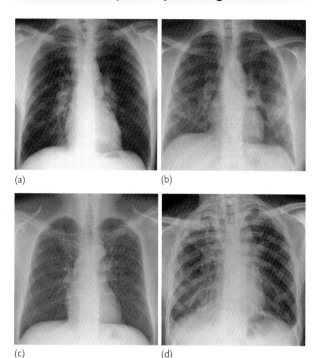

(a)

(b)

(c)

(d)

Fig. 6.4 CXRs in four patients showing radiographic stages of sarcoidosis. (a) Stage I: bilateral symmetrical hilar lymph node enlargement with no evidence of parenchymal infiltration. (b) Stage II: there is bilateral hilar lymph node enlargement and a reticulonodular infiltrate in the mid and lower zones of both lungs. (c) Stage III: there is fine reticulation in the upper zones bilaterally. The hilar contours are normal. (d) Stage IV: there is a coarse reticular pattern in both upper zones with elevation of the hila. These features indicate established fibrosis.

CT findings

CT is rarely indicated in patients with a 'typical' clinicoradiographic presentation and uncomplicated disease as it adds no clinically-relevant additional information. The specific indications for CT in patients with sarcoidosis are listed in the box.

Specific indications for CT in sarcoidosis

- In patients with a normal CXR but in whom there is a strong clinical suspicion of the diagnosis
- In patients with atypical clinico-radiographic presentations
- As a guide to biopsy in atypical disease
- To explain the morphological basis of sometimes complex physiological impairment (e.g. combined restrictive and obstructive deficits)
- To detect complications (e.g. mycetoma formation, infection, fibrosis)
- To identify large airway disease (e.g. stenosis, bronchiectasis)
- Pre-transplant assessment
- In patients with unusual symptoms (e.g. haemoptysis—rare in sarcoidosis) or suspected concurrent disease (e.g. lung cancer)

Typical CT appearances (Figs. 6.5–6.7)

- Lymph node enlargement
  - The distribution of nodal enlargement mirror those seen on CXR.
  - Nodal enlargement at other sites (e.g. supraclavicular fossa, axilla), not easily visible on CXR, may be also demonstrated.
  - CT is of value for the detection, distribution and pattern of nodal calcification. This may aid in the distinction from post-tuberculous nodal enlargement: in contrast to tuberculosis, calcification in sarcoid lymph nodes tends to be i) more focally sited with nodes (as opposed to complete replacement) and ii) more often bilateral. Calcification in sarcoid lymph nodes often has a delicate 'icing sugar' type of appearance. Occasionally a pattern of 'egg-shell' calcification may be seen but this is relatively uncommon.

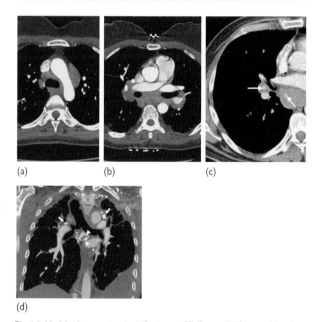

Fig. 6.5 Nodal enlargement and calcification on CT. Targeted CT images (a) at the level of the aortic arch and (b) below the carina (in the same patient as (a)), showing enlarged precarinal nodes, para-aortic nodes, symmetrical hilar, and subcarinal nodes. (c) Targeted image in another patient shows delicate ('icing sugar') calcification in enlarged right hilar and subcarinal nodes (arrows). (d) Coronal CT reconstruction in another patient showing calcification in bilateral hilar and mediastinal nodes (arrows). There is also 'egg-shell' calcification (arrowheads) in enlarged subcarinal nodes.

- Parenchymal disease (reversible changes)
  - Micronodules and nodules—well-defined, soft tissue density lesions (due to conglomerate granulomata) are the most common CT manifestation and represent potentially—but not invariably—reversible disease. Micronodules (≤3mm diameter) and nodules (measuring up to 1cm in diameter) are generally bilateral, subpleural (N.B. including fissural), in a peri-bronchovascular distribution (the latter giving rise to the appearance of 'bronchovascular beading') and along interlobular septa. Nodules are most prevalent in the mid and upper zones.
  - Ground-glass opacities—due to granulomatous infiltration and thickening of the interstitium. This pattern is also believed to be a potentially reversible manifestation of parenchymal sarcoidosis.
  - Interlobular septal thickening—this may be smooth or nodular. Septal thickening may or may not regress with corticosteroid therapy.

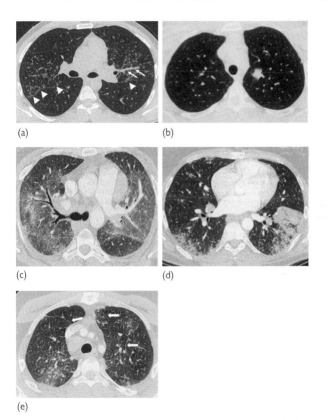

(a) (b)

(c) (d)

(e)

Fig. 6.6 CT patterns of reversible parenchymal disease in sarcoidosis. (a) Multiple micronodules in a bronchocentric and subpleural distribution; there is bronchovascular beading on the left (arrows) and nodular thickening of the oblique fissures (arrowheads) bilaterally. (b) CT through the upper zones demonstrating a large (1 cm diameter) bronchocentric nodule on the left. (c) Widespread ground-glass opacification due to interstitial infiltration. (d) CT showing an 'air space' pattern of sarcoidosis. (e) Thickening of interlobular septa (arrows) and small nodules in a patient with biopsy-confirmed sarcoidosis.

- Consolidation—also called 'air space' sarcoidosis. At histopathological examination, this pattern is usually caused by extensive interstitial thickening but manifests as a pattern of consolidation because of the complete displacement of air from the air spaces. The typical finding is that of bilateral, peripheral areas of consolidation; usually associated with intrathoracic lymph node enlargement and nodular parenchymal infiltrates.
- Parenchymal disease (irreversible changes)
  - Coarse linear or reticular pattern (± honeycombing, ± traction bronchiectasis/bronchiolectasis)—these patterns indicate established fibrosis. Fibrosis is typically bronchocentric and most pronounced in the mid and upper zones, usually 'streaming' off the hila. Bronchovascular structures are characteristically displaced posteriorly by fibrosis. As this progresses, fibrocavitary areas may develop and these may subsequently be colonized by aspergillus.

Less common CT manifestations and complications of sarcoidosis (Fig. 6.8)

- Small airways disease—areas of decreased density in a mosaic attenuation pattern; there is a reduction in the number and/or calibre of pulmonary vessels in regions of reduced attenuation. Air-trapping may be seen on expiratory CT images. May be present at any radiographic stage of sarcoidosis.
- Large airway disease—distortion and stenoses of the larger airways (larynx, trachea, and bronchi) due to fibrosis or endobronchial nodules. Large airway abnormalities may be optimally demonstrated on multiplanar CT reconstructions. In some patients there is evidence of bronchiectasis distal to (obstructive) peribronchial fibrosis or endobronchial sarcoid nodules.

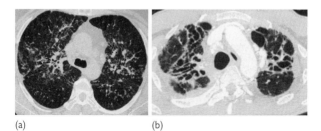

(a)   (b)

Fig. 6.7 CT patterns of irreversible parenchymal disease in two patients with sarcoidosis. (a) CT through the upper zones demonstrating signs of fibrosis. There is distortion of parenchymal structures, ground-glass opacification and dilatation of segmental/subsegmental airways. (b) Coarse bronchocentric fibrosis in the upper zones with honeycomb destruction of lung.

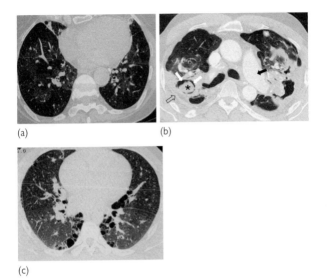

(a) (b)

(c)

Fig. 6.8 Unusual CT manifestations/complications of sarcoidosis. (a) Small airways disease: expiratory CT through the lower zones shows widespread air-trapping—there are areas of decreased density in which there is a reduction in the number/calibre of pulmonary vessels. (b) Mycetoma in fibrocavitary disease: there is a characteristic mass (black asterisk) in a pre-existing upper lobe 'cavity' (white arrows) surrounded by a crescent of (air) lucency. Some thickening and retraction of the adjacent pleura (open arrow) is present and there is prominence of the left main pulmonary artery (black arrow) suggesting pulmonary hypertension. (c) Lower zone fibrosis resembling a pattern of usual interstitial pneumonia in a biopsy-proven case of sarcoidosis. There are multiple subpleural honeycomb cysts bilaterally.

- Mycetomas—fibrocavitary disease in the upper zones predisposes patients with sarcoidosis to fungal colonization (most commonly by *Aspergillus* species). The typical CT appearance of a mycetoma is that of a mobile intracavitary mass, often sponge-like; the classical air-crescent is easily demonstrated on CT.
- Pulmonary hypertension—occurs in nearly one quarter of patients with sarcoidosis at rest, and is more common with advanced CXR stage. The CT signs of pulmonary hypertension are discussed elsewhere 📖 Vascular diseases/Pulmonary hypertension, p298.
- Atypical fibrosis—a pattern which superficially resembles usual interstitial pneumonia may be seen.

Connective tissue disease-related DPLD

- Lung involvement is common in patients with connective tissue diseases (CTDs) and may precede—sometimes by years—the onset of systemic or joint manifestations. Lung disease in CTD patients is an important cause of morbidity and mortality.
- Interpretation of CXR and HRCT findings is aided by knowledge of the likely range of pathological patterns and their variable prevalence in different CTDs.
- The patterns of interstitial lung disease broadly mirror the patterns seen in the idiopathic interstitial pneumonias (see 🕮 Diffuse parenchymal lung diseases/Idiopathic interstitial pneumonias, p234).
- In addition to DPLD, airways diseases (e.g. in rheumatoid arthritis and Sjögren's syndrome), vasculopathy and serosal inflammation (e.g. systemic lupus erythematosus) are recognized complications in different CTDs. Lung disease may also be the consequence of treatment of the underlying rheumatological disorder (see 🕮 Diffuse parenchymal lung diseases/Drug-induced DPLD, p206).

Table 6.5 Principal pathological patterns associated with individual CTDs

Connective tissue disease	Pathological patterns*
Rheumatoid Arthritis	UIP >NSIP, LIP, DAD, OP, OB, FB, exudative bronchiolitis, necrobiotic nodules
Systemic sclerosis	NSIP >UIP, DAD
Polymyositis/ dermatomyositis	OP, NSIP, UIP, DAD
Systemic lupus erythematosus	DAD, diffuse pulmonary haemorrhage, serositis, (pleural/ pericardial effusions), OP
Sjögren's syndrome	NSIP, LIP, bronchiectasis, OB, lymphoma

*Note: UIP = usual interstitial pneumonia; NSIP = non-specific interstitial pneumonia; LIP = lymphoid interstitial pneumonia; DAD = diffuse alveolar damage; OP = organizing pneumonia; OB = (constrictive) obliterative bronchiolitis; FB = follicular bronchiolitis; > = more prevalent than.

Imaging in CTD

The radiological features of lung disease in the CTDs vary according to the underlying pathological process(es) (Table 6.5). The CXR and HRCT features of the interstitial lung diseases are, to a greater or lesser degree, identical to those seen in the context of the idiopathic interstitial pneumonias and are covered in detail in relevant sections; some illustrative examples are shown below (Fig. 6.9).

Indications for HRCT in CTD-related lung disease

- To confirm a clinical suspicion of lung disease in patients with an established CTD but a normal CXR
- For a 'histospecific' diagnosis of the pattern(s) of ILD
- As part of 'baseline' in routine clinical evaluation—In many patients with CTDs there is an expectation of lung disease and HRCT may be performed to either exclude or identify 'early' involvement.
- To quantify the extent of lung abnormality—Accurate quantification on HRCT may be of value for stratification in clinical studies.
- To identify complications of CTD and/or their treatment—Iatrogenic or otherwise; important complications include opportunistic infection, pulmonary drug-toxicity or the development of malignancy (e.g. lymphoma in Sjögren's syndrome).

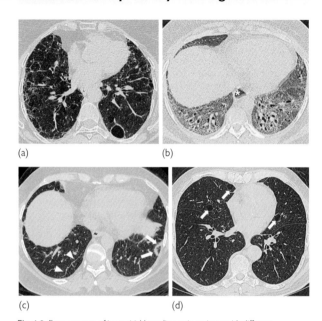

Fig. 6.9 Four patterns of interstitial lung disease in patients with different connective tissue diseases. (a) Usual interstitial pneumonia pattern in rheumatoid arthritis: HRCT shows subpleural reticulation with honeycombing; (b) Non-specific interstitial pneumonia in systemic sclerosis: there is widespread ground-glass opacification and traction bronchiolectasis. Note the dilated oesophagus (asterisk); (c) organizing pneumonia in systemic lupus erythematosus: there is peri-lobular consolidation in the left lower lobe (arrows) and a peripheral linear opacity on the right (arrowheads) and (d) lymphoid interstitial pneumonia in rheumatoid arthritis: there is subtle ground-glass opacification and multiple bilateral thin-walled lung cysts (arrows).

Hypersensitivity pneumonitis

- Hypersensitivity pneumonitis (HP; synonymous with extrinsic allergic alveolitis) is an immune-mediated hypersensitivity reaction related to repeated exposure to inhaled organic (but sometimes chemical) allergens.
- The range of antigens known to be associated with HP is large (a few of the recognized causes are listed below (Table 6.6)). NB In around one-third of patients, a causative antigen may not be identified.
- Because of the variable influence of individual immunity, host, and exposure factors the true prevalence is difficult to guage.
- Three broadly distinct phases of HP are recognized (acute, subacute, and chronic) and reflected in the imaging findings.

Table 6.6 Common causes of HP

Disease	Antigen	Typical Source
Bird fancier's lung	Avian precipitins	Bird feathers/droppings
Farmer's lung	*Aspergillus* sp. Thermophilic *Actinomyces*	Mouldy hay, compost
Hot tub lung	MAI complex	Hot tubs
Isocynate HP	Isocyanates	Paint sprays, plastic

MAI = *Mycobacterium avium-intracellulare* HP = hypersensitivity pneumonitis

Imaging of HP

The imaging features of HP do not always correlate with the duration of symptoms and overlap between the three phases may occur.

Acute HP

The imaging features of acute HP are poorly documented. The CXR may show diffuse ground-glass opacification, a nodular or reticulonodular pattern. In some instances, particularly with heavy antigen exposure there is widespread pulmonary consolidation. The HRCT features mirror the CXR changes.

CXR findings (Figs. 6.10 and 6.11)

The CXR appearances of subacute HP are non-specific. In some patients, the CXR may be completely normal. The CXR features of HP include:

- Ground-glass opacification—usually widespread.
- Ill-defined nodules—small and sometimes more pronounced in the upper zones.

CT findings (Figs. 6.10, 6.12, and 6.13)

The typical HRCT features include:

- Ground-glass opacification—generally widespread but with apparent 'sparing' of individual pulmonary lobules.
- Centrilobular nodules—small (3–4mm diameter), ill-defined; may have an upper lobe distribution.
- Mosaic attenuation pattern (on inspiratory sections) and evidence of air-trapping (on end-expiratory images).
- Scattered lung cysts—in ~10% (see 📖 Diffuse parenchymal lung diseases/Lymphoid interstitial pneumonia, p248).

CXR findings

In many patients, disease appears to be most pronounced in the upper zones. (NB on HRCT disease may be more marked in the mid/lower zones). The CXR signs include:

- Ground-glass opacification
- Reticular pattern ± honeycombing
- Volume loss with pulmonary distortion.

CT findings (Fig. 6.14)

With experience and recognition of the typical features, a confident (and accurate) diagnosis of chronic HP can be made on HRCT. The extent and combination of abnormalities (which has been called the 'head cheese' sign) varies but includes:

- Ground-glass opacification (± traction bronchiectasis/bronchiolectasis) with lobular areas of 'sparing' which show air trapping on end-expiratory scans—a key ancillary sign.
- Reticular pattern ± variable severity of honeycombing. The appearances may resemble the pattern of usual interstitial pneumonia (see 📖 Diffuse parenchymal lung diseases/Usual interstitial pneumonia, p236).
- Thin-walled cysts.

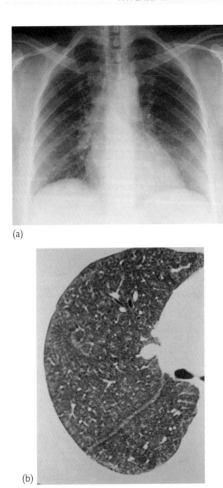

(a)

(b)

Fig. 6.10 (a) Normal CXR in a patient with subacute HP. (b) Contemporaneous HRCT in the same patient shows widespread ground-glass opacities with ill-defined centrilobular nodules.

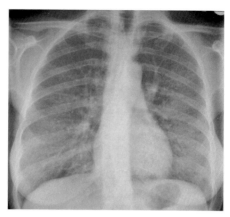

Fig. 6.11 CXR in subacute HP with diffuse ground-glass opacification.

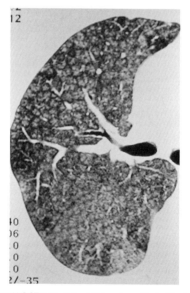

Fig. 6.12 Targeted HRCT through the right lung in a patient with subacute HP showing multiple acinar nodules.

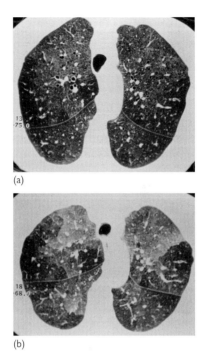

(a)

(b)

Fig. 6.13 (a) Inspiratory and (b) end-expiratory HRCT in a patient with subacute HP showing mosaic attenuation and air-trapping on the end-expiratory images.

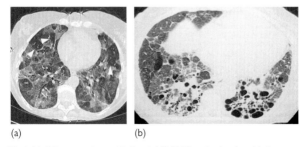

(a)   (b)

Fig. 6.14 CT in two patients with chronic HP. (a) There is a 'patchwork' of ground-glass opacification (reflecting lymphocytic/plasma cell interstitial infiltration ± fibrosis; there is dilatation of a subsegmental airway in the right lower lobe (arrows)) and lobular regions of apparently spared lung parenchyma (arrowheads) denoting small airways obstruction. (b) CT through the lower lobes showing honeycombing destruction, particularly on the left. Patchy ground-glass opacification and areas of lobular low attenuation, similar to (a), are also present.

Drug-induced DPLD

- The reported prevalence of drug-induced lung disease varies considerably according to the specific drug, the index of clinical suspicion, and the methods used to identify such complications. A detailed discussion is beyond the scope of this book but a useful source is *http://www.pneumotox.com*.
- Histopathological confirmation of a specific drug-induced lung disease is rarely obtained because the patterns of pulmonary injury do not differ from those of other causes (Tables 6.7 and 6.8); therefore, the role of biopsy is often to exclude other causes.

Table 6.7 Histopathological mechanisms and patterns of drug-induced DPLD

- **Direct lung toxicity**
  - Diffuse alveolar damage
  - Organizing pneumonia
  - Chronic interstitial pneumonia
- **Hypersensitivity reactions**
  - Eosinophilic pneumonia
  - Asthma
  - Hypersensitivity pneumonitis
  - Autoimmune reactions
  - Vasculitis
- **Granulomatous reactions**
  - Sarcoidosis
  - Lipoid pneumonia
- **Humoral/neural mechanisms**
  - Pulmonary oedema
- **Miscellaneous**
  - Pleural effusions and pleural fibrosis
  - Pulmonary haemorrhage
  - Vasospasm
  - Thromboembolism
  - Pulmonary calcification
  - Obliterative bronchiolitis

Imaging of drug-induced lung disease

The radiological manifestations of drug-induced lung disease are highly variable but broadly reflect the different histopathological patterns. The radiological features (Figs. 6.15 and 6.16) of some of the more commonly encountered drug-induced lung diseases are discussed briefly below.

Amiodarone

CXR findings

- Reticular pattern—usually bilateral
- Consolidation (diffuse, patchy, or peripheral).

Table 6.8 Specific drugs associated with the more common histopathological patterns of lung injury

- **Organizing pneumonia**
  - Bleomycin, methotrexate, amiodarone, gold, sulphasalazine, cyclophoshamide, penicillamine
- **Chronic interstitial pneumonia**
  - Amiodarone, nitrofurantoin, methotrexate, bleomycin, carmustine (BCNU)
- **Diffuse alveolar damage**
  - Bleomycin, carmustine, busulphan, gold, cyclophospamide, amiodarone
- **Pulmonary haemorrhage**
  - Anticoagulants
- **Eosinophilic pneumonia**
  - Sulphasalazine, penicillamine, NSAIDs, nitrofurantoin, amiodarone

CT findings
- Consolidation—peripheral or peribronchial, bilateral.
- Ground-glass opacities—bilateral with associated reticular pattern.
- Increased lung attenuation (80–175 HU)—usually associated with increased density of the liver parenchyma (due to high iodine content). These features are not common now because of the lower doses that are generally used.
- Pleural effusions.

Bleomycin

CXR findings
- Reticular or reticulonodular pattern—often peripheral and bibasal but becoming progressively diffuse.

CT findings
- Ground-glass opacity ± consolidation (reflecting a pathological pattern of diffuse alveolar damage).
- Ground-glass opacity with reticular pattern ± traction bronchiectasis (due to NSIP).
- Consolidation—patchy and peripheral (either reflecting a pattern of organizing pneumonia or pulmonary eosinophilia).

Busulphan

CXR findings
- Reticular or reticulonodular pattern—lower lobe predominance or diffuse.

CT findings
- Ground-glass opacity with a reticular pattern.

Nitrofurantoin

Clinical presentation may be acute or chronic (but median onset is typically two years after the start of treatment). The imaging features reflect the presence of an interstitial pneumonia often with a component of organizing pneumonia.

CXR findings

- Septal lines—resembling those seen in pulmonary oedema
- Pleural effusions (acute)
- Bilateral reticular pattern—bilateral, diffuse, upper or lower zone distribution (chronic).

CT findings

- Ground-glass opacity with reticular pattern (NB may be reversible when it represents an unusual manifestation of organizing pneumonia), less commonly subpleural or peribronchial consolidation.

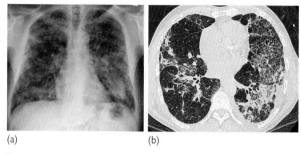

(a)   (b)

Fig. 6.15 (a) CXR and (b) CT in a patient with amiodarone-induced lung disease. There are ground-glass opacities and focal areas of consolidation. Parenchymal distortion is readily demonstrated on CT.

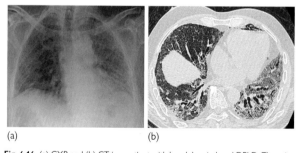

(a)   (b)

Fig. 6.16 (a) CXR and (b) CT in a patient with busulphan-induced DPLD. There is volume loss, ground-glass opacification and a fine reticular pattern in the left lower zone. On CT, marked traction bronchiectasis is seen. The appearances are likely to be due to NSIP.

Imaging of lung diseases related to illicit drugs

Illicit drugs may be inhaled or injected and lead to a variety of pulmonary complications (Table 6.9). The imaging of lung complications related to some illicit drugs is described below but the radiological features of specific complications (e.g. pulmonary oedema, haemorrhage, aspiration etc) are covered elsewhere. What follows is a brief account of the imaging abnormalities which occur because of the abuse of some common illicit drugs (Figs. 6.17–6.20).

Table 6.9 Known complications of illicit drug abuse

- Cardiogenic pulmonary oedema
- Non-cardiogenic (permeability) pulmonary oedema
- Pulmonary haemorrhage
- Septic embolus
- Pneumonia
- Aspiration
- Talcosis
- Emphysema
- Mycotic aneurysms
- Pulmonary hypertension

Cocaine (including 'crack' cocaine)

The list of possible complications associated with the misuse of cocaine includes:

- Pulmonary oedema
- Haemorrhage
- Organizing pneumonia
- Eosinophilic vasculitis
- Pneumothorax, pneumomediastinum, and pneumopericardium
- Tracheal stenosis
- Asthma and obliterative bronchiolitis
- Talcosis
- Acute aortic dissection
- Pulmonary veno-occlusive disease

Heroin and opiates

- Pulmonary oedema
- Aspiration pneumonia
- Septic emboli (associated with right-sided endocarditis)
- Pneumothorax, haemothorax, and pyothorax

Marijuana

- Emphysema—sometimes bullous.

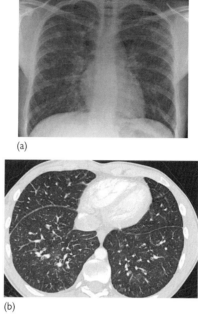

(a)

(b)

Fig. 6.17 Pulmonary oedema caused by crack-cocaine abuse. (a) CXR and (b) CT 24 hours later. There is perihilar ground-glass opacification on CXR. On CT there is interlobular septal thickening and subtle ground-glass opacification.

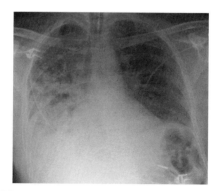

Fig. 6.18 CXR in a patient with a severe aspiration pneumonia following a drug overdose.

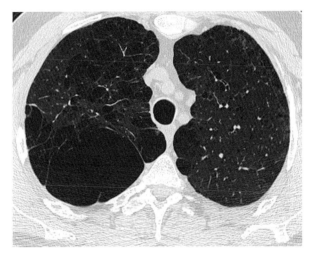

Fig. 6.19 CT through the upper lobes in a 43-year-old known to have smoked marijuana heavily. There is extensive bullous and centrilobular emphysema.

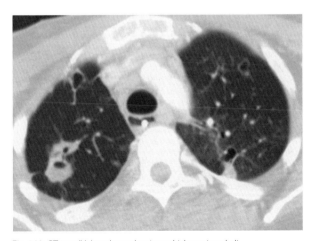

Fig. 6.20 CT in an IV drug abuser showing multiple septic emboli.

Radiation-induced lung disease

- Radiation-induced lung injury is most likely with fractionated *total* doses of over 60Gy (NB rare with doses <20Gy); injury is usually restricted to the irradiated field.
- Multiple factors are believed to contribute to the variable severity/extent of radiation-induced lung injury (Table 6.10).
- The characteristic temporal sequence of histopathological events following radiation are oedema and lymphocyte infiltration into the bronchial mucosa. There is lymphoid follicle degeneration (after 24–48 hrs), followed by acute radiation pneumonitis (after 1–6 months) and, finally, interstitial fibrosis (after 6–12 months).
- Patients are usually asymptomatic for the first 24–48hrs and may not complain of respiratory symptoms if there is mild fibrosis but dyspnoea may be disabling with extensive injury.

Table 6.10 Putative factors contributing to severity of radiation-induced lung injury

- Age and performance status
- Pre-existing lung disease (e.g. emphysema)
- Volume of lung irradiated
- Radiation dose (including fractionation)—a single large dose is more damaging
- Host susceptibility
- Previous radiotherapy
- Concurrent treatment with cytotoxic drugs (e.g. bleomycin, vincristine)

Imaging of radiation-induced lung injury

The typical CXR and CT features of radiation-induced lung injury are discussed below. It should be noted that newer techniques such as intensity-modulated radiotherapy (IMRT), three-dimensional conformal radiotherapy (3-D CRT) and fractional techniques may result in radiological features that differ from those expected with more conventional radiotherapy protocols.

CXR findings (Fig. 6.21)
- Normal within 48 hrs of exposure.
- *Early*—hazy opacification usually confined to radiation field (geometric shapes with sharp linear margins), pleural effusions (within six months).
- *Late*—reticular opacities, consolidation, volume loss.

CT findings (Figs. 6.22–6.24)

- *Early*—(within a few weeks) ground-glass opacification and consolidation confined to radiation portal, sometimes small nodules.
- *Late*—consolidation, cicatricial atelectasis, traction bronchiectasis and well-demarcated fibrosis. An organizing pneumonia-like syndrome is reported in women after radiotherapy for breast cancer.
- IMRT and 3D-CRT may result in conventional, 'scar-like' or even 'mass-like' patterns and may deliver dose to unexpected areas.
- Breast cancer treatment may result in characteristic tangential anterolateral, subpleural distribution of fibrosis.
- Mantle radiotherapy for lymphoma leads to a typical paramediastinal distribution of fibrosis.

Approximate time course of lung injury following radiotherapy

- Imaging abnormalities generally appear within 4–8 weeks
- Peak 3–4 months after treatment completion
- Post-radiation fibrosis can progress for 6–12 months after the end of treatment but usually stabilizes by 18 months

^{18}FDG-positron emission tomography (PET) or ^{18}FDG-PET/CT (Fig. 6.24)

- Acute radiation pneumonitis may result in increased FDG uptake which persists for up to 18 months.
- High negative predictive value in acute radiation pneumonitis—can be useful and may differentiate radiation-induced injury from disease recurrence.
- False-positive studies are common in the context of radiation pneumonitis and PET/CT should be performed at least six months after end of treatment.

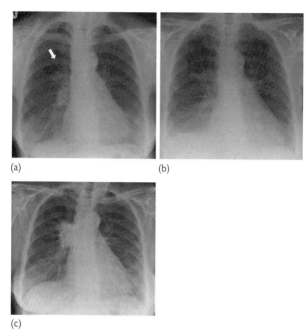

(a)   (b)

(c)

Fig. 6.21 Sequence of CXR changes following radiotherapy for treatment of lung cancer. (a) Pre-treatment CXR shows a right upper lobe non-small cell lung cancer (arrow). (b) Early CXR changes post-radiotherapy: there is hazy increased density and a right pleural effusion. (c) Late radiographic appearances of radiation fibrosis 12 months following treatment. Note the increased right hilar density and distortion in the right hemithorax.

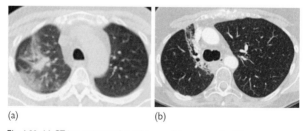

(a)   (b)

Fig. 6.22 (a) CT in a patient with a right upper lobe non-small cell lung cancer showing diffuse ground-glass opacification in the right lung around the tumour 4 weeks following radiotherapy. (b) CT in a different patient 18 months post-radiotherapy for lung cancer demonstrating volume loss, increased density and traction bronchiectasis. Note the well-defined lateral margin demarcating the zone of radiation fibrosis from normal lung.

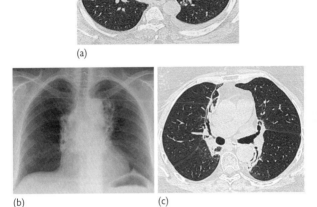

Fig. 6.23 Classical distributions of radiation-induced fibrosis. (a) CT showing characteristic fibrosis in the anterolateral subpleural lung (note also the left mastectomy), following tangential-beam radiotherapy for breast cancer. (b) CXR and (c) CT in patient with fibrosis following mantle mediastinal radiotherapy for lymphoma. The margins between fibrosed and normal lung are well-demarcated on CXR and CT.

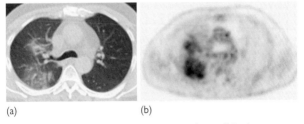

Fig. 6.24 (a) CT showing right lung ground-glass opacification (following radiotherapy) and (b) ^{18}FDG-PET showing mild increased radioisotope uptake in the same region.

Pneumoconioses

Asbestosis

- Asbestosis is defined as diffuse interstitial fibrosis caused by the inhalation of asbestos fibres.
- Asbestos is a naturally occurring fibrous hydrous silicate with unique heat resistant properties: fibre types can be divided into amphiboles (needle-shaped) and serpentines (curly).
- Heavy and prolonged exposure to asbestos generally precedes the development of asbestosis; there is a characteristically long latency (typically 20–30 years) between exposure and onset of asbestos-related lung disease.
- The diagnosis of asbestosis is confirmed by one or more clinical or laboratory findings combined with a history of *non-trivial* asbestos exposure; an appropriate time interval (usually a minimum of 15 years) is also regarded as an essential for diagnosis.

Imaging of asbestosis

The typical CXR and HRCT appearances of asbestosis are illustrated.

CXR findings (Fig. 6.25)

Chest radiography is relatively specific in the context of a combination of pleural and parenchymal disease in an individual with an appropriate history of asbestos exposure and may be sufficient for diagnosis in advanced cases. However, CXR is insensitive in early disease (NB extensive asbestosis at presentation is increasingly rare and CXR is often normal or only subtly abnormal).

- Reticulonodular pattern—characteristically bilateral and basal but upper zone fibrosis has been described.
- Small rounded and small irregular opacities.
- Honeycombing—a feature of advanced disease.
- Septal lines—not a consistent finding.
- Irregular cardiac outline—because of adjacent fibrosis.
- Basal volume loss—as judged by the depression of the horizontal fissure and/or the hila.
- Pleural plaques (± calcification) and bilateral blunting of the costophrenic angles related to diffuse visceral pleural thickening are common (but may be mild and asymmetric).

CT findings (Fig. 6.25)

No individual HRCT feature is specific for asbestosis: however, a constellation of features which are bilateral and multifocal, with an appropriate occupational history, is considered diagnostic. In advanced disease, apart from pleural disease, the features are indistinguishable from UIP (see 📖 Diffuse parenchymal lung diseases/Usual interstitial pneumonia, p236). The findings on HRCT which indicate a diagnosis of asbestosis include:

- Normal—in early disease.
- Subpleural centrilobular 'dots' or branching structures—the earliest HRCT sign of asbestosis representing peribronchiolar fibrosis; over time, subpleural dots become larger and more confluent.
- Thickened interlobular septa and intralobular lines.
- Subpleural curvilinear lines (NB once believed to be pathognomonic for asbestosis but not considered so now).
- Ground-glass opacification.
- Traction bronchiectasis/bronchiolectasis.
- Honeycombing.
- Enlarged reactive mediastinal lymph nodes.
- Pleural disease (plaques or diffuse pleural thickening). NB Common (>90%) but not invariable.

Ancillary CT features

HRCT demonstrates abnormalities other than asbestosis in patients with previous asbestos exposure. These include:

- Pleuro-parenchymal bands—representing the effects on adjacent lung which occur in the context of diffuse pleural thickening (a *forme fruste* of folded lung) and not 'asbestosis' (see 📖 Pleural diseases/'Folded' lung and pleuro-parenchymal bands, p383).
- 'Hairy' pleural plaques—due to mechanical effects of plaques on adjacent pulmonary parenchyma (analogous to the appearances sometimes seen in lung adjacent to thoracic osteophytes); should be differentiated from fibrosis seen in lung not adjacent to plaques (see 📖 Pleural diseases/Pleural plaques, p378).

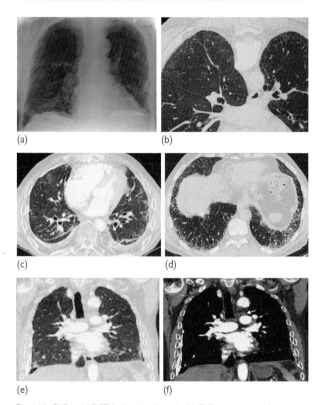

(a)

(b)

(c)

(d)

(e)

(f)

Fig. 6.25 CXR and HRCT findings in asbestosis. (a) CXR in a patient with asbestosis showing a bibasal reticulonodular pattern. There are also bilateral calcified pleural plaques. (b) Targeted HRCT in another patient showing peripheral branching 'X' and 'Y-shaped' dots, representing peribronchiolar fibrosis caused by asbestos fibres. (c) HRCT showing bilateral posterior subpleural curvilinear lines (representing fibrosing bronchioalveolitis) in a patient with asbestosis. (d) HRCT in a patient with asbestosis: there is a bilateral subpleural reticular pattern with honeycombing. Note the calcified pleural plaque on the right hemidiaphragm. Coronal CT on (e) lung and (f) mediastinal window settings in a patient with benign asbestos-related pleuro-parenchymal disease and reactive mediastinal lymph node enlargement (arrow).

Silicosis and coal worker's pneumoconiosis

- Silicosis is a lung disease caused by inhalation of significant amounts of silica and coal worker's pneumoconiosis (CWP) is caused by inhalation of carbonaceous material (anthracosis). The radiological features of silicosis and coal worker's pneumoconiosis are similar and best considered together.
- Occupations which increase the risk of silicosis include quarrying, tunnelling, mining, and sandblasting. Underground coal miners are particularly at risk of CWP.
- Silica exposure may cause acute silicoproteinosis, accelerated silicosis, or 'classic' silicosis. Simple coal worker's pneumoconiosis is characterized by the deposition of coal dust and pigmented macrophages around respiratory bronchioles whereas complicated CWP occurs when there is continued exposure.

Imaging in silicosis and CWP

Acute silicoproteinosis

The imaging features resemble those seen in pulmonary alveolar proteinosis.

CXR findings

- Ground-glass opacities.
- Septal lines.

CT findings (Fig. 6.26)

- 'Crazy-paving' pattern—sharply demarcated (i.e. 'geographic') areas of ground-glass opacification and thickened interlobular septa and intralobular lines.

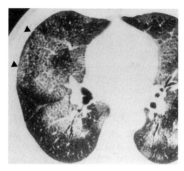

Fig. 6.26 HRCT of a quarry worker with acute silicoproteinosis showing a 'crazy-paving' pattern, indistinguishable from alveolar proteinosis (arrowheads). Reproduced with permission from Kim K-I, Kim CW, Lee MK et al. Imaging of Occupational Lung Disease. *RadioGraphics* 2001:**21**;1371–1391. Copyright RSNA Publications.

Accelerated silicosis, classic silicosis, and CWP
The imaging features of these pneumoconioses are indistinguishable and are detailed below.

CXR findings (Figs. 6.27 and 6.28)
- Small (1–5mm diameter) nodules—rounded upper, mid zone, and posterior; nodules may calcify (in ~20%) or coalesce to form conglomerate masses (progressive massive fibrosis (PMF)) sometimes with surrounding emphysematous destruction initially in the outer lung but, over time, migrating centrally.
- 'Egg-shell' calcification of mediastinal lymph nodes.

CT findings (Figs. 6.29–6.31)
- Small centrilobular or subpleural nodules—at least soft tissue density, variable size.
- Nodules—may calcify, increasing their conspicuity on CT.
- Subpleural nodules or 'pseudoplaques' in CWP.
- 'Egg-shell' calcification of mediastinal lymph nodes.
- Emphysema—develops in a significant proportion of lifelong non-smokers exposed to silica and may be functionally significant.
- Progressive massive fibrosis.

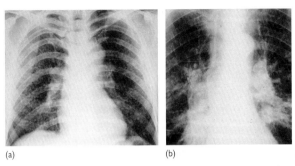

(a)   (b)

Fig. 6.27 CXRs in two patients with exposure to silica. (a) CXR in a patient with simple silicosis. There are multiple small nodules in both lungs. Reproduced with permission from Kim K-I, Kim CW, Lee MK et al. Imaging of Occupational Lung Disease. *RadioGraphics* 2001:**21**;1371–1391. Copyright RSNA Publications and (b) Coned chest radiograph of an individual with simple silicosis showing egg-shell calcification of mediastinal lymph nodes. Reproduced with permission from *Self-assessment Colour Review of Thoracic Imaging*, SJ Copley, DM Hansell and NL Müller. Manson Publishing Ltd, 2005.

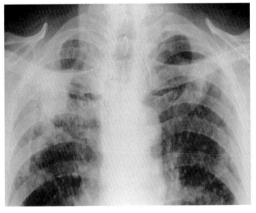

Fig. 6.28 Coned CXR of the upper lung zones in an individual with complicated coal worker's pneumoconiosis showing bilateral upper lobe densities (progressive massive fibrosis) on a background of smaller pulmonary nodules.

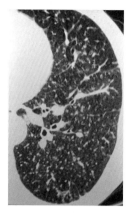

Fig. 6.29 Targeted CT in simple silicosis. There are multiple small well-defined pulmonary nodules in a random distribution.

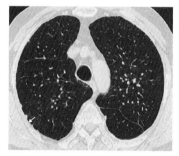

Fig. 6.30 CT through the upper lobes in a patient with simple coal worker's pneumoconiosis showing pseudoplaques (arrow) in a subpleural distribution mimicking pleural plaques.

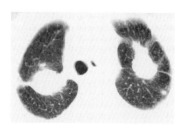

Fig. 6.31 CT through the upper lobes in patient with bilateral progressive massive fibrosis.

Uncommon pneumoconioses

A brief synopsis of the imaging appearances in uncommon pneumoconioses is given below.

Berylliosis

- Exposure to beryllium occurs in light bulb manufacture, the aerospace and ceramic industries, and in dentistry.
- The histopathological changes in berylliosis are indistinguishable from those seen in sarcoidosis.

CXR/CT findings (Fig. 6.32)

The appearances of berylliosis on CXR and CT are the same as for pulmonary sarcoidosis (see 📖 Diffuse parenchymal lung diseases/Granulomatous DPLD: sarcoidosis, p190).

Hard metal lung disease

- A rare pneumoconiosis related to exposure to 'hard metal' (i.e. an alloy of tungsten carbide and cobalt to which other metals [e.g. titanium, nickel, chromium] may be added).
- Hard metal exposure may cause asthma, hypersensitivity pneumonitis, or fibrosis. The characteristic pathological finding is multinucleated giant cells in the airspaces or interstitium (previously termed 'giant cell interstitial pneumonia').

CXR findings

- Small irregular opacities—mid and lower zone predominance
- Diffuse reticulonodular pattern.
- Ground-glass opacification.

CT findings (Fig. 6.33)

In general the appearances are non-specific and may resemble NSIP or UIP.

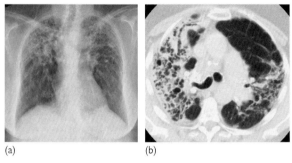

(a)   (b)

Fig. 6.32 CXR and CT features in berylliosis. (a) CXR in a female patient with berylliosis caused by occupational exposure. There is bilateral upper zone fibrosis and volume loss; the appearances are strikingly similar to those seen in pulmonary sarcoidosis. (b) CT in another patient with berylliosis. There is asymmetrical upper lobe fibrosis and calcification of mediastinal and hilar lymph nodes.

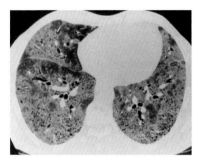

Fig. 6.33 CT in a patient with lung disease caused by hard-metal exposure. There is bilateral ground glass opacification, a reticular pattern and honeycombing with traction bronchiectasis. Reproduced with permission from *Occupational Disorders of the Lung*. Hendrick, Burge, Beckett and Churg (eds). WB Saunders Harcourt Publishers, London 2002.

Aluminium pneumoconiosis

- Pneumoconiosis related to occupational exposure to aluminium and aluminium oxides. (NB interstitial fibrosis related to the inhalation of aluminium fumes is rare).
- On histopathological sections there is interstitial fibrosis and a granulomatous pneumonitis with giant cells. The patterns of desquamative interstitial pneumonitis and alveolar proteinosis have also been described.

CXR findings

- May be normal.
- Bilateral hazy ground-glass opacities or small nodules with an upper and mid zone predominance.
- Basal emphysema—in advanced cases.
- Reticular pattern.
- Honeycombing.

CT findings

- Variable (may mimic silicosis, sarcoidosis, NSIP or UIP).
- Nodular densities in the upper lobes.
- Ground-glass opacification, reticular pattern, and honeycombing— diffuse or upper lobe distribution.
- Increased attenuation of mediastinal lymph nodes.

Welder's pneumoconiosis (siderosis)

- Pneumoconiosis related to inhalation of iron oxide particles. (NB Inhalation of iron oxide dust is also a risk factor for the development of lung cancer.)
- The histopathological findings are often of a limited interstitial fibrosis with iron-dust laden macrophages.

CXR findings

- Small nodules—in the mid (i.e. perihilar) or lower zones. Resolution of abnormalities after cessation of exposure.

CT findings (Fig. 6.34)

- Bilateral ill-defined centrilobular micronodules (mimicking hypersensitivity pneumonitis (see 📖 Diffuse parenchymal lung diseases/Hypersensitivity pneumonitis p201)).
- Fine reticular pattern—honeycombing is rare.
- Diffuse distribution.
- Emphysema.
- Ground-glass opacification.
- Masses with high attenuation—related to the iron content.

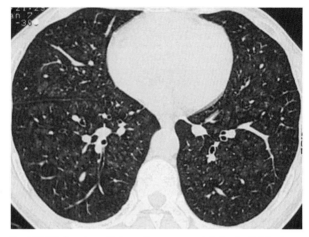

Fig. 6.34 CT of a patient with Arc-welder pneumoconiosis showing ill-defined bilateral small centrilobular nodules. Reproduced with permission from Kim K-I, Kim CW, Lee MK et al. Imaging of Occupational Lung Disease. *RadioGraphics* 2001: **21**;1371–1391. Copyright RSNA Publications.

Lung disease caused by aspiration

Aspiration of solids or liquids into the lungs may result in a chemical or bacterial pneumonitis; inert substances may also be aspirated. A distinction is sometimes made between aspiration pneumonia and aspiration pneumonitis. Other forms of aspiration include near-drowning and lipoid pneumonia.

Aspiration pneumonia

- Aspiration pneumonia results from aspiration of bacteria-laden secretions (both anaerobic and aerobic) from the upper aerodigestive tract. The effect on the lung depends on the type and quantity of aspirated material, and also on the frequency of aspiration.
- Factors which predispose to aspiration pneumonia are summarized in Table 6.11.
- Histopathological features depend on the type and volume of material aspirated but include oedema, polymorphonuclear cell infiltration and haemorrhage with foreign body granulomas. The distribution of pneumonia depends on patient's position at the time of aspiration: when supine, aspiration typically occurs in the posterior segments of the upper lobes and the superior segments of the lower lobes.
- Clinical presentation varies significantly from sub-clinical asymptomatic aspiration to life-threatening acute lung injury. Aspiration may be 'silent' in the context of an intubated patient or in the elderly.

Table 6.11 Factors predisposing to an increased risk of aspiration

- Old age
- Swallowing disorders
- Loss of consciousness
- Alcoholism
- Oesophageal/pharyngeal abnormalities—e.g. cancer, benign strictures, diverticula, congenital or acquired tracheo-oesophageal stricture
- Upper airway or oropharyngeal instrumentation—e.g. tracheal intubation
- Dementia
- Poor dental hygiene—infection with *Actinomyces* species

Imaging in aspiration pneumonia

The CXR and CT findings are non-specific. CT may be of value in identifying complications (e.g. abscess formation, parapneumonic effusion/empyema).

CXR findings

- Unilateral or bilateral consolidation—in general aspirated material will affect the lung that is most dependent at the time of aspiration.
- Complications of aspiration—lung abscess, empyema.

CT findings (Fig. 6.35)

- Consolidation—unilateral or bilateral, patchy or confluent; most pronounced in the region of lung that was dependent at the time of aspiration.
- Centrilobular nodules—an uncommon finding except in patients with a variety of benign and malignant oesophageal diseases (e.g. achalasia, oesophageal cancer) and in lentil aspiration pneumonia. When present, these branching centrilobular (tree-in-bud) nodules indicate an inflammatory bronchiolitis.
- Complications of aspiration: lung abscess, empyema possibly UIP.

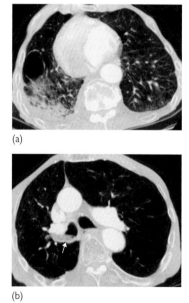

(a)

(b)

Fig. 6.35 CT in a patient with motor neurone disease showing (a) right basal consolidation and volume loss caused by aspiration. (b) Aspirated material is seen in the right main bronchus (arrow).

Aspiration pneumonitis

- Aspiration pneumonitis is an acute lung injury secondary to the aspiration of pneumotoxic substances (e.g. mineral oil, gastric acid). The term Mendleson syndrome refers specifically to the aspiration of large quantities of gastric acid.
- Any cause of decreased consciousness is a risk factor for the aspiration of gastric contents. Some gastrointestinal disorders also predispose to aspiration (Table 6.12).
- The cardinal histopathological abnormality in aspiration pneumonitis is diffuse alveolar damage, identical to that seen in acute respiratory distress syndrome (see 📖 Air space diseases/Miscellaneous causes of pulmonary oedema, p130).
- Mortality rates may be as high as 60%.

Table 6.12 Factors predisposing to an increased risk of aspiration pneumonitis

- **Decreased consciousness**
  - Cerebrovascular accident
  - Drug overdose
  - Epilepsy and seizures
- **Gastrointestinal disorders**
  - Hiatus hernia
  - Achalasia
  - Gastro-oesophageal reflux
  - Vomiting

Imaging of apiration pneumonitis

The CXR is the mainstay of the diagnosis of aspiration pneumonitis. CT will demonstrate the extent of abnormality more accurately and may be of value for 'problem-solving' when CXR appearances are difficult to interpret.

CXR findings (Fig. 6.36)

- Bilateral ground-glass opacification/consolidation—typically perihilar in distribution; in uncomplicated cases, there is improvement over several days. Radiographic deterioration may indicate superadded (nosocomial or ventilator-associated) bacterial infection. (NB In patients with pneumonitis caused by contrast aspiration, there may be characteristic high density material in a bronchographic pattern).
- Absence of cardiomegaly or features of pulmonary venous hypertension (comparison with cardiogenic pulmonary oedema).

CT findings

- The CT features are identical to those seen in acute respiratory distress syndrome (see 📖 Air space diseases/Miscellaneous causes of pulmonary oedema, p130).

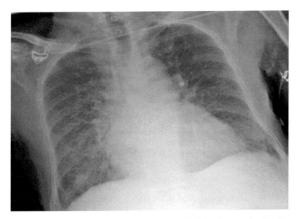

Fig. 6.36 CXR in a patient with aspiration pneumonitis following a stroke showing increased perihilar density.

Near-Drowning

- Near-drowning results in the aspiration of large amounts of water. The clinical syndrome of near drowning is characterized by hypoxia, pulmonary oedema, and acidosis.

Imaging in near drowning

Aspiration of large volumes of water results in radiological features which are indistinguishable from those seen in cardiogenic pulmonary oedema (see 📖 Air space diseases/Pulmonary oedema p126).

Lipid aspiration/lipoid pneumonia

- Lung disease related to the repeated inhalation or aspiration of mineral oil resulting in an 'exogenous' lipoid pneumonia.
- The commonest cause of exogenous lipoid pneumonia in adults is mineral oil ingestion (commonly occurring because of self-medication for constipation or over-the-counter oily nose drops). Aspiration is often silent over significant periods of time. In children, aspiration of milk may cause exogenous lipoid pneumonia.
- Exogenous oily substances incite a foreign body reaction in the lung. Microscopically, there are lipid-laden macrophages in the alveoli and interstitium together with an inflammatory infiltrate.
- Subjects are often asymptomatic and lipoid pneumonia may be an incidental finding on CT.

Imaging of lipoid pneumonia (Figs. 6.37 and 6.38)
CXR findings
- Multifocal ground-glass opacification.
- Consolidation.
- Focal mass—sometimes mimicking lung cancer.

CT findings
- Characteristic focal areas of consolidation containing components of fat attenuation—typically −30 to −120 HU.
- 'Crazy-paving' appearance—a rare manifestation of lipoid pneumonia.

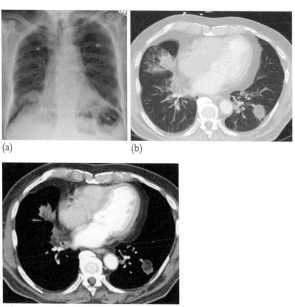

(a)

(b)

(c)

Fig. 6.37 CXR and CT in an elderly male patient with lipoid pneumonia caused by olive oil used to moisten his nasal mucosa. (a) CXR shows opacities in both lower lobes. CT through the lower zones photographed on (b) lung and (c) soft-tissue window settings show multifocal consolidation in the middle and both lower lobes. Images on soft-tissue settings confirm the presence of low (fat) attenuation within these foci.

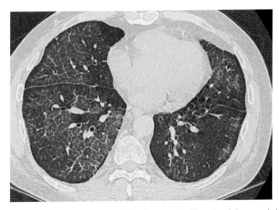

Fig. 6.38 The crazy-paving pattern in lipoid pneumonia. There is subtle ground-glass opacification with thickening of interlobular septa and intralobular lines best seen in the right lung.

Idiopathic interstitial pneumonias

The idiopathic interstitial pneumonias (IIPs) are a separate group of DPLD that share many features but are sufficiently different to one another to be regarded as separate disease entities (Table 6.13).

- Each pattern of IIP may be idiopathic or secondary to a recognizable cause (e.g. DPLD related to connective tissue disease or drug toxicity).
- The diagnosis of a specific IIP is best made by review of clinical, imaging, and/or pathological data. A consensus approach has been shown to improve diagnostic accuracy.
- In clinical practice, the two commonest patterns of IIP are usual interstitial pneumonia (UIP) and non-specific interstitial pneumonia (NSIP).
- The distinction between the patterns of IIPs is important because of differences in prognosis: a pattern of UIP is generally associated with poor survival in contrast to other IIPs; thus, the most important task is to identify individuals with a UIP pattern from those with other IIPs.

Important imaging considerations in IIPs

- Classification of the IIPs is based on histologic criteria and each histologic pattern is associated with a more or less characteristic imaging pattern.
- Differential diagnosis of IIPs always includes underlying connective tissue disease and inhalational exposures.
- Typical CT features of each IIP are distinct but there is some overlap.
- CT features of UIP are diagnostic in about half of cases.
- CT features of organizing pneumonia may be diagnostic in the correct clinical context.
- CT features of NSIP, DIP, RBILD, and LIP are less specific.
- CT features of AIP are similar to that of ARDS from any cause.
- Radiologists must distinguish patients with typical features of UIP, who will usually not require biopsy, from those with other lung diseases.
- Clinical evaluation must prove that an interstitial pneumonia is idiopathic and exclude a recognizable cause or association (e.g. connective tissue disease).

Table 6.13 Summary of patterns of the idiopathic interstitial pneumonias

Morphologic pattern	Histologic features	Typical imaging features	Imaging differential diagnosis
UIP	Spatial and temporal heterogeneity, dense fibrosis, fibroblastic foci, honeycombing, with interspaced normal lung	Basal, subpleural predominance, often patchy, reticular pattern *with* honeycombing	CTD-related, asbestosis, chronic HP
NSIP	Spatially and temporally homogeneous lung fibrosis or inflammation	Basal predominance, ground-glass opacification, reticular pattern with limited or no honeycombing	CTD-related, chronic HP, DIP
COP	Polypoid plugs of loose organizing connective tissue (with or without endobronchiolar intraluminal polyps); preserved lung architecture	Bilateral patchy consolidation	Lymphoma, adenocarcinoma, chronic eosinophilic pneumonia, infection
DIP	Diffuse macrophage accumulation in alveoli	Basal, peripheral predominance; ground-glass attenuation; occasional cysts	Subacute HP, NSIP
RB/RBILD	'Dusty brown' bronchiolocentric alveolar macrophages; mild fibrosis	Centrilobular nodules, ground-glass opacities; thickened interlobular septa and mild emphysema	DIP, subacute HP, NSIP
AIP	Diffuse alveolar damage with oedema and hyaline membranes in acute phase and alveolar septal fibrosis and type II pneumocyte hyperplasia during recovery	Diffuse ground-glass attenuation and consolidation	ARDS, infection, diffuse pulmonary haemorrhage
LIP	Diffuse lympho-plasmacytic infiltration of alveolar septa	Ground-glass attenuation, cysts	DIP, NSIP, HP

Adapted from Müller NL, Colby TV. Idiopathic interstitial pneumonias: high-resolution CT and histologic findings. *RadioGraphics* 1997; **17**:1016–1022.
UIP = usual interstitial pneumonia; NSIP = non-specific interstitial pneumonia;
COP = cryptogenic organizing pneumonia; DIP = desquamative interstitial pneumonia;
AIP = acute interstitial pneumonia; LIP = lymphoid interstitial pneumonia; CTD = connective tissue disease; HP = hypersensitivity pneumonitis; ARDS = acute respiratory distress syndrome
RB/RBILD = respiratory bronchiolitis/respiratory bronchiolitis interstitial lung disease

Usual interstitial pneumonia

- The commonest of the IIPs and associated with the worst prognosis (~50% 5-year survival).
- UIP is the histopathological pattern associated with the clinical syndrome of idiopathic pulmonary fibrosis (IPF) (formerly known as cryptogenic fibrosing alveolitis) or as a pattern of 'lung injury' secondary to other known causes (e.g. connective tissue diseases). (Table 6.14).
- Patients with IPF are usually male, aged over 65 years who present with progressive breathlessness and cough; symptoms are usually present for ~6 months before presentation.
- The key histopathological lesion in UIP is the fibroblastic focus.

Table 6.14 Clinical conditions associated with a UIP pattern

- Idiopathic pulmonary fibrosis
- Connective tissue diseases
- Chronic hypersensitivity pneumonitis
- Asbestosis
- Familial idiopathic pulmonary fibrosis
- Hermansky–Pudlak syndrome

Adapted from American Thoracic Society/European Respiratory Society International Multidisciplinary Consensus Classification of the Idiopathic Interstitial Pneumonias. *Am J Respir Crit Care Med* 2002; **165**:277–304.

Imaging in UIP

CXR findings

The CXR is usually abnormal at presentation but a confident diagnosis of the UIP pattern can rarely be made on the basis of CXR features alone. The characteristic CXR appearances include:

- Reticular pattern—mid and lower zones and peripheral.
- Volume loss—NB relative preservation of lung volumes is seen in patients with coexistent emphysema.
- Enlarged mediastinal lymph nodes—'reactive' and more readily demonstrated on CT.

CT findings (Figs. 6.39 and 6.40)

The presence of the typical HRCT features will permit a confident and accurate diagnosis of the UIP pattern to be made, obviating surgical biopsy. NB Atypical appearances (most commonly resembling NSIP (see 🔲 Diffuse parenchymal lung diseases/Non-specific interstitial pneumonia, p238)) occur in ~30–50% of patients and so, HRCT cannot *exclude* the diagnosis. The characteristic HRCT appearances of UIP include:

- Reticular pattern—bilateral and most pronounced in the basal and subpleural lung. With progression, reticulation increases in extent and appears to 'creep' cranially and anteriorly to involve the anterior aspects of the upper lobes.

- Honeycombing—may be microcystic (<4mm diameter) or macrocystic. The extent and severity of honeycombing tends to increase slowly over time.
- Ground-glass opacification—is often seen on HRCT but is never more extensive than reticulation. Over time the extent of ground-glass opacification generally decreases. A sudden increase in the extent of ground-glass opacification, coupled with rapid clinical deterioration, may be due to an accelerated phase or acute exacerbation of IPF but might indicate another complication (opportunistic infection, pulmonary oedema/fluid overload).
- Ancillary features: traction bronchiectasis/bronchiolectasis; architectural distortion; volume loss (particular with advanced fibrosis; there may be relative preservation of volumes with coexistent emphysema); 'reactive' mediastinal lymph node enlargement; lung cancer (the reported frequency ranges from 10–15%).

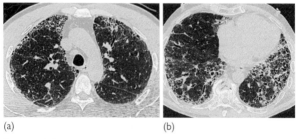

(a) (b)

Fig. 6.39 HRCT in a patient with IPF. Image (a) at the level of the aortic arch and (b) through the lower zones. There is a reticular pattern with honeycombing in the subpleural lung. Disease is more pronounced in the lower zones.

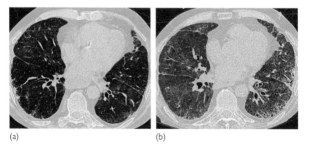

(a) (b)

Fig. 6.40 HRCT performed (a) before and (b) following a period of rapid clinical deterioration in a patient with biopsy proven UIP. In (b) there is a generalized increase in lung attenuation (reflecting a pattern of diffuse alveolar damage) consistent with accelerated IPF.

Non-specific interstitial pneumonia

- After UIP, this is the commonest pattern of interstitial fibrosis. However, in contrast to UIP, this pattern is associated with a significantly better prognosis.
- Most commonly presents in 5th–6th decades; ♂:♀ ≈ 1:1 for idiopathic disease (although slightly higher in females for NSIP occurring on a background of a connective tissue disease).
- As with UIP, the pattern of NSIP may be idiopathic or it occurs on a clinical background of other disorders (Table 6.15).

Imaging in NSIP

Table 6.15 Clinical settings associated with a pattern of NSIP

- Idiopathic
- Connective tissue diseases—*systemic sclerosis, rheumatoid arthritis, polymyositis/dermatomyositis, Sjögren's syndrome*
- Drug-induced lung disease
- Infection
- Immunodeficiency states (HIV infection)

Adapted from American Thoracic Society/European Respiratory Society International Multidisciplinary Consensus Classification of the Idiopathic Interstitial Pneumonias. *Am J Respir Crit Care Med* 2002; **165**:277–304 and Schwartz DA et al. Determinants of progression in idiopathic pulmonary fibrosis *Am J Respir Crit Care Med* 1994; **149**:444–449.

CXR finding
- Ground-glass opacification—most commonly in the mid and lower zones bilaterally.
- Reticular pattern.

CT findings (Fig. 6.41)
The HRCT features of NSIP are more variable than those of UIP.
- Ground-glass opacification—the major HRCT feature in NSIP. Usually bilateral and symmetrical. Most pronounced in the lower zones in >90%; NSIP may be asymmetric or diffuse. In the axial plane, disease may be peripheral/subpleural, diffuse, or peribronchovascular. As with UIP, a sudden increase in the extent of ground-glass opacities may signal an acute exacerbation. Over time the extent of ground-glass opacities tend to decrease and reticulation may increase.

- Reticulation—usually present and associated with ground-glass opacification. The extent of a reticular pattern may remain stable or increase in extent at follow-up (as the extent of ground-glass opacification decreases). On serial HRCT, a pattern indistinguishable from UIP may develop.
- Volume loss.
- Traction bronchiectasis/bronchiolectasis.
- Honeycombing—much less prevalent than in UIP.

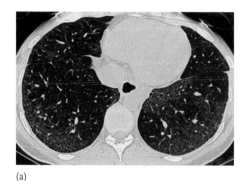

(a)

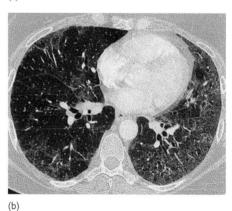

(b)

Fig. 6.41 HRCT in two patients with NSIP. a) CT through the lower zones shows patchy ground-glass opacification with superimposed reticulation. There is no honeycombing (b) Image through the lower zones showing bilateral ground-glass opacification, and a fine reticular pattern.

Organizing pneumonia

- A pattern of idiopathic interstitial pneumonia which predominantly affects the air spaces.
- Patients are usually 50–60 years of age; σ:φ ≈ 1:1. More frequent in nonsmokers.
- Prognosis in cryptogenic disease is usually good with response to corticosteroid treatment but relapses are common; the clinical associations of the OP pattern are summarized below (Table 6.16).

Table 6.16 Clinical settings in which an OP pattern is known to occur

- Idiopathic (i.e. cryptogenic organizing pneumonia)
- Diffuse alveolar damage
- Infection
- Distal to obstruction
- Aspiration
- Drug toxicity, fume, and toxic exposures
- Connective tissue disease—*rheumatoid arthritis, polymyositis/dermatomyositis*
- Inflammatory bowel disease
- Miscellaneous (as a reparative reaction)—*Wegener's granulomatosis, tumours, abscesses.*

Adapted from American Thoracic Society/European Respiratory Society International Multidisciplinary Consensus Classification of the Idiopathic Interstitial Pneumonias. *Am J Respir Crit Care Med* 2002; **165**:277–304.

Imaging in organizing pneumonia

CXR findings

- Consolidation—patchy, bilateral or unilateral, peripheral, and in the lower zones. May progress over time. With corticosteroid therapy there may be dramatic resolution.
- Nodules.
- Reticulonodular pattern.
- Solitary pulmonary mass—mimicking a neoplasm.

CT findings (Figs. 6.42 and 6.43)

In most patients, the HRCT features of OP are not specific; areas of air space opacification are a feature of many respiratory diseases. The recognized CT appearances of OP include:

- Consolidation—bilateral or unilateral, more frequently in the lower zones either in a subpleural or a peribronchial distribution, the latter is sometimes a feature of OP in polymyositis/dermatomyositis. A distinctive peri-lobular pattern of consolidation is recognized. Another pattern is one in which there are 'rings' of consolidation surrounding ground-glass opacification (the 'Atoll' or 'reverse halo' sign).
- Band-like opacities containing an air bronchogram. Resolution of linear opacities with treatment is the norm.
- Ground-glass opacification—usually associated with consolidation.
- Reticular pattern—less common than consolidation and ground-glass opacification. May indicate fibrosis (a known complication, particularly in patients with connective tissue disease-related OP).
- Nodules—less common manifestation of OP; measuring up to 1cm in diameter. May be multiple or solitary and can mimic malignancy.

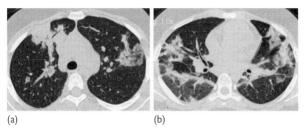

Fig. 6.42 Typical HRCT appearances in two patients with organizing pneumonia. (a) HRCT through the upper and (b) the lower zones. There is patchy, multifocal consolidation in both patients.

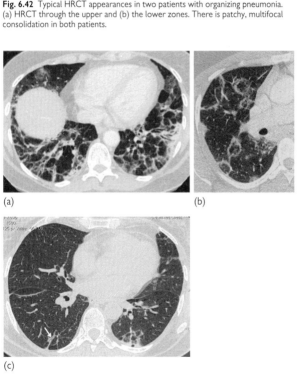

Fig. 6.43 Different HRCT patterns in organizing pneumonia. (a) Perilobular: there is an arcade-like appearance caused by consolidation around multiple pulmonary lobules. (b) Reverse-halo sign: targeted image through the right lung shows multiple rings of consolidation with central ground-glass opacification and (c) band-like: two linear bands of opacification are shown in the right lower lobe. In one of these, a subsegmental airway is shown (arrow). There is also perilobular consolidation in the left lower lobe.

Acute interstitial pneumonia

- Acute interstitial pneumonia (AIP) is a rare and rapidly progressive form of interstitial pneumonia, associated with a poor prognosis.
- AIP occurs overs a wide age range. ♂:♀ ≈ 1:1. A preceeding 'viral-type' upper respiratory illness is often reported but is followed by marked breathlessness progressing over days.
- The outlook is poor with a mortality of ~50%.

Imaging in AIP

CXR findings (Fig. 6.44)

- Ground-glass opacification and consolidation—bilateral and diffuse; sparing of the costophrenic recesses is occasionally seen.

CT findings (Fig. 6.44)

The HRCT appearances are generally the same as those seen in ARDS (see Air space diseases/Miscellaneous causes of pulmonary oedema, p130) and include:

- Ground-glass opacification—seen in all patients. Typically bilateral and diffuse involving all zones (may be more prevalent in upper or lower zones in some patients). Patchy foci of normally aerated lung parenchyma may be present. There may be thickened interlobular septa in areas of ground-glass opacification giving rise to a 'crazy-paving' appearance.
- Consolidation—common but less pronounced than ground-glass opacities.
- Traction bronchiectasis/bronchiolectasis—in areas of ground-glass opacity or consolidation. Associated with a poorer survival.
- Architectural distortion.

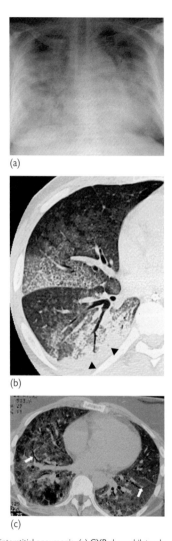

Fig. 6.44 Acute interstitial pneumonia. (a) CXR shows bilateral symmetrical air space opacities in a patient with severe breathlessness and hypoxia. (b) Targeted HRCT through the right lung in the same patient shows widespread ground-glass opacification and dependent dense parenchymal opacification (arrowheads). (c) CT in another patient with acute interstitial pneumonia. Within areas of ground-glass opacification, there are dilated subsegmental airways (arrows), a poor prognostic feature.

Desquamative interstitial pneumonia

- Desquamative interstitial pneumonia (DIP) is a rare interstitial pneumonia.
- DIP typically presents in patients aged 30–40 years. ♂ : ♀ ≈ 2:1. There is a strong (but not consistent) relationship with smoking (see 📖 Diffuse parenchymal lung diseases/Respiratory bronchiolitis and respiratory bronchiolitis interstitial lung disease, p246).
- Prognosis is generally good with smoking cessation and corticosteroid treatment leading to remission in the majority.

Imaging in DIP

CXR findings

- Ground-glass opacification—patchy, bilateral, and most pronounced in the mid/lower zones.

CT findings (Fig. 6.45)

- Ground glass opacification—the principal CT abnormality. Most commonly in the mid/lower zones with a peripheral (in ~60%) or random distribution.
- Irregular linear opacities/reticular pattern—less common.
- Cysts.

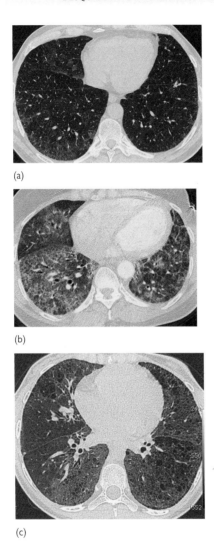

(a)

(b)

(c)

Fig. 6.45 HRCT appearance in three patients with DIP. (a) Image through the lower zones show subtle peripheral ground-glass opacification. This is most obvious on the right. (b) HRCT through the lower zones in another patient shows widespread ground-glass opacities with superimposed fine reticulation. (c) Image shows bilateral ground-glass opacities and multiple thin-walled cysts in both lungs.

Respiratory bronchiolitis and respiratory bronchiolitis interstitial lung disease

- Respiratory bronchiolitis (RB)—of variable severity—is an invariable but clinically-silent histopathological finding in cigarette smokers.
- Respiratory bronchiolitis interstitial lung disease (RBILD) is the clinical manifestiation of interstitial lung disease in patients with the pathological lesion of RB.
- Most patients with RBILD are young (aged 30–40 years). $\male : \female \approx 2:1$.
- Although the 'lesion' of RB can persist, the prognosis is generally favourable following smoking cessation.

Imaging of **RBILD**

CXR findings
- Ground-glass opacification.
- Reticular or reticulonodular pattern.

CT findings (Fig. 6.46)
The CT features of RBILD bear some resemblance to those seen in subacute hypersensitivity pneumonitis (see 📖 Diffuse parenchymal lung diseases/Hypersensitivity pneumonitis, p201).

- Centrilobular nodules.
- Ground-glass opacification—focal and patchy.
- Lobular decreased attenuation—reflecting the bronchiolitic component of RBILD.
- Thickened interlobular septa—rarely extensive.
- Emphysema—upper zones but usually of limited extent.

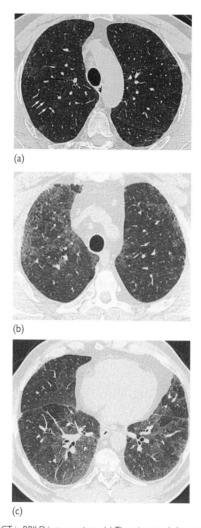

(a)

(b)

(c)

Fig. 6.46 HRCT in RBILD in two patients. (a) There is ground-glass opacification and ill-defined centrilobular nodules (arrows) in the upper lobes of a heavy cigarette smoker. (b) HRCT through the upper lobes in another patient shows ground-glass opacities but also subtle centrilobular emphysema of limited extent. (c) Image through the lower zones in the same patient as in (b) shows lobular decreased attenuation (best seen in the left lower lobe) and thickened interlobular septa, in addition to ground-glass opacities.

Lymphoid interstitial pneumonia

- A recognizable pattern of interstitial pneumonia distinct from other known patterns of IIP and malignant lymphocytic infiltrations.
- Idiopathic LIP is uncommon. ♀ > ♂.
- Despite its classification as an IIP, LIP frequently occurs on a background of other disorders (i.e. connective tissue diseases, immunodeficiency and autoimmune conditions (Table 6.17)).

Table 6.17 Associations of a LIP pattern

- Idiopathic
- Connective tissue diseases—*Sjögren's syndrome, rheumatoid arthritis, systemic lupus erythematosus*
- Immunodeficiency—*HIV-related, severe immunodeficiency, common variable immunodeficiency, multicentric Castleman's disease*
- Immunological/autoimmune state—*autoimmune-haemolytic anaemia, myasthenia gravis, pernicious anaemia, Hashimoto's thyroiditis, primary biliary cirrhosis*
- Drug-induced/toxic exposure
- Infections—*Pneumocystis jiroveci pneumonia, hepatitis B, Epstein–Barr virus*

From American Thoracic Society/European Respiratory Society International Multidisciplinary Consensus Classification of the Idiopathic Interstitial Pneumonias. *Am J Respir Crit Care Med* 2002; **165**:277–304.

Imaging in LIP

CXR findings
- Ground-glass opacification—typically bilateral and mid/lower zones.
- Reticulonodular pattern.

CT findings (Fig. 6.47)
- Ground-glass opacification—present in all patients. Usually bilateral and diffuse. Patchy distribution and sub-pleural disease are less common.
- Centrilobular nodules—poorly defined, bilateral, and diffuse distribution in the majority.
- Small nodules—sub-pleural. Present in >85% of patients.
- Thickened interlobular septa.
- Cysts—random distribution; present in ~70% of patients.

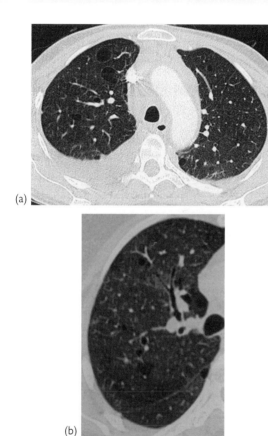

Fig. 6.47 HRCT in two patients with LIP. (a) There is subtle ground-glass opacification and multiple thin-walled cysts. There are bilateral pleural effusions and enlarged lymph nodes in this patient undergoing investigation for suspected lymphoma. (b) Targeted image through the right lung showing ground-glass opacification and scattered cysts.

Miscellaneous interstitial lung diseases

Langerhans' cell histiocytosis

- Langerhans' cell histiocytosis (LCH) is a disease of unknown aetiology characterized by histiocyte proliferation. Several synonyms including histiocytosis X, eosinophilic granuloma, and Langerhans' cell granulomatosis have been used in the past but the term Langerhans' cell histiocytosis (appended with the particular organ(s) involved [e.g. lung LCH or bone LCH]) is now preferred.
- Pulmonary LCH is very strongly associated with cigarette smoking and usually occurs in the absence of other organ involvement. $\male : \female \approx 1:1$
- There is proliferation of CD1a-positive histiocytes: there is an initial cellular infiltrate around the small airways followed by increasing interstitial infiltration. The archetypal lesion is a 'stellate' nodule which eventually cavitates and then forms a thin-walled cyst. In end-stage disease, there is fibrosis and emphysema-like destruction.

Imaging in Langerhans' cell histiocytosis

CXR findings (Fig. 6.48)

- The CXR may be entirely normal in early disease.
- Nodular or reticulonodular pattern—in the upper/mid zones. The reticulonodular pattern is due to the presence of multiple thin-walled cysts which, on a 2-dimensional CXR, are summated to create the impression of criss-crossing lines.
- Cavities/cysts—nodules eventually cavitate and finally form cysts.
- Preserved or increased lung volumes.
- Honeycombing and parenchymal distortion—in advanced disease, (may be impossible to distinguish from advanced emphysema on CXR).
- Ancillary features include: pneumothorax, signs of pulmonary hypertension.

CT findings (Figs. 6.49–6.51)

- Multiple small nodules (usually <1cm diameter)—in early disease with an upper and mid lung predominance; sparing of the costophrenic angles and anterior tips of the lingula and middle lobe is an important diagnostic clue.
- Larger nodules—unusual; very rarely there is a solitary pulmonary nodule.
- Cavitating nodules—cavities may be odd-shaped and, later thin-walled and more eccentric with coalescence in more advanced disease.
- Cysts—a combination of cysts and nodules is common. Cysts typically have bizarre outlines. NB Both nodules and cysts may regress with smoking cessation.
- In end stage, there is extensive parenchymal destruction and honeycombing.

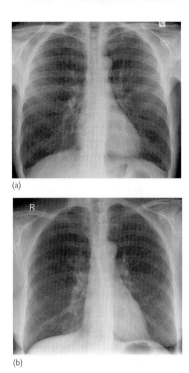

(a)

(b)

Fig. 6.48 Targeted CXRs in two patients with LCH. (a) Subtle small nodules are present in both lungs. (b) Widespread fine reticulonodular pattern in both lungs.

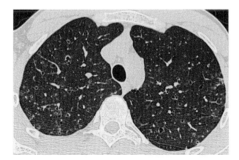

Fig. 6.49 HRCT through the upper lobes in a patient with pulmonary LCH showing bilateral cavitating nodules.

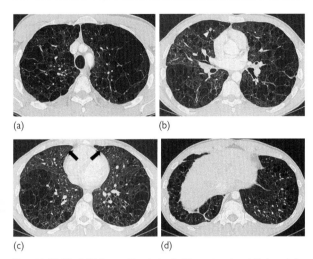

(a)   (b)

(c)   (d)

Fig. 6.50 HRCT in LCH. Images (a) at the level of the aortic arch and (b) through the mid zone shows multiple thin-walled cysts many of which have odd (non-spherical) outlines; there is a nodule in the middle lobe (arrowhead). Lower sections show (c) relative sparing of the anterior tip of the middle lobe and lingula (arrows) and (d) the costophrenic recesses.

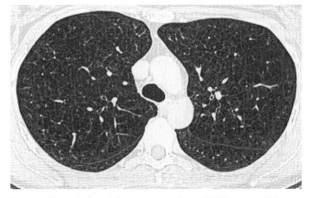

Fig. 6.51 CT in a patient with biopsy-proven end-stage LCH showing multiple cysts which are indistinguishable from emphysema.

Lymphangioleiomyomatosis

- Lymphangioleiomyomatosis (LAM) is a rare disease of unknown aetiology characterized by smooth muscle cell proliferation around airways, blood vessels, and lymphatics.
- LAM almost exclusively affects females of childbearing age; the prevalence of sporadic LAM (i.e. sole manifestation of disease) is approximately 1 per million population.
- There is an association with tuberous sclerosis (see 📖 Diffuse parenchymal lung diseases/Tuberous sclerosis, p255) and mutations in the TSC1 gene are recognized in LAM.

Imaging in lymphangioleiomyomatosis

CXR findings (Fig. 6.52)

- Nodular, reticular, or reticulonodular opacities—fine, bilateral, and symmetrical.
- Preserved or increased lung volumes.
- Enlargement of central pulmonary arteries in end-stage disease indicating cor pulmonale.
- Pleural effusions.

CT findings (pulmonary) (Fig. 6.53)

- Thin-walled cysts—well-defined and of roughly uniform size (~5–15mm in diameter but may be as large as 5cm; the intervening lung is normal. Cysts are uniformly distributed throughout the lungs (see 📖 Diffuse parenchymal lung diseases/Langerhans' cell histiocytosis, p250) with *no* sparing of the costophrenic angles and anterior tips of the lingula/middle lobe.
- (Chylous) pleural effusion—unilateral or bilateral and recurrent.
- Pneumothoraces—unilateral or bilateral and recurrent. May be a presenting feature in ~50% of patients.
- Lymph node enlargement.

CT findings (abdominal)

- Renal and hepatic angiomyolipomas.
- Lymphangiomyomas.
- Chylous ascites.
- Retroperitoneal lymph node enlargement.
- Dilatation of the thoracic duct or cisterna chili.

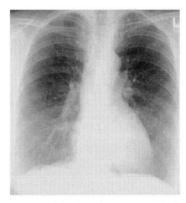

Fig. 6.52 CXR in a patient with lymphangioleiomyomatosis. The lungs are slightly increased in volume. Reproduced with permission from *Self-assessment Colour Review of Thoracic Imaging*, SJ Copley, DM Hansell and NL Müller. Manson Publishing Ltd, 2005.

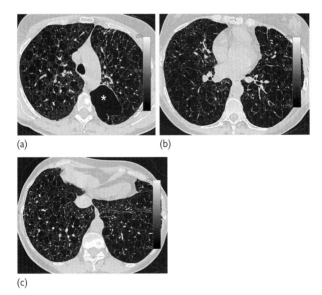

(a)   (b)

(c)

Fig. 6.53 HRCT images at (a) the level of the aortic arch, (b) the pulmonary venous confluence and (c) through the lower lobes. There is a uniform distribution of thin-walled cysts with no sparing of the tip of the middle lobe/lingula or the lower zones. An encysted pneumothorax (asterisk) is seen in the left upper zone.

Tuberous sclerosis

- Tuberous sclerosis complex (TSC) is a rare autosomal dominant neurocutaneous disorder.
- ♂:♀ ≈ 1:1 (NB Lung involvement is more common in women and is histopathologically identical to LAM).

Imaging in tuberose sclerosis

CXR findings (Fig. 6.54)

- Nodular, reticular, or reticulonodular opacities—bilateral, symmetrical; nodules measuring 1–2mm in diameter. May be diffuse or basally predominant.
- Honeycombing/cysts—with advancing disease.
- Preserved or large volume lungs.
- Pneumothorax.
- Central pulmonary artery dilatation—caused by pulmonary hypertension in advanced disease.

CT findings (Fig. 6.54)

- Thin-walled cysts—uniformly distributed; usually <2cms in diameter with normal intervening lung. The appearances are broadly comparable to those in LAM.
- Nodules—presumably reflecting Type II pneumocyte hyperplasia. (NB Uncommon in LAM).
- Bony lesions—sclerotic ribs/vertebral bodies.

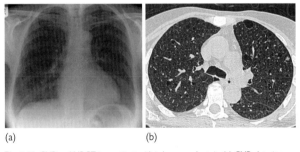

(a)   (b)

Fig. 6.54 CXR and HRCT in a patient with tuberous sclerosis. (a) CXR showing subtle reticulonodular opacities. (b) HRCT clearly demonstrates bilateral lung cysts and small nodules.

Neurofibromatosis (Type I)

- An autosomal dominant neurocutaneous syndrome characterized by peripheral nerve sheath tumours (schwannomas and neurofibromas), skin pigmentation (café au lait spots), optic gliomas, and hamartomas of the iris.
- Type I neurofibromatosis occurs in approximately 1 in 3000 live births; ♂:♀ ≈ 1:1.
- The commonest pulmonary manifestation is diffuse interstitial fibrosis and bullae: lung fibrosis occurs in ~10% whereas bullae are demonstrated in ~20%.
- On histopathological examination, the features are similar to diffuse interstitial pneumonias of other causes. A variably severe fibrosis and chronic inflammation is seen predominantly in the subpleural regions.

Imaging in Type I neurofibromatosis

CXR findings (Fig. 6.55)

In neurofibromatosis, the extra-pulmonary manifestations probably outnumber the lung abnormalities. The manifestations of Type I neurofibromatosis on CXR include:

- Skin nodules—multiple and creating the impression of intra-pulmonary nodules.
- Extrapleural soft tissue density mass—due to intercostal nerve tumours with pressure effects (e.g. rib notching or 'twisted ribbon' rib deformities).
- Kyphoscoliosis and other vertebral body anomalies—e.g. posterior scalloping of vertebral bodies on a lateral projection.
- Posterior mediastinal masses—due to neural tumours, phaeochromocytomas or lateral thoracic meningocoeles.
- Middle mediastinal masses (vagus and phrenic nerve sheath tumours).
- Bilateral basal reticular pattern (± septal lines)—may progress to honeycombing ± bullae.
- Preserved lung volumes—despite the presence of apparently extensive 'interstitial lung disease'.

CT findings (Fig. 6.56)

The CT features mirror those seen on CXR and include:

- Skin nodules—typically multiple and readily demonstrated at CT.
- Extrapleural soft tissue mass due to intercostal nerve tumours with rib notching or other rib abnormalities.
- Kyphoscoliosis and other vertebral body abnormalities.
- Posterior mediastinal masses—neural tumours, phaeochromocytomas (smooth, well-defined soft tissue masses demonstrating a variety of enhancement patterns post IV contrast) or lateral thoracic meningocoeles (usually right sided, fluid attenuation and may be associated with rib and vertebral body abnormalities with enlargement of adjacent intervertebral foramen).

- Middle mediastinal masses—due to vagus or phrenic nerve sheath tumours, plexiform neurofibromas.
- Reticular pattern—bilateral and basal (sometimes with interlobular septal thickening) which may progress to honeycombing ± bullae.
- Rarely parenchymal nodules due to neurilemmomas or neurofibromas.

MRI findings (Fig. 6.57)
- Imaging method of choice for evaluating nerve sheath tumours and lateral thoracic meningocoeles; CT is better at demonstrating calcification.
- Neurofibromas have variable signal characteristics. Sometimes high on T1, low on T2-weighted images and may demonstrate 'dumb-bell' extension into spinal canal with widening of intervertebral foramina.
- Lateral thoracic meningoceles are of fluid signal (low on T1, high on T2-weighted images) with extension into the spinal canal and enlargement of the intervertebral foramen.

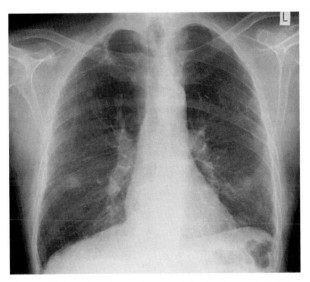

Fig. 6.55 CXR in a patient with neurofibromatosis Type I. Note the left-sided rib deformity and multiple skin nodules.

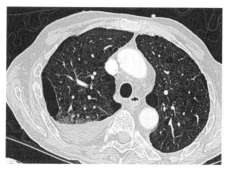

Fig. 6.56 CT in a patient with neurofibromatosis. There is a right pleural effusion and multiple pulmonary bullae. Note the small skin nodules on the anterior chest wall.

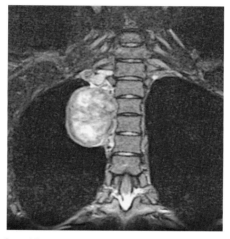

Fig. 6.57 Coronal T2-weighted MRI in a patient with neurofibromatosis Type I showing a paraspinal neurofibroma with heterogeneous signal characteristics.

Pulmonary vasculitides

- A rare group of systemic disorders characterized by the inflammatory destruction of large, medium, and/or small blood vessels.
- Vascular destruction is caused by granulomatous, neutrophilic, lymphoplasmacytic or eosinophilic infiltration.
- Lung involvement can occur in all types (Table 6.18) but is most common in the primary (idiopathic) small vessel vasculitides which includes Wegener's granulomatosis, microscopic polyangiitis, and Churg–Strauss syndrome. The small vessel vasculitides are characterized by the presence of circulating antineutrophil cytoplasmic antibodies (ANCA).

Table 6.18 Classification of systemic vasculitides

- **Primary (idiopathic)**
  - *Small vessel*—Wegener's granulomatosis, Microscopic polyangiitis, Churg-Strauss syndrome, isolated pauci-immune pulmonary capillaritis
  - *Medium vessel*—Polyarteritis nodosa, Kawasaki disease
  - *Large vessel*—Giant cell arteritis, Takayasu's arteritis
- **Primary (immune complex-mediated)**
  - Goodpasture's syndrome
  - Henoch–Schönlein purpura
  - Behçet's disease
  - IgA nephropathy
- **Secondary**
  - Autoimmune—SLE, rheumatoid arthritis, polymyositis/dermatomyositis, systemic sclerosis, antiphospholipid syndrome
  - Drug-induced
  - Infection
  - Paraneoplastic
  - Inflammatory bowel disease

Adapted from Brown KK. Pulmonary vasculitis. *Proc Am Thorac Soc* 2006; **3**:48–57.

Imaging in pulmonary vasculitides

The radiological appearances of individual primary vasculitides are discussed below but the signs which, in the appropriate clinical context, may suggest a diagnosis of a pulmonary vasculitis are:

- Nodules—generally multiple and bilateral (± cavitation); may be transient or migratory.
- Consolidation—patchy, peripheral (± cavitation); transient or migratory.
- Ground-glass opacification—may be widespread and usually reflects diffuse alveolar haemorrhage.

Primary (idiopathic) pulmonary vasculitides

Wegener's granulomatosis

- A multisystem disease characterized by a necrotizing predominantly small vessel vasculitis with granulomatous necrosis and elements of acute and chronic inflammation.
- More common in Caucasian races. ♂:♀ ≈ 1:1; wide age range (from childhood to >70 years) but typically diagnosed around 40–55 years of age.
- Wegener's granulomatosis (WG) classically affects the respiratory tract and kidneys but any organ system is susceptible including the central nervous system, gastrointestinal tract, the heart and lymph nodes. A 'limited' form of WG which affects the lungs alone (± upper respiratory tract) is recognized.
- No known aetiology but there is a strong association with the cytoplasmic staining pattern of anti-neutrophil cytoplasmic antibodies (c-ANCA); c-ANCA directed against proteinase-3 (PR3) is present in 70–90% of patients with active WG (NB PR3-ANCA is also positive in microscopic polyangiitis, polyarteritis nodosa, and Churg–Strauss syndrome but less prevalent). Putative link between *Staphylococcus aureus* infection (in the upper/lower respiratory tracts) and relapse of WG.

Imaging in Wegener's granulomatosis

The spectrum of CXR and CT findings in WG is broad and often non-specific. An additional difficulty (at follow-up), is the distinction between the radiological changes related to WG and those due to intercurrent infection or therapy-related complications.

CXR findings (Fig. 6.58)

The CXR is abnormal in ~75% of patients at presentation. Common manifestations include:

- Nodules or mass-like lesions—usually bilateral (but occasionally solitary) ± cavitation. Nodules/masses range in size from small (2–3 cm in diameter) to large (up to 10 cm); no zonal predilection. Nodules regress with treatment (but may take 1 month or longer for complete radiographic resolution); nodules may recur at relapse and sometimes at the same site.

- Consolidation ± cavitation—Typically pleurally-based. Less common than nodules in adults but consolidation is more common than nodules in children.

Less common CXR manifestations:
- Ground-glass opacities (localized or diffuse; the latter is seen in WG patients presenting with diffuse pulmonary haemorrhage caused by capillaritis); hilar/mediastinal lymph node enlargement (not seen in isolation); pleural effusions and pneumothorax; interstitial fibrosis.

CT findings (Figs. 6.58 and 6.59)
- Nodules/masses—seen in up to 90% of patients; multiple and bilateral in the majority. Often subpleural with lobulated or spiculated margins. Cavitation is present in 15–25% (generally seen in larger nodules). Cavities may have a thin wall. A 'feeding' vessel may be seen.
- Consolidation—present in around 30% of patients; often pleurally-based and wedge-shaped.
- Subglottic, tracheal, and bronchial stenosis—stenoses may be focal or diffuse.
- Bronchial wall thickening—affecting the segmental and subsegmental airways. Mild cylindrical bronchiectasis is common.

Less common CT manifestations:
- Ground-glass opacities—patchy or diffuse, the latter distribution is a feature of diffuse pulmonary haemorrhage.
- 'Halo' sign or 'reverse-halo' sign—nodules with surrounding ground-glass opacification or the reverse (i.e. ground-glass opacification surrounded by a rim of consolidation).
- Other minor features: hilar/mediastinal lymph node enlargement, pleural effusions, atelectasis, thickened interlobular septa, and interstitial fibrosis.

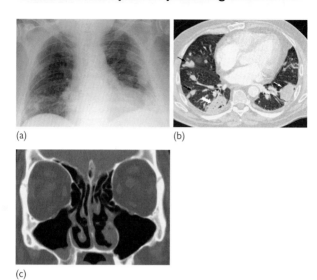

(a)

(b)

(c)

Fig. 6.58 45-year-old male patient with Wegener's granulomatosis. (a) CXR shows multiple nodules of varying size in both lungs. (b) HRCT through the lower zones also demonstrates multiple bilateral well-defined nodules (thin arrows); in addition there is cavitating consolidation in the right lower lobe (thick arrow) and (c) coronal CT through the sinuses showing mucosal thickening at the base of the right maxillary antrum.

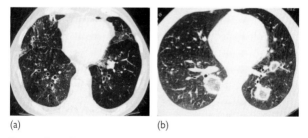

(a)

(b)

Fig. 6.59 Other CT manifestations of Wegener's granulomatosis. (a) Airways disease: CT through the mid/lower zones demonstrating cylindrical bronchiectasis in both lower lobes. There is a nodule in the left lower lobe and focal consolidation in the middle lobe. (b) 'Reverse-halo' sign: three lesions have central ground-glass opacification and a halo of more dense parenchymal opacification.

Microscopic polyangiitis

- A necrotizing small vessel systemic vasculitis affecting venules, capillaries, arterioles, and arteries which involves the kidneys (100%) and lungs (10–30%). A lung-localized form of microscopic polyangiitis (called idiopathic pauci-immune pulmonary capillaritis (typically ANCA negative)) is known to occur.
- In contrast to PR3-ANCA in WG, most patients (75–80%) with microscopic polyangiitis have circulating ANCA directed to myeloperoxidase (MPO-ANCA). Lung involvement most commonly presents with diffuse pulmonary haemorrhage (caused by capillaritis).

CXR findings (Fig. 6.60)

- Normal—if the severity/extent of intra-alveolar bleeding is mild
- Widespread bilateral ground-glass opacification.

CT findings (Fig. 6.60)

- Widespread ground-glass opacification/consolidation
- Centrilobular nodules.

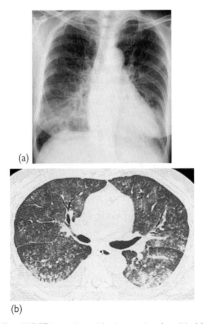

(a)

(b)

Fig. 6.60 CXR and HRCT in a patient with microscopic polyangiitis. (a) There is bilateral lower lobe ground-glass opacification due to pulmonary haemorrhage. (b) HRCT image below the level of the carina (performed one day after CXR) shows more extensive ground-glass opacities with dense parenchymal opacification in the lower lobes.

Churg–Strauss syndrome (allergic granulomatosis and angiitis)

- A small vessel vasculitis characterized by six clinico-pathological criteria (NB at least four needed for diagnosis): i) asthma, ii) blood eosinophilia (>10% of the white cell count), iii) migratory or transient lung infiltrates, iv) paranasal sinus disease, v) mono- or polyneuropathy and vi) extravascular eosinophils on biopsy of affected tissues.
- Slight male preponderance with a wide age range (15–70 yrs); MPO-ANCA positive in 35–75% patients.
- Lung involvement is common but pulmonary haemorrhage is less common than in WG and microscopic polyangiitis.

CXR findings (Fig. 6.61)
- Normal.
- Consolidation or ground-glass opacities—peripheral or patchy distribution; may be transient or migratory.
- Bronchial wall thickening ± dilatation.
- Nodules ± cavitation—up to 3.5cm in diameter.
- Minor features include: pleural effusions, septal lines (may be due to pulmonary oedema because of cardiac involvement).

CT findings (Fig. 6.61)
- Normal.
- Consolidation or ground-glass opacities—peripheral or patchy. Typically in the mid- to lower zones.
- Nodules ± cavitation—measuring anything from 5mm up to 3.5cm.
- Bronchial wall thickening.
- Thickened interlobular septa (indicating interstitial oedema).

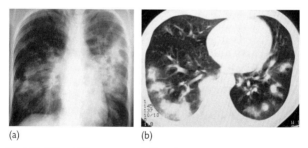

(a)   (b)

Fig. 6.61 CXR and CT in a patient with Churg–Strauss syndrome. (a) CXR showing bilateral asymmetric consolidation, predominantly in the mid-zones. (b) CT demonstrates multifocal consolidation in the lower lobes

Eosinophilic lung diseases

- A heterogeneous group of diseases characterized by pulmonary eosinophilic infiltration usually (but not invariably) associated with a peripheral (blood) eosinophilia.
- Eosinophilic lung infiltration may be idiopathic or of a known cause (Table 6.19).
- Diagnosis is based on one of three features: i) the demonstration of pulmonary opacities in the presence of peripheral eosinophilia, ii) an increased percentage (typically >10%) of eosinophils in bronchoalveolar lavage fluid or iii) the pathological demonstration lung eosinophilia on biopsy.
- A confident and correct radiological (i.e. CT) diagnosis is made in only 1/3 of cases.

Table 6.19 Causes and associations of pulmonary eosinophilia

- **Idiopathic pulmonary eosinophilia**
  - Simple pulmonary eosinophilia (Löffler syndrome)
  - Chronic pulmonary eosinophilia
  - Acute eosinophilic pneumonia
  - Hypereosinophilic syndrome
- **Pulmonary eosinophilia of known cause or association**
  - Immunological
    Wegener's granulomatosis
    Churg-Strauss syndrome
    Rheumatoid arthritis
  - Drug-induced (NSAIDs, 'crack' cocaine)
  - Infection
    Parasitic (ascariasis, tropical eosinophilia)
    Fungal
  - Miscellaneous associations
    Lymphoma
    Pneumocystis jiroveci infection
    Excessive dust exposure (e.g. 9/11 survivors)

Adapted from Jeong YJ et al. *RadioGraphics* 2007; **27**:617–639.

Imaging in eosinophilic lung diseases

The findings on CXR and CT in patients with pulmonary eosinophilia vary depending on cause. However, the imaging features which raise the suspicion of an underlying eosinophilic lung disease include:

- Flitting and migratory foci of consolidation and/or ground-glass opacification.
- Predominantly peripheral distribution.
- Predominantly upper zone involvement.
- Non-segmental opacities.
- Central bronchiectasis ± mucoid impaction (in the case of allergic bronchopulmonary aspergillosis).

Idiopathic eosinophilic lung diseases

Simple pulmonary eosinophilia (Löffler syndrome)

- Löffler syndrome is either idiopathic or related to an underlying cause (e.g. parasitic infection, drugs)
- Characterized by self-limiting (<1 month) minor constitutional symptoms, migratory and transient radiographic opacities, and peripheral eosinophilia.

CXR findings

- Flitting and migratory non-segmental areas of consolidation and/or ground-glass opacification.
- Predominantly peripheral involvement.

CT findings

- Patchy ground-glass opacities ± consolidation—typically in the periphery of the mid and upper zones bilaterally but may be randomly distributed.
- Nodules.
- Bronchial wall thickening.
- Less common findings: mediastinal/hilar lymph node enlargement, bronchiectasis, interlobular septal thickening.

Chronic pulmonary eosinophilia

- A disorder of unknown aetiology which is generally more protracted (i.e. >1 month) and severe than simple pulmonary eosinophilia.
- Response to corticosteroid treatment is often dramatic but relapse can occur.
- The radiological findings may be characteristic and allow a confident diagnosis to be made.

CXR findings (Fig. 6.62)

- Consolidation/ground-glass opacification—patchy and non-segmental; typically the opacities are peripheral and appear to be parallel to the chest wall (an appearance called the 'photographic negative of pulmonary oedema').

CT findings (Fig. 6.62)

- Ground-glass opacities (± interlobular septal thickening) and/or dense confluent consolidation.
- Band-like sub-pleural increased attenuation.
- Peripheral in the majority and usually in the mid/upper zones but may be random.
- Less common findings: nodules or mass-lesions, volume loss, pleural effusions, bronchial wall thickening/bronchiectasis, mediastinal/hilar lymph node enlargement.

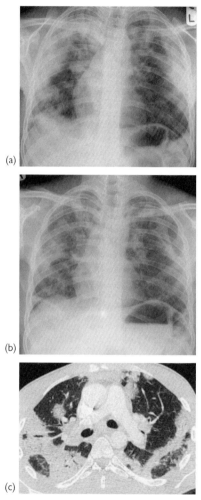

Fig. 6.62 CXRs and CT in chronic pulmonary eosinophilia. (a) CXR demonstrates typical peripheral, upper zone opacities aligned parallel to the chest wall. (b) CXR one week after commencing corticosteroid treatment shows a striking reduction in the extent of consolidation; the CXR requested at clinic follow-up, one month later, was normal. (c) pre-treatment CT through the upper zones shows 'band-like' peripheral and non-segmental areas of consolidation. There are also enlarged hilar lymph nodes.

Acute eosinophilic pneumonia

- A disorder of unknown aetiology, affecting young adults (♂ > ♀), leading to respiratory failure but with an excellent prognosis (with critical supportive care) and no relapse following recovery. Two-thirds of patients are smokers.
- The criteria for a diagnosis of acute eosinophilic pneumonia are: i) acute onset (typically developing over a few days and <1 month), ii) hypoxaemia (PaO_2<60mmHg or O_2 saturation <90% on room air), iii) lavage fluid with >25% eosinophils or eosinophilic pneumonia on lung biopsy, iv) bilateral consolidation on CXR infiltrates and v) absence of a known cause of pulmonary eosinophilia.

CXR findings (Fig. 6.63)

- Diffuse bilateral ground-glass opacification—± superimposed reticulation; no particular zonal predilection (specifically, abnormalities are *not* confined to the lung peripheries).
- Pleural effusion (uni- or bilateral)—common and seen at some time during the course in the majority of patients.

CT findings

- Diffuse bilateral ground-glass opacification ± consolidation.
- Smooth thickening of interlobular septa.
- Pleural effusions.
- Nodules.
- Less common findings: mediastinal/hilar lymph node enlargement, bronchiectasis.

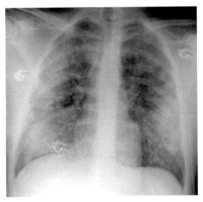

Fig. 6.63 Acute eosinophilic pneumonia. CXR in a patient presenting with rapidly progressive dyspnoea leading to respiratory failure. There are bilateral, symmetrical air space opacities.

Lung calcification

- Calcification occurs in abnormal (termed 'dystrophic' calcification) or otherwise normal lung (called 'metastatic' calcification), the latter usually occuring in conditions of abnormal calcium metabolism.
- The causes of pulmonary calcification are listed below (Table 6.20); the distribution of calcification may be focal and relatively localized (e.g. post-tuberculous) or diffuse (as in alveolar microlithiasis or metastatic pulmonary ossification).

Table 6.20 Causes of localized and diffuse lung calcification

- **Focal or relatively localized**
  - Tuberculous or other granuloma
  - Calcification in metastatic lung nodules—typically osteosarcoma
  - Bronchial carcinoid tumour
  - Sclerosing haemangioma
  - Hamartoma
- **Diffuse**
  - Alveolar microlithiasis
  - Metastatic pulmonary calcification
  - Diffuse pulmonary ossification—dendriform or nodular
  - Silicosis/silicoproteinosis
  - Post viral infection—chickenpox pneumonia, histoplasmosis

Miscellaneous causes of diffuse lung calcification

Alveolar microlithiasis

- A disorder characterized by the deposition of small stones ('calcipherites', composed of calcium phosphate) within alveoli.
- Rare diffuse lung disease which occurs worldwide but, for unknown reasons, higher prevalence in Japan and Turkey. ♂:♀ ≈ 1:1; typically presenting in 3rd to 5th decades. The aetiology is unclear but a genetic background is suspected: a mutation in a gene (SLC34A2) that codes for sodium-dependent phosphate transport has been identified; inheritance is probably autosomal recessive.
- The characteristic lesions of alveolar microlithiasis are alveolar concretions (measuring 250–750μm) with a concentric laminated ('onion skin') appearance. With chronic disease, fibrosis may ensue.
- Despite apparently extensive disease at presentation, around 50% of patients are asymptomatic.

Imaging in alveolar microlithiasis

CXR findings (Fig. 6.64)

- Bilateral high-density (calcific) micronodules—most pronounced in the mid and lower zones. With extensive disease, there is widespread infiltration (a 'snow storm' appearance) which obscures the cardiac and diaphragmatic outlines.
- Black sub-pleural line of spared lung.
- Thickening and beading of the fissures.
- Less common findings include: apical bullae/blebs, signs of fibrosis, septal (Kerley B) lines.

CT findings (Fig. 6.64)

- Bilateral calcified micronodules—most pronounced in the postero-basal lung. Where there are nodules in close proximity these may manifest as ground-glass opacification and/or consolidation.
- Calcific micronodular thickening of interlobular septa and bronchovascular bundles.
- Bullae and blebs—more readily demonstrated than on CXR. Bullae and blebs may be seen at the apices or sub-pleurally.
- Paraseptal emphysema.

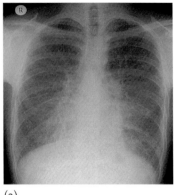

(a)

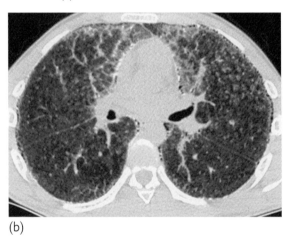

(b)

Fig. 6.64 CXR and HRCT in pulmonary alveolar microlithiasis. (a) There is diffuse micronodular infiltration predominantly in the mid and lower zones. The horizontal fissure is thickened and there are some basal septal lines (best appreciated on the left). (b) HRCT through the mid-zones showing multiple small dense pulmonary nodules. Dense nodular thickening of interlobular septa is present in the non-dependent lung and there are small sub-pleural cysts.

Metastatic pulmonary calcification

- Deposition of calcium in otherwise normal lung parenchyma.
- Most commonly associated with abnormal calcium metabolism or hypercalcaemic states (e.g. in chronic renal failure, following renal transplantation, primary hyperparathyroidism, multiple myeloma, metastatic bone disease, idiopathic hypercalcaemia).
- Most patients are asymptomatic but respiratory failure is a recognized complication.

CXR findings (Fig. 6.65)

- Normal—with limited disease, the CXR may show no abnormality.
- Nodules—multiple, poorly defined, measuring 3–10mm; calcification may or may not be visible. Variable distribution (upper zone, lower zone, or diffuse).

CT findings (Fig. 6.65)

- Nodules—multiple, poorly defined ('fluffy'); calcification seen in most.
- Ground-glass opacities.
- Consolidation.
- Calcification in the vessels of chest wall or heart.

Diffuse pulmonary ossification

- Metaplastic bone formation (ossification) in the interstitium or air spaces is a rare and usually incidental pathological and radiological finding: the two main types of ossification are dendriform and nodular.
- Dendriform ossification occurs principally in the interstitium and is usually seen on a background of interstitial fibrosis. Nodular ossification is found in the air spaces and occurs in conditions of venous congestion (classically mitral valve stenosis). In either case, the foci of calcification tend to be small (1–5mm in diameter).

CXR findings (Fig. 6.66)

- 'Normal'—signs of the underlying disorder (pulmonary fibrosis, mitral valve stenosis) may be present but because of the dimensions of calcified lesions in the lung, these may not be resolved on CXR.
- Focal calcific opacities—more prevalent in the lower zones. The branching pattern (characteristic of dendriform ossification) is not appreciated on CXR.

CT findings (Fig. 6.66)

- Branching or focal calcification—most pronounced in the lower zones and, in the case of the dendriform pattern, a subpleural distribution. CT signs of the underlying lung disease (e.g. a pattern of usual interstitial pneumonia or cardiac chamber enlargement) may be seen.

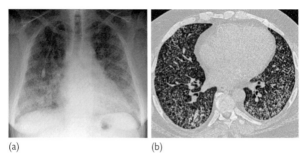

(a)   (b)

Fig. 6.65 CXR and HRCT of metastatic pulmonary calcification in a patient with end-stage renal failure requiring haemodialysis. (a) CXR shows multiple high-density (calcified) micronodules throughout both lungs. There is no particular zonal predilection. (b) HRCT also demonstrates multiple micronodules throughout the lungs.

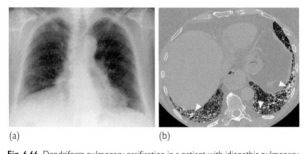

(a)   (b)

Fig. 6.66 Dendriform pulmonary ossification in a patient with idiopathic pulmonary fibrosis. (a) Calcification on CXR, best seen in the left lower zone. However, the branching morphology is difficult to discern. (b) CT demonstrates a reticulonodular pattern in the mid/lower zones bilaterally. There are subtle foci of higher density through the costophrenic recesses (photographed on modified window settings) showing branching calcific opacities within areas of established fibrosis.

Pulmonary amyloidosis

- A heterogeneous group of diseases (systemic or localized) caused by the extracellular deposition of insoluble plasma proteins.
- All amyloid proteins have strikingly similar morphology: there is a precursor protein (Table 6.21) coupled with a common plasma glycoprotein (serum amyloid P (SAP)). Amyloid proteins are uniquely stable because of the anti-parallel β-pleated sheet structure.
- Amyloidosis is categorised according to i) the type of amyloid protein and ii) the anatomical distribution of deposits. Amyloid may be localized to the respiratory tract and is then most commonly of AL type. The morphological types of respiratory system amyloid are: laryngeal, tracheobronchial, parenchymal (nodular or alveolar septal), and intrathoracic nodal.

Table 6.21 Examples of amyloid proteins and their associations

Amyloid type	Precursor protein (*origin/associations*)
AL	Immunoglobulin light chains (*multiple myeloma, macroglobulinaemia; AL is the commonest cause of clinically-significant lung disease*)
AA	Serum amyloid A (*any cause of chronic inflammation including respiratory causes (e.g. bronchiectasis, TB, cystic fibrosis)*)
Aß₂M	Amyloid β_2 microglobulin (*normal constituent of plasma which cannot be cleared during haemodialysis—occasionally causes systemic disease*)
ATTR	Plasma transthyretin (*associated with cardiac involvement*)

Imaging in pulmonary amyloidosis

In addition to conventional radiology, radiolabelled iodine[123]-serum amyloid protein (SAP) (which localize amyloid deposits) may be used.

Laryngeal and tracheobronchial amyloidosis

- Both forms of amyloid deposition are uncommon but potentially important because of the propensity to cause airway obstruction and related symptoms (i.e. stridor, dyspnoea, cough).
- Deposition of amyloid may be focal or diffuse; in the larynx, the supraglottic region is the most common site.

CXR findings
The CXR has limited utility for the diagnosis of major airway involvement by amyloid.

CT findings (Fig. 6.67)
- Nodules—focal or diffuse submucosal lesions ± calcification.
- Circumferential thickening/narrowing—may be associated with distal lung atelectasis or collapse depending on severity.

Nodular parenchymal amyloidosis
- The most common form of respiratory system amyloidosis, usually localized and of AL type.
- Amyloid deposits of varying size (ranging from a few millimetres to 10cm)

CXR findings
- Nodules—bilateral, peripheral and most prevalent in the mid/lower zones; calcification may be seen in nodules. Varying sizes and potential for slow growth over time. Occasionally there may be a solitary amyloid nodule.

CT findings (Fig. 6.68)
- Nodules—bilateral, subpleural, and in the mid/lower zones ± calcification (in 30–50%) and cavitation. The margins of nodules may be smooth or spiculated.
  NB In rare instances, amyloid nodules ± calcification coexist with a lymphoid interstitial pneumonia (usually on a background of Sjögren's syndrome). In these patients there is ground-glass opacification, thin-walled cysts and signs of obliterative bronchiolitis on HRCT.

Alveolar septal amyloidosis
- Less common than the nodular parenchymal form of amyloid; usually associated with systemic AL amyloidosis
- Characterized histopathologically by amyloid deposition in the interstitium and along small vessels.

CXR findings
- Reticular or reticulonodular pattern—most prevalent in the mid/lower zones
- Prominent septal lines

CT findings (Fig. 6.69)
- Reticular pattern/interlobular septal thickening.
- Micronodules—2–4mm in diameter. Always seen in association with evidence of interstitial amyloid infiltration.
- Less common findings: ground-glass opacification, traction bronchiectasis/bronchiolectasis, and honeycombing.

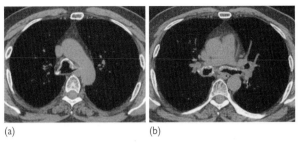

(a)   (b)

Fig. 6.67 Tracheobronchial amyloidosis in a 63-year-old male patient. CT demonstrates nodular and almost circumferential calcified thickening of (a) the trachea and (b) right and left main bronchi.

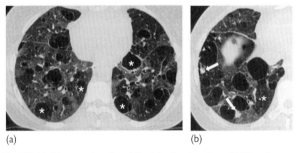

(a)   (b)

Fig. 6.68 Nodular parenchymal amyloidosis in a female patient with Sjögren's syndrome. (a) HRCT through the mid zones demonstrates multiple thin-walled cysts (asterisks) and diffuse ground-glass opacification. (b) Targeted HRCT through the right lung shows two irregular nodules (arrows), representing amyloid deposition adjacent to cysts. There is evidence of accompanying small airways disease with a region of decreased lung attenuation (asterisk) in which there is a reduction in the number and calibre of pulmonary vessels.

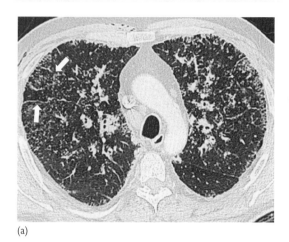

(a)

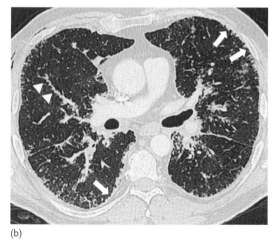

(b)

Fig. 6.69 Alveolar septal amyloidosis in a 50-year-old male patient who presented with a spontaneous right pneumothorax. (a) CT at the level of the aortic arch demonstrates septal thickening (arrows) and multiple small nodules. (b) CT below the carina shows innumerable micronodules which have a subpleural (arrows) and peribronchovascular (arrowheads) distribution.

Pulmonary alveolar proteinosis

- Pulmonary alveolar proteinosis is a diffuse lung disease characterized by alveolar and interstitial accumulation of a periodic acid-Schiff (PAS)-positive phospholipoprotein derived from surfactant.
- Rare with a prevalence of ~4 per million population. May be idiopathic (most common form), secondary (related to inhalation of variety of antigens (silica dust, aluminium), haematological malignancies or immunodeficiency (including HIV infection)) or congenital.
- The key problem is abnormal/altered surfactant production caused by a reduction in surfactant proteins or abnormal granulocyte-macrophage-colony stimulating factor. Analysis of bronchoalveolar lavage fluid may demonstrate PAS-positive granular acellular eosinophilic proteinaceous material and elevated levels of surfactant proteins A and D.

Imaging in pulmonary alveolar proteinosis

CXR findings (Fig. 6.70)

- Air space opacities—ground-glass opacification and/or consolidation ± air bronchograms. Bilateral and roughly symmetrical opacification with a perihilar predominance with relative sparing of the apices and lower zones. A random distribution is common.
- Reticular or reticulonodular pattern.
- Relevant negative findings: normal heart size, no pleural effusions (these features help to differentiate pulmonary alveolar proteinosis from pulmonary oedema).

CT findings (Fig. 6.71)

- 'Crazy-paving' pattern—geographical areas of ground-glass opacification within which there are thickened interlobular septa and intralobular lines. Bilateral and diffusely distributed, with no specific zonal predilection.
- In rare cases, significant interstitial fibrosis may develop.

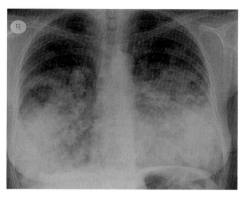

Fig. 6.70 CXR in a patient with alveolar proteinosis. There is bilateral air-space opacification with a predominantly basal distribution.

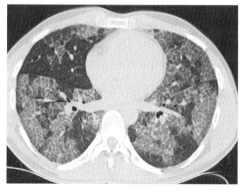

Fig. 6.71 Typical HRCT appearances in pulmonary alveolar proteinosis. There are patchy but well demarcated areas of ground-glass opacification with superimposed thickened interlobular septa—the crazy-paving pattern.

Erdheim–Chester disease

- A rare multisystem (non-Langerhans' cell) histiocytic disorder.
- Typically presenting in patients aged >40 years; ♂ : ♀ ≈1:1.
- Patients usually present with bone disease (symmetrical osteosclerosis of metaphyses of long bones); mediastinal infiltration is more common than lung disease.
- Mediastinal and pulmonary infiltration by CD68-positive histiocytes containing eosinophilic cytoplasm is the key histopathological finding. There is infiltration around major mediastinal structures, the visceral pleura, interlobular septa and bronchovascular bundles.

Imaging of Erdheim–Chester Disease

CXR findings

- Reticular/reticulonodular pattern—bilateral and involving all zones (may be in upper zones).
- Thickening of fissures.
- Interlobular septal thickening.
- Pleural/pericardial effusions.

CT findings (Figs. 6.72 and 6.73)

- Mediastinal infiltration—circumferential soft-tissue around the thoracic aorta, its major branches (including the coronary arteries), the intercostal arteries and the heart.
- Interlobular septal thickening—seen in the majority of patients. Symmetrical and smooth. Variable zonal distribution. Related to interstitial infiltration by histiocytes/macrophages ± mild fibrosis.
- Ground-glass opacification—present in the majority.
- Centrilobular nodules—diffuse or localized.
- Isolated thin-walled cysts—present in a minority of patients.
- Fissural thickening.
- Pleural/pericardial effusions or thickening.

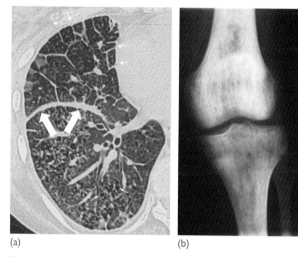

(a) (b)

Fig. 6.72 Erdheim–Chester disease in a 50-year-old female patient presenting with progressive dyspnoea and a restrictive lung function deficit. a) CT at the level of the right inferior pulmonary vein showing smooth thickening of interlobular septa (arrows) and the right oblique fissure (thick arrows). There are multiple scattered thin-walled lung cysts in the lower lobe (thin arrows). b) Radiograph of the left knee showing characteristic widespread sclerosis. Images courtesy of Professor J Remy and Professor M Remy-Jardin, Hospital Calmette, University Centre of Lille, France. Image 2a reproduced with kind permission from Springer Science+Business Media: *European Radiology*, Pulmonary involvement in Erdheim-Chester disease: high-resolution CT findings, **3**: 1993, 389–382, Remy-Jardin, M., Remy, J., Gosselin, B., Caparros, D., Wallaert, B., and Tonnel, A.-B.

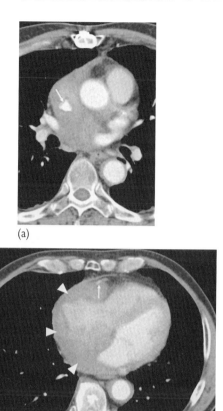

(a)

(b)

Fig. 6.73 Mediastinal disease on CT in a 66-year-old male patient with Erdheim–Chester disease. a) Targeted CT image shows extensive soft-tissue infiltration of the mediastinal structures; there is complete encasement of the superior vena cava (arrow). b) Image at a lower level showing infiltration around the heart (arrowheads). The right coronary artery (arrow) is displaced anteriorly from its normal position in the atrio-ventricular groove.

Vascular diseases

Acute pulmonary embolism

- Acute pulmonary embolism (PE) is an important compliction of venous thrombosis and is potentially life-threatening.
- The estimated incidence of acute PE is 60–70 cases/100,000; nearly half of cases are hospital in-patients or individuals in long-term care.
- Predisposing risk factors include any cause of decreased mobility (e.g. after major surgery, long-haul air-travel), late pregnancy/Caesarean section, malignancy, and a history of venous thromboembolism (VTE); the majority of PEs originate from lower limb deep venous thrombosis.
- The clinical features are highly variable and usually non-specific.
- Validated clinical probability scores (e.g. the Wells, Geneva, and Pisa scores) should be used to determine the clinical pre-test probability before requesting radiological tests.

Imaging of acute PE/VTE

The main imaging tests that are variably brought to bear in the investigation of patients with suspected acute PE are listed below. NB Invasive (catheter-based) angiography is almost never offered as a test by UK radiology departments. Interested readers are also referred to the recommendations of the British Thoracic Society (BTS Standards of Care Committee. Pulmonary embolism guideline development group. *Thorax* 2003; **58**:470–483) and the Fleischner Society (Remy-Jardin M. et al. Management of suspected aciate pulmonary embolism in the era of CT angiography: a statement of the Fleischner Society. Radiology 2007; **245**: 315–329).

- CXR
- CT pulmonary angiography
- Ventilation perfusion (V/Q) scintigraphy
- Lower limb/pelvic Doppler ultrasound
- Echocardiography
- Magnetic resonance angiography.

CXR findings (Figs. 7.1 and 7.2)

CXR is insensitive and non-specific and cannot accurately confirm or exclude the diagnosis. The main role of CXR is in the exclusion of alternative diagnoses (e.g. pneumonia or pneumothorax) which mimic the clinical features, or as a 'triage' tool (prior to V/Q scintigraphy) to exclude patients with significant cardiopulmonary disease in whom the likelihood of an intermediate probability result is high. The recognized (indirect) CXR signs of acute PE include:

- Oligaemia—beyond the occlusion (the Westermark sign).
- Vascular 'cut-off' sign and pulmonary artery enlargement proximal to the occlusion (the Fleischner sign).
- Elevated hemidiaphragm.
- Linear atelectasis.
- Consolidation—related to pulmonary haemorrhage; typically multifocal, peripheral and lower zone. The consolidation may have a rounded apex directed towards the hilum (called Hampton's hump). Cavitation is relatively rare and denotes infarction.
- Pleural effusion.

CT findings (Figs. 7.3–7.5)

CT pulmonary angiography (CTPA) is the recommended initial imaging modality in patients with suspected acute PE and the signs (direct and

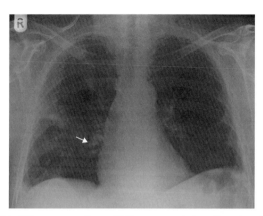

Fig. 7.1 CXR in a patient with acute PE. There is a vascular 'cut-off' sign (arrow) and a peripheral wedge-shaped density within the right midzone.

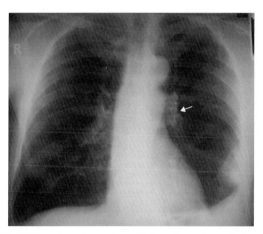

Fig. 7.2 CXR in another patient with acute PE. Note the prominent left pulmonary artery (arrow) and the peripheral density in the left lower zone (Hampton's hump). There is also a left pleural effusion.

indirect) are readily seen. CTPA has a sensitivity of 83–100% and a specificity of 89–97%. The added advantage is that other causes (with a similar clinical presentation) may be identified. The signs of accute PE or CTPA are:

- Filling defect within an opacified pulmonary artery—giving rise to a 'polo mint' appearance.
- Focal consolidation—typically peripheral (pleurally-based) triangular consolidation with haemorrhage, rarely cavitation.

- Pleural effusion(s).
- Variations in calibre of segmental and subsegmental pulmonary arteries.

Potential pitfalls in CT diagnosis of acute PE (Figs. 7.6 and 7.7)

Appearances on CTPA which may lead to false negative or positive diagnoses include:

- False negative diagnoses
  - Suboptimal contrast opacification—due to suboptimal technique or, less commonly, the presence of arterio-venous shunting.
  - Cardiac and respiratory motion artefacts.
  - Large pleural effusion, extensive consolidation, or interstitial fibrosis—may render the arterial branches poorly visualized.
- False positive diagnoses
  - Hilar lymph nodes—when closely related to arterial branches may lead to the impression of filling defects.
  - Mucus-filled airways—may create the impression of filling defects. However, analysis of the anatomical arrangement and differentiation of airways from vessels (on lung window settings) will help distinguish these.
  - Pulmonary veins—flow-related 'filling defects' are more commonly seen in veins and may be interpreted as emboli. Knowledge of the normal anatomical disposition of veins should prevent this error.

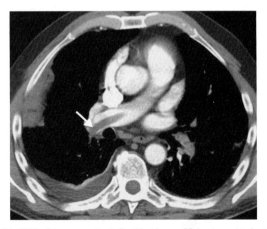

Fig. 7.3 CTPA of the same patient in Fig. 7.1 with acute PE showing an intraluminal filling defect (arrow) and lack of opacification of the left lower lobe arteries. There is also a small right pleural effusion and peripheral consolidation.

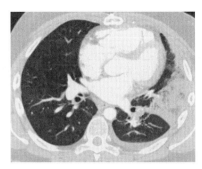

Fig. 7.4 CTPA shows peripheral consolidation, caused by haemorrhage, in a patient with an acute PE. There are filling defects in the left lower lobe pulmonary artery.

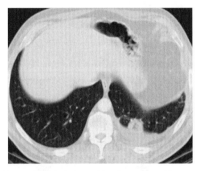

Fig. 7.5 CTPA image through the lower lobes in a patient with an acute PE. There is a small left pleural effusion and peripheral air-space opacity.

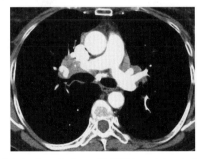

Fig. 7.6 Pitfalls in the diagnosis of acute PE. CTPA image below the level of the carina shows right hilar lymph node enlargement which might be mistaken for a filling defect in the right main pulmonary artery.

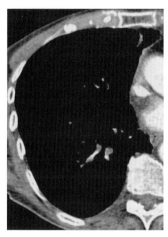

Fig. 7.7 Targeted CTPA image in a patient with bronchiectasis in the right lower lobe. On the mediastinal window settings the appearances were initially mistaken for filling defects in the segmental arterial branches; review of the images on lung window settings confirmed that this was due to dilated mucus-filled airways.

Ventilation-perfusion (V/Q) scintigraphy (Fig. 7.8)

An advantage of V/Q scanning is the relative widespread availability in most hospitals. In the appropriate clinical setting, a normal or high probability V/Q scan result effectively excludes or confirms (respectively) the diagnosis of acute PE. The disadvantages include the lack of an 'out-of-hours' facility and the high rate of 'indeterminate' probability results. A V/Q mismatch (i.e. patchy defects in perfusion without a corresponding abnormality of ventilation) is the cardinal finding in acute PE. The appearances on V/Q scans are categorized as normal, near-normal, low, intermediate, or high probability of PE.

MRI

Specific imaging sequences may be used in the diagnosis of acute PE; clinically acceptable sensitivities and specificities for MR pulmonary angiography have been reported. However, the lack of widespread availability of dedicated MR hardware and software is a limitation. Other problems with MR include, the lower spatial resolution of MR angiography (compared to CTPA), the longer acquisition times, poor demonstration of the lung parenchyma and the problems of monitoring potentially unstable patients in the MR scanner.

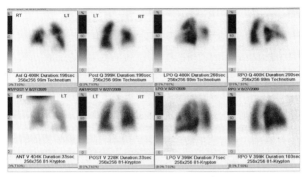

Fig. 7.8 A high probability V/Q scan showing multiple photopenic areas on the perfusion images (top row) not matched by any abnormality on the ventilation scans (bottom row).

Imaging of suspected PE in pregnancy

Pregnancy is a risk factor for PE; the incidence of venous thromboembolism is 5–12/10,000 during pregnancy and 37/10000 post-partum. There are no established guidelines for investigation of PE in pregnancy. One approach would be to use Doppler ultrasound in patients with signs suggestive of lower limb deep venous thrombosis. If this is positive, no further imaging is required. In the absence of such signs, the choice is between CTPA and V/Q scintigraphy. The latter might be preferred first because a normal or near normal V/Q rules out the diagnosis of PE and has the advantage of a lower maternal radiation dose. CTPA might then be reserved for patients with an intermediate probability V/Q or those with a high probability study but in whom the clinical pre-test probability was low.

Chronic thromboembolic disease

- Chronic thromboembolic disease is a rare disorder that results from incomplete resolution of thrombi and vascular remodelling; pulmonary hypertension may result if there is occlusion of a significant proportion of the pulmonary arterial tree.
- A source of recurrent emboli is only occasionally demonstrable.
- Underlying pathophysiological mechanism is poorly understood: however, mechanical obstruction and vasoconstriction are believed to play a role. Thrombotic occlusion of the microvasculature may also contribute to pulmonary hypertension.
- On histopathological examination, both elastic and muscular pulmonary arteries show organized thrombus; plexiform lesions are absent (in contrast to primary pulmonary arterial hypertension).

Imaging in chronic thromboembolic disease

CTPA is the most commonly requested radiological investigation and other tests are often used in a 'supporting' role. The imaging findings in chronic thromboembolic disease are detailed and illustrated below.

CXR findings (Fig. 7.9)
- Rarely normal.
- Central/proximal pulmonary arteries enlarged with peripheral oligaemia.
- Cardiomegaly—due to right ventricular dilatation.
- Parenchymal or pleural scars.

Conventional (invasive) pulmonary angiography (Fig. 7.10)
- Filling defects—due to thrombi in lobar and segmental arteries in conjunction with proximal arterial occlusions. Thrombus may be laminated along arterial walls; 'web-like' defects are rarely identifiable.
- Dilatation of central pulmonary arteries with distal tapering ('pruning').
- Out-pouching of arteries—due to complete or partial occlusion.

CT findings (Figs. 7.11–7.13)

The differentiation between acute and chronic thrombus is not always straightforward. The recognized CT angiographic findings in chronic thromboembolic disease include:

- Filling defects in pulmonary arteries—may be laminated/crescentic and adherent to vessel walls or web-like.
- Right heart 'strain'—right ventricular dilatation ± convex bulging of the interventricular septum; an increase in the right ventricle to left ventricular diameter ratio. Reflux of contrast into the inferior vena cava/hepatic veins.
- Central/proximal pulmonary arterial dilatation—'out-pouchings' and aneurysmal dilatation is uncommon.
- Hypertrophied bronchial arteries—the bronchial arteries arise from the descending thoracic aortic and are variable in number. Normal bronchial arteries are generally not identifiable.
- Pulmonary artery strictures and irregularities—there may be regional alterations in calibre of distal pulmonary arteries.
- Mosaic attenuation pattern—there is a reduction in the number and/or calibre of pulmonary vessels in the regions of decreased attenuation.
- Basal peripheral linear opacities—representing areas of previous pulmonary infarction.
- Segmental/subsegmental bronchial dilatation (± occasional air-trapping)—may be due to the phenomenon of 'hypoxic bronchodilatation'.
- Lymph node enlargement—a reported finding (possibly due to vascular transformation of lymph node sinuses).
- Pleural effusion(s).

Ventilation-perfusion (V/Q) scintigraphy findings

- Multiple mismatched ventilation and perfusion defects—may be indistinguishable from a high probability study due to acute PE.

MRI findings

The pulmonary vascular and cardiac abnormalities seen at MR are broadly analogous to those seen at CT. However, MR has the additional benefit of providing data about right heart function.

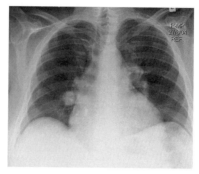

Fig. 7.9 CXR in a patient with chronic thromboembolic disease: there is enlargement of the central pulmonary arteries and cardiomegaly.

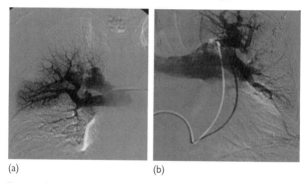

(a)   (b)

Fig. 7.10 Conventional digital subtraction pulmonary angiogram of (a) the right and (b) left lungs showing strictures and marked distal tapering of vessels.

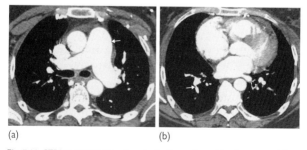

(a)   (b)

Fig. 7.11 CTPA in chronic thromboembolic disease shows (a) enlargement of the main pulmonary artery (arrow) by comparison with the transverse diameter of the ascending aorta and (b) arterial stricturing (arrow).

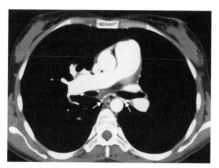

Fig. 7.12 CTPA in a patient with chronic thromboembolic disease showing hypertrophied bronchial arteries (arrows). Bronchial arteries are usually too small to visualize on CT in healthy individuals.

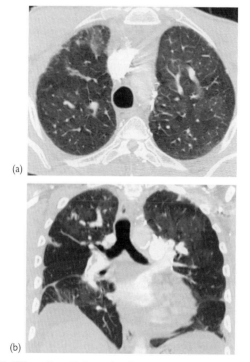

(a)

(b)

Fig. 7.13 CT in a patient with chronic thromboembolic disease showing (a) a mosaic attenuation pattern and b) coronal reconstructions demonstrating peripheral foci of scarring (presumed to be a consequence of previous infarction).

Tumour embolism

- A very rare cause of pulmonary hypertension.
- Common tumours associated with tumour embolization include: renal cell carcinoma, breast, hepatoma, adenocarcinoma, gastric carcinoma, prostatic malignancy and choriocarcinoma.
- Tumour emboli are malignant microdeposits that lodge in pulmonary arteries. Rarely, tumour emboli in the pulmonary arteries elicit a florid fibrocellular proliferation and subsequent thrombosis/luminal occlusion—termed thrombotic microangiopathy.

Imaging of tumour embolism

CXR findings

- A diagnosis of tumour embolization is rarely, if ever, made on CXR, which typically shows no abnormality.
- Peripheral consolidation—may be present and represent areas of pulmonary infarction.

CT findings (Fig. 7.14)

- Pulmonary arterial irregularity and dilatation—due to expansion by tumour emboli.
- Multifocal consolidation—representing areas of infarction.
- 'Vascular' tree-in-bud pattern—a widespread increased conspicuity of small distal pulmonary arteries due to fibrocellular proliferation, arterial thrombosis, and occlusion.

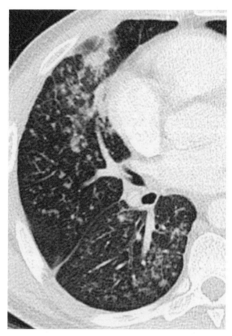

Fig. 7.14 CT in a patient with metastatic adenocarcinoma and thrombotic microangiopathy. There are multiple tiny nodules, some of which are branching, resembling a tree-in-bud pattern but caused by tumour emboli within the vessel eliciting a fibroproliferative response.

Pulmonary hypertension

- A condition in which mean pulmonary artery pressure (PAP) is increased to ≥25mmHg, as measured by right heart catheterization (NB normal mean PAP at rest = 14±3 mmHg).
- Pulmonary hypertension can be classified according to the principal anatomical site of abnormality in the pulmonary circulation (i.e. pre-capillary or post-capillary) and recognizable clinical 'groupings' (Table 7.1).

Table 7.1 Causes/classification of pulmonary hypertension

Pre-capillary	Post-capillary
1. Pulmonary arterial hypertension	**2. Left heart diseases**
Idiopathic	Systolic dysfunction
Heritable (genetic)	Diastolic dysfunction
Drug/toxin-induced	Valvular disease
Other disorders:	
Congenital heart disease	
Connective tissue diseases	
Portal hypertension	
HIV infection	
1' Veno-occlusive disease/capillary haemangiomatosis	
3. Lung diseases/hypoxaemia	
Chronic obstructive pulmonary disease	
Interstitial lung diseases	
Chronic exposure to high altitude	
4. Chronic thromboembolism	
5. Unclear or multifactorial mechanisms	
Myeloproliferative disorders	
Langerhans' cell histiocytosis	
Lymphangioleiomyomatosis	
Fibrosing mediastinitis	

Adapted from The ESC/ERS guidelines: guidelines for the diagnosis and treatment of pulmonary hypertension *Eur Heart J*, 2009; **30**:2493–2537; and Simonneau G et al. Updated clinical classification of pulmonary hypertension *J Am Coll Cardiol* 2009; **54**:S43–S54.

Imaging in pulmonary hypertension

The CXR and CT (HRCT and/or CTPA) are the mainstays of radiological investigation. Additional imaging tests—ventilation/perfusion (V/Q) scanning, echocardiography, ultrasound, magnetic resonance imaging—may be required for further evaluation of pulmonary hypertension or as a means of identifying specific underlying causes (e.g. V/Q scanning in suspected chronic thromboembolism, HRCT for the diagnosis of diffuse parenchymal lung disease or abdominal ultrasound in chronic liver disease).

CXR findings (Fig. 7.15)

The likelihood that abnormalities will be seen on CXR increases with the severity of pulmonary hypertension. The CXR signs of pulmonary hypertension include:

- Dilatation of central pulmonary arteries.
- Attenuation ('pruning') of peripheral arterial branches.
- Pulmonary artery calcification—in patients with intracardiac shunts and generally associated with prolonged and marked pulmonary hypertension.
- Cardiomegaly—because of enlargement of right-sided cardiac chambers.

CT findings

The CT features believed to indicate pulmonary hypertension can be divided into those which directly indicate elevated pulmonary artery pressure and the signs which indirectly suggest the diagnosis.

Direct (vascular) CT signs (Figs. 7.15 and 7.16)

- Increased main pulmonary artery (PA) diameter—there is a broad correlation between mean PAP and main PA diameter but the correlation is generally stronger with more severe pulmonary hypertension. Absolute measurements of what constitutes a 'normal' upper limit of main PA diameter (ranging from >25 to >36 mm) are quoted. However, increased PA diameter may be seen in patients with normal PA pressure and the size of the PA may be dependent on other factors including patient size and the presence of underlying lung disease (e.g. pulmonary fibrosis).
- Increased ratio of the diameters of the main PA to the ascending aorta (AAo)—a PA/AAo ratio >1 is highly specific for PHTx. The PA/AAo ratio is also a stronger predictor of mean PAP in patients with pulmonary fibrosis.
- The 'egg and banana' sign—the main PA is usually not visible on axial images at the level of the aortic arch. However, as the main PA enlarges, it may be seen at the same level as the arch.
- Enlargement of segmental pulmonary arteries—dilatation of segmental PA branches (as compared to the (outer) diameter of the accompanying segmental bronchus).
- Small peripheral serpiginous arterioles—originating from centrilobular arterioles and believed to reflect neovascularity.

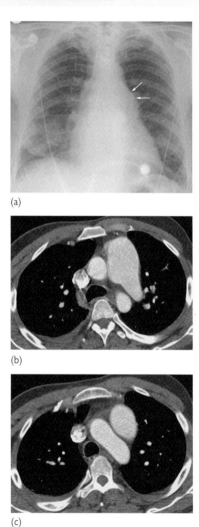

(a)

(b)

(c)

Fig. 7.15 CT signs of pulmonary hypertension on CXR and CT. (a) CXR shows enlargement of the central pulmonary artery; the aortopulmonary window is filled-in (arrows) (b) CT showing enlargement of the main pulmonary trunk. There is a clear increase in the ratio (i.e. >1) of the transverse diameters of the pulmonary trunk to the ascending aorta (c) the 'egg and banana' sign due to enlargement of the pulmonary trunk (the 'egg') so that it is seen at the same anatomical level as the aortic arch (the 'banana').

Indirect or ancillary CT signs

- Bronchial artery hypertrophy—tortuous vessels (measuring >1.5mm in diameter) arising variably from the proximal descending thoracic aorta. This sign is more commonly encountered in pulmonary hypertension related to chronic thromboembolic disease.
- Contrast reflux into the inferior vena cava and hepatic veins—a reflection of tricuspid valve regurgitation.
- The 'bikini bottom' sign—fluid in the anterior pericardial recess. The pathophysiological mechanism for pericardial fluid accumulation is not fully understood.
- Mosaic attenuation pattern ('mosaic oligaemia')—patchy areas of decreased attenuation ('black' lung) admixed with regions of normal or increased attenuation ('grey' lung). Vessels in black lung are reduced in number/calibre. Typically associated with chronic thromboembolic disease.
- 'Soft' centrilobular nodules—the cause of these nodules is not entirely clear. Such nodules (together with thickened interlobular septa) are a feature of pulmonary hypertension caused by veno-occlusive disease and pulmonary capillary haemangiomatosis.
- Pleurally-based areas of consolidation—indicating pulmonary infarction.

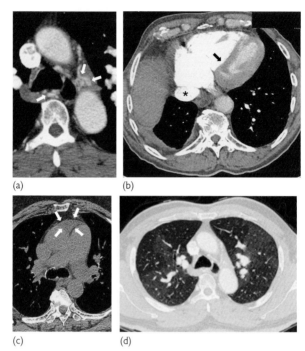

(a)   (b)

(c)   (d)

Fig. 7.16 Indirect CT signs of pulmonary hypertension. (a) Targeted CT shows multiple dilated, serpiginous bronchial arteries (arrows) in a patient with chronic thromboembolic pulmonary hypertension. (b) Contrast reflux into the inferior vena cava (asterisk). There is also bowing of the interventricular septum towards the left ventricle (arrow) because of elevated right heart pressure. (c) The 'bikini bottom' sign: there is a roughly triangular opacity (arrows) due to fluid in the anterior pericardial recess. (d) Mosaic oligaemia. There is heterogeneity of lung parenchymal attenuation; in regions of lower density (i.e. black) lung, the number/calibre of pulmonary vessels is significantly reduced. Note also the dilatation of the proximal subsegmental pulmonary arteries.

Specific causes of pulmonary hypertension

In the following sections, the imaging findings of two exceedingly rare causes of pulmonary hypertension (i.e. pulmonary veno-occlusive disease (PVOD) and pulmonary capillary haemangiomatosis (PCH)) are reviewed. The differentiation from other causes of pulmonary hypertension is important since vasodilator therapy may cause catastrophic pulmonary oedema in those with PVOD and PCH.

Pulmonary veno-occlusive disease (PVOD)

- Rare vascular disease caused by widespread fibrous intimal thickening and occlusion of venules and small pulmonary veins.
- Reported at all ages from neonatal to the 7th decade; ♂:♀ ≈ 1:1.
- The prognosis is poor.

CXR findings (Fig. 7.17)

- Dilatation of the main pulmonary artery.
- Thickened interlobular septa—caused by the thickening of interlobular septa by oedema.
- Normal heart size—specifically, the left atrial and left ventricular contours appear normal.
- Pleural effusions.
- Bilateral air space opacification—caused by intra-alveolar oedema or haemorrhage.

CT findings (Fig. 7.17)

(see also 📖 CT findings of Vascular diseases/Pulmonary hypertension, p299)

- Dilatation of the main and central pulmonary arteries.
- Thickened interlobular septa and fissures.
- Ground-glass opacification—diffuse or central/peribronchovascular.
- Enlarged right atrium/ventricle but normal-sized left cardiac chambers.
- Mosaic attenuation pattern.
- Small poorly circumscribed nodules—related to patchy bronchiolocentric alveolar septal thickening.
- Pleural effusions.

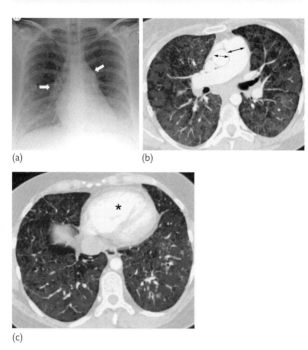

(a)

(b)

(c)

Fig. 7.17 CXR and CT appearances in pulmonary veno-occlusive disease in a 39-year-old female patient with dyspnoea and haemoptysis. (a) CXR shows enlargement of central pulmonary arteries (arrows). (b) CT through the mid zones shows widespread ground-glass opacification in both lungs. There is dilatation of the main pulmonary artery (solid arrow) by comparison with the transverse diameter of the ascending aorta (dashed arrow). (c) CT through the lower zones showing ground-glass opacities and smooth thickening of interlobular septa; there is enlargement of the right-sided cardiac chambers (asterisk).

Pulmonary capillary haemangiomatosis (PCH)

- Rare disorder related to the abnormal proliferation of capillaries in the alveolar and interlobular septa, peribronchovascular interstitium and in the pleura.
- Can present at any age; ♂ : ♀ ≈ 1:1.

CXR findings

- Dilatation of the main pulmonary artery.
- Widespread nodular or reticulonodular pattern.

CT findings (Fig. 7.18)

- Dilatation of the main and central pulmonary arteries.
- Ill-defined centrilobular nodules.
- Less common features: thickening of interlobular septa (less frequent than in PVOD), pleural and pericardial effusions.

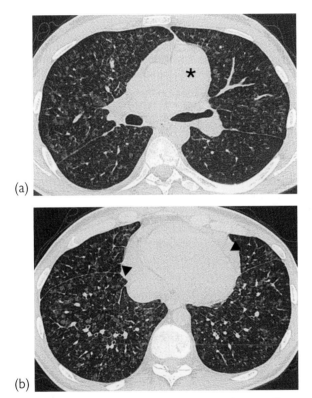

Fig. 7.18 CT in 35-year-old male patient with biopsy-proven pulmonary capillary haemangiomatosis. (a) Image just below the level of the carina demonstrates multiple 'soft' centrilobular nodules. There is marked enlargement of the main pulmonary artery (asterisk; by comparison to the transverse diameter of the ascending aorta) (b) Image through the lower zones showing extensive centrilobular nodules and some thickening of interlobular septa. There is a moderate sized pericardial effusion (arrowheads).

Congenital abnormalities

Congenital lung anomalies

Congenital lung anomalies may be encountered as incidental findings on imaging tests. Their clinical presentation and severity varies widely. Prenatal ultrasound testing may detect lung anomalies but a precise diagnosis is often only made in the post-natal period. In recent years, there has been increasing enthusiasm for the use of fetal MRI (including volumetric assessment and lung spectroscopy) to identify abnormal fetal lung growth.

The CXR is usually the initial imaging test in the immediate post-natal period. CT and CT-angiography may be requested to confirm/support a diagnosis, provide further characterization, or for pre-operative evaluation.

Congenital lung anomalies

- **Congenital cystic pulmonary lesions**
  - Congenital pulmonary adenomatoid malformation
  - Bronchopulmonary sequestration
  - Bronchial atresia
  - Bronchogenic cysts
- **Congenital lobar emphysema**
- **Pulmonary underdevelopment disorders**
  - Pulmonary agenesis
  - Pulmonary hypoplasia
  - Hypogenetic lung (scimitar) syndrome

Congenital cystic pulmonary lesions

Congenital cystic lesions of the lung comprise congenital pulmonary adenomatoid malformations, bronchopulmonary sequestrations, bronchial
atresia, and bronchogenic cysts; the latter are usually mediastinal in location and discussed elsewhere. This group of anomalies are a result of some
disruption in lung/airway embryogenesis. The typical imaging features are
described below but overlap exists and 'hybrid' lesions exhibiting the anatomic and histologic features of different anomalies are well described.

Congenital pulmonary adenomatoid malformation (CPAM)

- CPAMs (previously called congenital cystic adenomatoid malformations)
  encompass a wide array of hamartomatous anomalies thought to
  result from abnormal branching of immature bronchioles during lung
  morphogenesis.
- The quoted incidence is 1:25,000—1:35,000 live births. Lesions occur
  with equal frequency in the right and left lungs (unilobar > multilobar
  disease; lower > upper lobes).
- CPAMs communicate with the tracheobronchial tree and derive their
  arterial blood supply and venous drainage from normal pulmonary
  circulation. Hybrid lesions have pulmonary and systemic arterial supply.
  Presentation is usually during the newborn period or infancy with
  symptoms of respiratory distress or recurrent infections.
- Three principal subtypes of CPAM (Types I–III) have been previously
  recognized; two additional subtypes (Types 0 and IV) have recently
  been added.

Recognized subtypes of CPAM

Type 0 (1–3% of total)—Solid tissue with bronchial-type airways, containing cartilage, smooth muscle, and glands, separated by abundant
mesenchymal tissue. This subtype is considered incompatible with life.

Type I (60%)—Comprising single or multiple cysts (3–10cm diameter)
surrounded by smaller cysts and compressed normal lung parenchyma.

Type II (10%)—Consisting of numerous smaller cysts (0.5–2.0cm).

Type III (5%)—Solid-appearing lesion due to the presence of microscopic cysts (<2mm in diameter). The mass effect of Type III lesions may
cause mediastinal shift in utero and lung hypoplasia.

Type IV (15%)—Comprised of large thin-walled cysts lined by flattened
epithelium; this subtype may demonstrate histopathological overlap
with pleuropulmonary blastoma.

Imaging of CPAM
CXR findings (Figs. 8.1 and 8.2)

- Unilateral mass—solid or containing air-filled cystic spaces. Air fluid
  levels may be present; Type I and II lesions may initially appear solid
  (i.e. in the time before the fetal lung fluid has drained).
- Mass effect—e.g. mediastinal displacement, compression of adjacent
  lung, flattening of the ipsilateral diaphragm.

CT findings (Figs. 8.1 and 8.2)

- Unilateral mass—as with CXR, Type I and II lesions manifest as a mixture of solid and cystic elements with or without air/air-fluid levels. NB The appearance of Type II and Type III CPAM may be difficult to distinguish from bronchopulmonary sequestration.

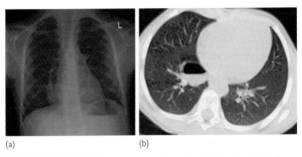

(a)　　　　　　　　　　　(b)

Fig. 8.1 CPAM I. (a) CXR demonstrates an abnormal well-defined opacity in the right lower lobe. (b) CT confirms the presence of a cyst with an air-fluid level.

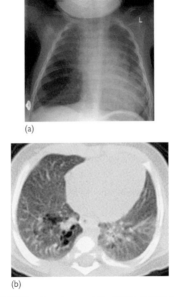

(a)

(b)

Fig. 8.2 CPAM II. (a) Discrete cysts are not identifiable on CXR but there is an area of increased lucency within the right lower zone. (b) CT demonstrates multiple small cysts.

Bronchopulmonary sequestration
- The sequestration 'spectrum' has been used to describe malformations (congenital or acquired) characterized by an abnormal non-functioning and dysplastic pulmonary tissue without the normal bronchial connections and a systemic arterial supply.
- Two subtypes: extralobar (accounting for 25% of bronchopulmonary sequestrations; ♂ > ♀, 4:1 and typically diagnosed in childhood) and intralobar (accounting for 75%, ♂ ≈ ♀ and diagnosed later in life).
- Extralobar sequestrations have a separate visceral pleural covering; intralobar sequestrations are covered by the normal visceral pleura of the affected lung.
- Extralobar sequestrations are associated with other congenital abnormalities (e.g. congenital diaphragmatic hernia).
- Intralobar sequestrations drain into the pulmonary venous circulation whereas extralobar sequestrations have systemic venous drainage.
- Both types are more common in the left lung.

Imaging of bronchopulmonary sequestration
CXR findings (Fig. 8.3)
- Solid, focal lung opacity or mass—located in the lower lobes.
- Air-fluid levels—air may enter through a bronchial connection or, in the case of intralobar sequestration, by collateral ventilation.

CT findings (Fig. 8.3)
- Mass—soft-tissue density ± cysts, ± air-fluid levels.
- Hyperlucent lung.
- Anomalous systemic arterial supply—CT angiography with 3D-reconstruction is helpful for detecting anomalous arterial vessels from the lower thoracic or upper abdominal aorta and for evaluating anomalous veins
- Bronchiectasis—caused by recurrent infections.

Congenital bronchial atresia
- Congenital bronchial atresia refers to the atresia or obstruction of a segmental or subsegmental bronchus but with normal development of the distal airway.
- There are two proposed pathogenetic mechanisms: i) a loss of 'connection' at the tip of the bronchial bud but normal growth distal to the disconnection and ii) localized intrauterine interruption of the bronchial arterial supply again leading to bronchial disconnection.
- The majority of patients are asymptomatic; recurrent infections (related to mucus in the distal patent bronchus) rarely occur.

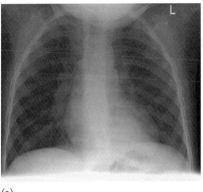

(a)

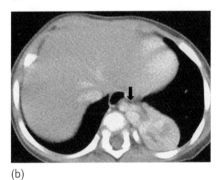

(b)

Fig. 8.3 Bronchopulmonary sequestration (a) Abnormal mass-like opacity is seen on the CXR projected behind the left heart simulating left lower lobe collapse. (b) On CT, there is a mass within the left lower lobe which has areas of fluid attenuation. The systemic arterial supply (solid arrow) arises from the aorta.

Imaging of bronchial atresia
CXR and CT findings (Fig. 8.4)

- Central mass-like opacity—usually with a tubular configuration.
- An air-fluid level—representing the obstructed, dilated, and mucus-filled airway may be seen on CXR or CT.
- Localized hyperinflation—due to collateral air drift and a relative paucity of vessels in the involved segment. This sign is unlikely to be seen on CXR.

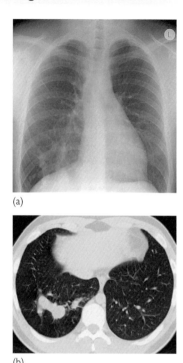

(a)

(b)

Fig. 8.4 Bronchial atresia (a) Branching, tubular opacities are present within the right lower lobe. (b) On CT, these structures are mucus-filled bronchocoeles reflecting mucus accumulation within the patent bronchus distal to the atretic segment. The distal lung is of low attenuation.

Congenital lobar emphysema

- Congenital lobar emphysema (CLE) is also known as congenital lobar overinflation (CLO) and is characterized by over-distension of histologically normal alveolar parenchyma thought to be due to central obstruction.
- Majority of patients present in the neonatal period. ♂ > ♀; symptoms vary in severity and include dyspnoea, cyanosis, wheezing, chest infection, and acute respiratory distress.
- No known cause in 50% but may be associated with congenital cartilage defect or any cause of bronchial obstruction. Recognized association with congenital heart disease.
- Left upper lobe is the most common site followed by the right upper and middle lobes.
- Can resolve spontaneously.

Imaging of congenital lobar emphysema
CXR findings (Fig. 8.5)

- Hyperlucent lung—most commonly in left upper lobe. In the immediate post-natal period, there may be a focal opacity due to retention of fetal lung fluid. There may be 'mass effect' with compression of adjacent lung. The affected lobe may cross the midline.
- Reduced vascularity.
- Widening of rib spaces.
- Flattening of the hemidiaphragm.

CT findings

- Hyperinflated lobe—multilobar involvement may be seen.
- Attenuated/displaced pulmonary vessels—CT is useful for diagnosis of multilobar involvement (rare) and for determining the extent of mass effect on the ipsilateral lung and mediastinal structures.

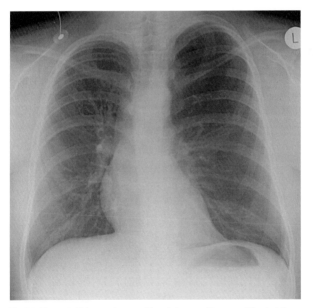

Fig. 8.5 Congenital lobar emphysema. There is increased lucency within the left upper zone in association with hyperinflation and mediastinal shift to the right.

Lung agenesis and hypoplasia (pulmonary underdevelopment)

Pulmonary underdevelopment may affect a single lobe or an entire lung, and may be categorized into three broad groups:

- Pulmonary agenesis—in which the bronchi and lung tissue are absent.
- Pulmonary aplasia—in which a rudimentary bronchus is present but this is limited to a blind-ending pouch and there is no associated lung tissue.
- Pulmonary hypoplasia—in which there is a variable reduction of lung tissue.

Pulmonary agenesis/aplasia

- A very rare congenital malformation in which there is complete absence of a lung or a lobe (including its bronchi and vascular supply).
- Agenesis of a lung or lobe is associated with other congenital (tracheobronchial, tracheo-oesophageal) anomalies.
- Agenesis of a lung is more common on the left, whereas lobar agenesis tends to occur more commonly on the right.
- Unilateral pulmonary agenesis is compatible with life and patients may be asymptomatic; NB increased mortality rate may be due to associated congenital anomalies (e.g. congenital heart disease, tracheo-oesophageal atresia and spinal or renal anomalies).

Imaging of pulmonary agenesis/aplasia
CXR findings
- CXR demonstrates an opacified hemithorax associated with marked mediastinal shift to that side.
- The contralateral lung is normal but demonstrates compensatory hyperinflation.
- Bony structures of the affected side can be hypoplastic.

CT findings
- Absence of pulmonary vessels on the affected side.

Pulmonary hypoplasia

- Pulmonary hypoplasia is defined as deficient or incomplete development of the lungs. The small lungs may be normal or abnormal in form but the alveoli are reduced in number and size.
- Small lungs may be an isolated finding with no underlying cause but are more usually associated with a variety of other malformations which directly or indirectly compromise the thoracic space available for lung growth (e.g. diaphragmatic defects, renal anomalies, extralobar pulmonary parenchymal malformations, and severe neuromuscular or musculoskeletal disorders).

Imaging
CXR findings (Fig. 8.6)
- Decreased aeration or homogeneous density of the affected hemithorax (more frequent in the right lung) and a small thoracic cage.
- Displacement of the mediastinum—to the side of the hypoplasia, accentuated during inspiration because of increased compensatory ventilation of the contralateral lung.

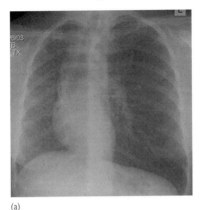

(a)

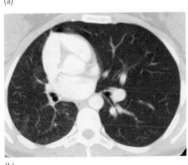

(b)

Fig. 8.6 Pulmonary hypoplasia. (a) Small right hemithorax with mediastinal shift to the right side of the hypoplasia. (b) There is a difference in attenuation of the lung parenchyma with the left (normal) side being of lower attenuation as a result of compensatory expansion.

Hypogenetic lung (scimitar) syndrome

- The scimitar (or 'venolobar') syndrome is a congenital cardiovascular anomaly involving the right lung (very rarely the left lung).
- In its complete form, the syndrome has the following features:
  - Anomalous pulmonary venous drainage—blood from the lungs returns to the right side of the heart; the anomalous pulmonary vein usually drains into the inferior vena cava, above or below the diaphragm. Occasionally, the anomalous veins may be multiple and drain into the right atrium, coronary sinus, or hepatic veins.
  - Hypoplasia of the right lung.
  - Dextroposition of the heart.
  - Hypoplasia of the right pulmonary artery.
  - A systemic arterial supply to the right lung from the subdiaphragmatic aorta or its main branches.
- The clinical significance and prognosis depend on the severity of the resulting left-to-right shunt; at least 40% of patients are asymptomatic. Clinical symptoms usually manifest in the 2nd to 3rd decade with fatigue and dyspnoea. Anomalous pulmonary venous connections are often narrow, and this may cause relatively mild pulmonary hypertension.

Imaging of the hypogenetic lung (scimitar) syndrome

CXR findings (Fig. 8.7)
- Abnormal band shadow—representing the abnormal pulmonary vein descending adjacent to the right cardiac border (likened to a 'scimitar')
- Small right hilum—related to pulmonary artery hypoplasia
- Cardiac dextroposition

CT and MR findings
- CT demonstrates reduction in size of the right hemithorax and pulmonary artery, bronchial anomalies, and the anomalous vein.
- MR angiography offers excellent visualization of the abnormal pulmonary vascular anatomy.

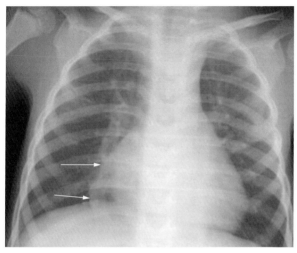

Fig. 8.7 Scimitar syndrome. CXR shows an abnormal tubular opacity (arrows) adjacent to the right heart border and extending inferiorly below the diaphragm. The opacity represents the anomalous pulmonary vein.

Lung tumours

Benign pulmonary lesions

Tuberculoma

- A focus of tuberculous infection demonstrating features of both repair and activity.

Imaging of tuberculomas

The CXR and CT features of tuberculomas are considered together below (Figs. 9.1 and 9.2). NB Tuberculomas are often [18]FDG-avid on PET imaging, as are all granulomatous lesions resulting in potential confusion with malignancy.

CXR/CT findings

- Nodule—often well-defined but may appear irregular or spiculated (because of adjacent fibrosis).
- Calcification—common (often apparent on CXR but readily seen at CT); calcification may be central, amorphous, laminar, or punctuate.
- 'Ring' enhancement or curvilinear central enhancement—following IV contrast injection on CT.
- Cavitation—rare; the presence of cavitation should suggest TB reactivation.

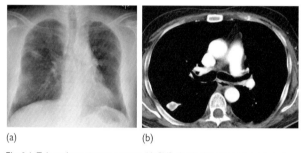

(a)   (b)

Fig. 9.1 Tuberculomas in two patients. (a) CXR clearly showing a tuberculoma in the right mid zone. (b) CT showing peripheral ring enhancement in a tuberculoma following injection of IV contrast; the central non-enhancing area is believed to correspond to caseous necrosis. The lesion remained unchanged over a two-year period.

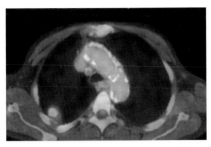

Fig. 9.2 Fused PET-CT image showing increased uptake in a pathologically-confirmed tuberculoma; the standardized uptake value (SUV) was 3.8 and this was considered malignant on initial assessment.

Hamartoma

- Hamartomas are benign lung tumours made up of an abnormal mixture of the *normal* components of lung (e.g. bronchial epithelium, cartilage and fat).
- Hamartomas are usually solitary but may be multiple. Multiple hamartomas occur in Carney's triad (comprising multiple pulmonary hamartomas, gastric leiomyoblastomas and functioning extra-adrenal paraganglionomas (phaeochromocytomas)).
- On histopathological examination, there is cartilage proliferation with clefts lined by fibromyxoid stroma and bronchial epithelium. Fat or fluid are also recognized components. Hamartomas are rarely endobronchial.

Imaging of hamartomas

Hamartomas are usually an incidental finding on CXR or CT. Further imaging is generally not necessary in the evaluation; hamartomas generally do not demonstrate ^{18}FDG uptake.

CXR findings (Fig. 9.3)

- Nodule/mass—well-defined, spherical with a lobulated or notched outline. Usually <4cm in diameter (rarely up to 10cm diameter) and can enlarge (slowly) over time.
- Calcification—in ~15%; calcification is commoner in larger lesions. Patterns of calcification vary but there may be characteristic 'popcorn' type.

CT findings (Fig. 9.4)
- Nodule/mass—Thin-section CT readily demonstrates fat and calcification which, when present in the same lesion, is diagnostic. Rarely, neither calcification nor fat is demonstrated. Enhancement following IV contrast may be seen.

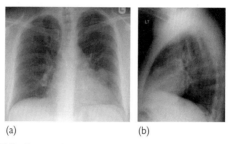

(a)   (b)

Fig. 9.3 CXR of benign pulmonary hamartoma. (a) Postero-anterior and (b) lateral projections showing a well-defined nodule anteriorly in the left lung.

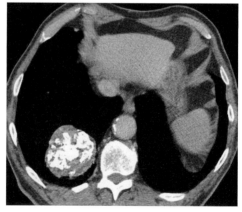

Fig. 9.4 Large hamartoma in the right lower lobe. CT shows extensive 'popcorn' calcification and areas of low density indicating fat.

Bronchial carcinoid
- Tumours of neuroendocrine origin which exhibit a spectrum of biological behaviour from slowly-growing, benign lesions to frankly malignant tumours.
- Account for <5% of lung neoplasms. ♂:♀ ≈ 1:1; occurring at any age from adolescence to old age.

- Broadly, two histopathological subtypes are recognized:
  - Typical carcinoids are the commonest subtype (85-90%) and are usually benign.
  - Atypical tumours account for 10–15%; may exhibit malignant features similar to small cell carcinoma.
  - Majority arise centrally at the carinas of bronchi.

Imaging of bronchial carcinoid tumours

The imaging features of pulmonary carcinoid tumours (Figs. 9.5–9.8) include:

CXR findings (Fig. 9.5)

- Segmental atelectasis or complete lobar collapse—the affected lobe may remain inflated or is overinflated because of a 'check valve' effect caused by the tumour. In this situation, there may be a paucity of vascular markings caused by underventilation.
- Hilar mass ± calcification—or less commonly a peripheral solitary pulmonary nodule.
- Bronchocoele—lobulated and 'branching' soft-tissue density opacity related to a small obstructing tumour.

CT findings (Figs. 9.6 and 9.7)

- Mass—well-defined, soft-tissue attenuation, commonly related to a central airway; the mass may be wholly intra- or largely extraluminal but protruding into the lumen (an appearance likened to an 'iceberg'). The airway proximal to the lesion may be slightly widened.
- Calcification—in 25–30%.
- Marked enhancement—following injection of IV contrast in some cases.
- Distal (mucous) plugging of the airways ± segmental atelectasis or lobar collapse—a small peripheral carcinoid may manifest only as a bronchocoele.

Other imaging tests

- MRI—avid enhancement following injection of IV gadolinium; small carcinoid lesions may be differentiated from adjacent vessels using specific MR sequences.
- ^{113}Indium-labelled octreotide (a somatostatin analogue) is highly sensitive for the detection of carcinoid tumours. However, false positive scans may occur in the context of inflammatory/infective diseases (Fig. 9.8).

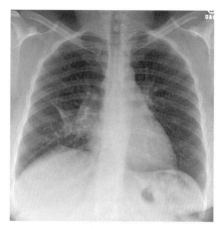

Fig. 9.5 CXR in a patient with a right hilar carcinoid tumour showing atelectasis in the right mid zone.

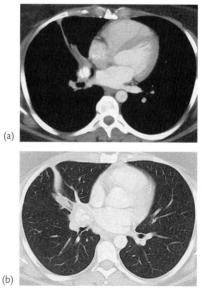

(a)

(b)

Fig. 9.6 CT of a right hilar carcinoid showing dense calcification on (a) mediastinal and (b) lung windows. Note the distal atelectasis.

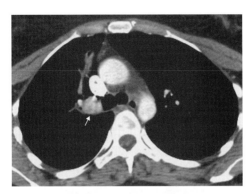

Fig. 9.7 Carcinoid tumour in the right main bronchus (arrow) showing enhancement on CT post-IV contrast.

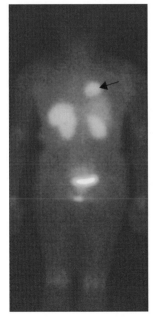

Fig. 9.8 Carcinoid tumour in the left midzone showing increased uptake on whole body ^{113}In-labelled octreotide scintigraphy (arrow).

Lung cancer

- Lung cancer is, by far, the commonest cause of death due to cancer in Western countries. In the UK, a little under 40,000 new cases are diagnosed each year and there are a similar number of deaths. A small but notable minority of patients are life-long non-smokers and around 4,000 deaths/year are caused by lung cancer in never-smokers.
- Median age at presentation ~70 years (NB slightly lower for small cell carcinoma). $\male:\female \approx 1.5:1$. The strong association between lung cancer and smoking is well known but other risk factors include: exposure to industrial carcinogens (e.g. radon, bis-chloromethyl ether, cadmium), interstitial fibrosis, HIV infection, and solid-organ (heart or heart-lung) transplantation.
- Four principal histopathological types: squamous carcinoma (accounting for 30–35% of all cases), small cell carcinoma (20%), adenocarcinoma (25–35%) and large cell carcinoma (10–15%). Mixed pathological subtypes occur.

Imaging tests used in lung cancer

Many imaging tests may be used in the diagnosis, staging, and follow-up of patients with lung cancer. The CXR and CT are the standard (and frequently, the only) tests needed for the initial diagnostic evaluation. ^{18}FDG-PET imaging has an important role (i.e. for diagnosis, staging, and follow-up).

CXR

The frontal CXR is often the first imaging test to reveal the presence of lung cancer. Additional features of potential staging significance (intrathoracic lymph node enlargement, pleural effusion, rib/chest wall erosion (see 📖 Lung tumours/Staging of lung cancer, p334) may be evident.

CT

Patients with suspected or confirmed lung cancer should be referred for CT which provides information about the morphological characteristics of the primary tumour and the extent/stage of the disease.

^{18}FDG-PET

Because it detects metabolically-active tissue, there has been an increasing dependence on ^{18}FDG-PET imaging in a wide variety of cancers. False positive (non-malignant, glucose-metabolizing cells) and false negative scans (for small lesions or tumours with low metabolic activity) are a problem.

MRI

Before the advent of multi-detector CT scanners and because of its ability to generate multiplanar imaging without ionizing radiation, it was thought that MRI would become the principal staging investigation in patients with lung cancer. However, MRI does not provide any greater clinically-significant information than modern CT machines.

Radionuclide scintigraphy

In specific circumstances, radionuclide imaging (e.g. bone scintigraphy for metastases, perfusion scanning for estimating potential lung 'reserve' following pneumonectomy), may be of value.

Ultrasound and endoscopic ultrasound

Ultrasound (US) has no major role in the diagnosis or staging of lung cancer. However, in some centres, US may be used to guide needle biopsy of peripheral tumours or, rarely, to confirm or exclude the possibility of chest wall invasion. US may also be used to guide needle biopsy of supraclavicular lymph nodes, particularly in patients with poor respiratory reserve. US may be used to evaluate a pleural effusion in patients with lung cancer by not only confirming its presence but also acting as a guide for diagnostic aspiration. More recently, US has been coupled with endoscopic probes and is proving useful for US-targeted fine needle aspiration of enlarged mediastinal lymph nodes as part of staging.

Imaging of lung cancer

The imaging features (direct and indirect) of lung cancer on CXR and CT will be considered together. The typical radiological features are listed and illustrated below.

Direct signs of lung cancer (Figs. 9.9 and 9.10)

- Intrapulmonary nodule or mass—the commonest radiological manifestation of lung cancer. In general, a peripheral lung cancer is a roughly rounded mass of soft-tissue density and variable size. The outline of the lesion may be umbilicated (i.e. a single 'notch' in an otherwise smooth margin), lobulated (multiple notches) or spiculated (multiple spicules emanating may give rise to the classical 'corona radiata' appearance). A 'tag' may extend from the tumour to the pleural surface.
- Cavitation—Seen in up to 15% of tumours. Most commonly associated with squamous cell carcinoma but may be seen in adenocarcinoma and large cell carcinoma. The cavity is usually eccentrically positioned and the wall of the cavity is typically irregular. An air-fluid level may be present.
- Calcification—rarely seen on CXR but present in up to 10% on CT. Calcification in lung cancers may be because of the incorporation of a pre-existing calcified granuloma or, alternatively, as a result of tumour necrosis (dystrophic calcification).
- Ground-glass opacities/focal consolidation—on CT, a focal nodule of ground-glass opacification alone ('non-solid') or a nodule with mixed ground-glass and higher attenuation ('part-solid') is a recognized finding of adenocarcinoma. An air bronchogram or bronchiologram may be seen. A focal area of consolidation (± air bronchogram or bronchiologram) is a finding in peripheral adenocarcinomas (see 📖 Air space diseases/Adenocarcinoma, p139).

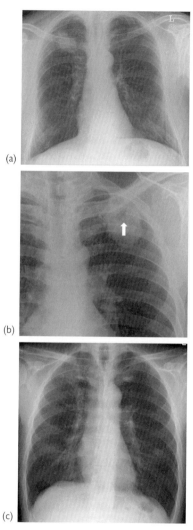

(a)

(b)

(c)

Fig. 9.9 Direct and indirect CXR signs of lung cancer. (a) CXR in a 67-year-old smoker with an irregular right upper lobe tumour. (b) Targeted image of the left upper lobe shows a lobulated left upper lobe tumour with cavitation (arrow). (c) Subtle and very ill-defined opacification at the right apex (compare with the opposite side) in a patient with squamous carcinoma; CXR 4 months later showed an obvious lesion at this site.

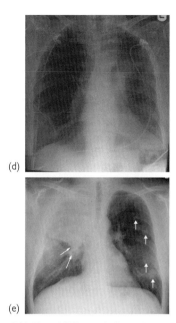

(d)

(e)

Fig. 9.9 (continued) (d) Classical CXR signs of left upper lobe collapse caused by a central tumour (proven at bronchoscopy). (e) Right upper lobe collapse in a patient with lung adenocarcinoma. There is homogeneous opacification in the right upper zone, demarcated inferiorly by the horizontal fissure which has a sigmoid configuration (Golden S sign); the slight 'bulge' of the fissure medially (long arrows) is caused by the central obstructing mass. Multiple nodules in both lungs indicate metastases (short arrows).

Indirect signs of lung cancer (Figs. 9.9 and 9.10)

With centrally situated tumours, the usual signs of the lung cancer itself may not be evident. The following features should raise the possibility of an underlying tumour, particularly in patients who have a smoking history:

- Lobar collapse—depending on the location a single or more than one lobe may be collapsed. In some patients, the lobe collapses 'around' the central mass and gives rise to a roughly, sigmoid- or S-shaped outline (the 'Golden S' sign).
- Distal consolidation—if consolidation is confined to a single lobe and particularly if this is persistent or recurrent, a central obstructing mass should be suspected. There may be associated volume loss or, occasionally, the affected lobe may be expanded.
- Increased hilar density—a unilateral dense hilum (on CXR) should raise the possibility of a central tumour. A lateral CXR projection will help to confirm that the mass is hilar (and not simply projected over the hilum) but CT will usually be requested to further evaluate this finding.

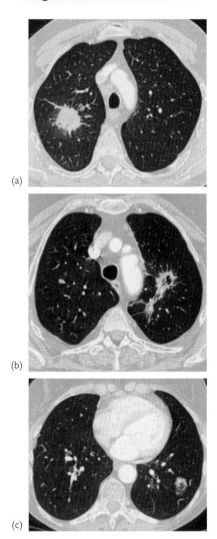

(a)

(b)

(c)

Fig. 9.10 Direct and indirect CT signs in lung cancer. (a) CT through the upper zones showing a spiculated right upper lobe tumour. (b) Cavitation in a left upper lobe squamous carcinoma. (c) CT through the lower lobes shows a part-solid (ground-glass with admixed dense opacification) peripheral left lower lobe lesion; biopsy confirmed the diagnosis of adenocarcinoma.

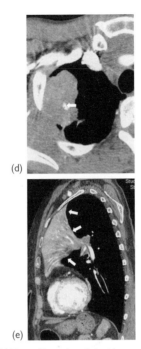

(d)

(e)

Fig. 9.10 (*continued*) (d) Targeted image through the right upper lobe shows a lobulated peripheral tumour with focal (dystrophic) calcification (arrow). (e) Sagittal CT shows collapse of the left upper lobe (bounded posteriorly by the oblique fissure (arrows)) caused by a central squamous cancer.

Associated findings in lung cancer

There are important ancillary features on CXR and CT that have diagnostic and staging significance. These include:

- Pleural effusion.
- Hilar/mediastinal/supraclavicular lymph node enlargement.
- Rib erosion or destruction ± chest wall invasion.
- Invasion of mediastinal fat and major mediastinal structures (vessels, pericardium, cardiac chambers).
- Signs of distant metastatic disease (lytic bone lesions, intrahepatic, adrenal, or CNS deposits).

Ancillary features

- Hypertrophic (pulmonary) osteoarthropathy.

Staging of lung cancer

Despite an increase in the number of treatment options, it remains a fact that surgical resection offers the only hope of cure from lung cancer. Therefore, pre-surgical staging is an important component of management. The key question which staging must answer is '*Which patients have operable disease?*'. For patients with extensive (inoperable) disease or in those with significant co-morbidity precluding surgery, staging tests may be used to judge whether the primary tumour can be captured within a radiotherapy field.

Pre-treatment staging provides information about the extent of loco-regional/distant tumour, guides treatment and has a bearing on prognosis (Tables 9.1–9.4). Imaging tests (principally CXR, CT, and [18]FDG-PET, supplemented in some patients with MRI) are important in staging but each has capabilities and limitations.

Table 9.1 5-year survival in relation to clinical stage for patients with non-small cell lung cancer (NSCLC)*

Stage based on TNM descriptors	5-year survival (%)
IA	50
IB	43
IIA	36
IIB	25
IIIA	19
IIIB	7
IV	2

*Reproduced with permission from: Goldstraw P. The IASLC lung cancer staging project: proposals for revision of the TNM stage groupings in the forthcoming (seventh) edition of the TNM classification of malignant tumours. *J Thorac Oncol* 2007; **2**:706–714, Wolters Kluwer Health.

The 'TNM' stage

Pre-operative staging of lung cancer is based on the Tumour-Nodes-Metastasis' (or TNM) system which describes the intrathoracic extent of tumour, the presence and distribution of nodal involvement, and the presence/absence of metastases. Based on the TNM descriptors, patients are assigned to a clinical stage from I to IV. The TNM system, particularly for describing the primary tumour, has recently been modified (Table 9.2).

The 'T' stage

The T component of the staging describes the primary tumour based on some key morphological characteristics which include the size of the primary tumour, its proximity to the tracheal carina and the presence/absence of visceral pleural, chest wall, or mediastinal invasion or the involvement of vital structures (e.g. heart and great vessels, vertebrae, trachea, recurrent laryngeal nerve).

Table 9.2 Characterization of the primary tumour*

TX

Primary tumour not assessable or proven tumour but not visualized on imaging studies or bronchoscopy.

T0/Tis

No evidence of primary tumour/carcinoma *in situ*.

T1 (T1a and T1b)

Tumour ≤3cm in longest dimension (subdivided as T1a = tumour ≤2cm; T1b = tumour >2 but ≤3cm in longest dimension, surrounded by lung or visceral pleura, without bronchoscopic evidence of invasion of the main bronchus).

T2 (T2a or T2b)

Tumour >3cm but ≤7cm in longest dimension (subdivided as T2a = tumour >3cm but ≤5cm; T2b = tumour >5cm but ≤7cm) OR tumour with involvement of the main bronchus ≥2cm from carina, invasion of visceral pleura OR atelectasis/obstructive pneumonia not involving the entire lung.

T3

Tumour >7cm or tumour invading the chest wall, diaphragm, phrenic nerve, mediastinal pleura, parietal pericardium OR tumour in main bronchus <2cm from (but not involving) carina OR atelectasis/obstructive pneumonia of whole lung OR separate tumour nodule(s) in same lung.

T4

Tumour of any size that invades the mediastinum, heart, great vessels, trachea, recurrent laryngeal nerve, oesophagus, vertebral body, carina OR separate tumour nodule(s) in a different but ipsilateral lobe.

*Reproduced with permission from: Goldstraw P. The IASLC lung cancer staging project: proposals for revision of the TNM stage groupings in the forthcoming (seventh) edition of the TNM classification of malignant tumours. *J Thorac Oncol* 2007; **2**:706–714, Wolters Kluwer Health.

The 'N' stage:

In the absence of distant metastatic disease, the extent of intrathoracic lymph node involvement is a key determinant of prognosis: pathologically-proven metastases in mediastinal lymph indicate N2 disease (Table 9.3) which shifts the patient from a potentially-operable to an inoperable stage.

Table 9.3 Staging of lymph nodes*

NX	Regional lymph nodes cannot be assessed
N0	No regional lymph node metastasis
N1	Metastasis in ipsilateral peribronchial and/or ipsilateral hilar lymph nodes and intrapulmonary nodes, including involvement by direct extension
N2	Metastasis in ipsilateral mediastinal and/or subcarinal lymph node(s)
N3	Metastasis in contralateral mediastinal, contralateral hilar, ipsilateral or contralateral scalene, or supraclavicular lymph node(s)

*Reproduced with permission from: Goldstraw P. The IASLC lung cancer staging project: proposals for revision of the TNM stage groupings in the forthcoming (seventh) edition of the TNM classification of malignant tumours. *J Thorac Oncol* 2007; **2**:706–714, Wolters Kluwer Health.

The 'M' stage:

The unequivocal identification of metastases indicates inoperable stage IV disease. The staging of metastatic disease is as in Table 9.4.

Table 9.4 Metastatic disease*

MX	Distant metastases cannot be assessed
M0	No distant metastasis
M1	Distant metastasis sub-categorized as: M1a (separate tumour nodule(s) in a contralateral lobe, tumour with pleural nodules, OR malignant pleural/pericardial effusion OR M1b (distant metastasis)

*Reproduced with permission from: Goldstraw P. The IASLC lung cancer staging project: proposals for revision of the TNM stage groupings in the forthcoming (seventh) edition of the TNM classification of malignant tumours. *J Thorac Oncol* 2007; **2**:706–714, Wolters Kluwer Health.

The value of radiological tests in staging lung cancer

A variety of imaging tests are used in the staging of lung cancer. Each has advantages and disadvantages:

CXR in staging

In patients with proven lung cancer, the CXR may provide some indication of tumour stage. However, it must be emphasized that this only applies when the radiographic signs are unequivocal (Table 9.5; Fig. 9.11).

Table 9.5 CXR features which have staging significance

CXR feature	Potential stage*
Tumour size (1 to >7cm)	T1–T3
Pleural/pericardial effusion	M1a
Contiguous chest wall invasion/rib destruction	T3
'Recent' elevation of the diaphragm	T3
Lobar atelectasis/consolidation	T2a or T2b
Collapse of whole lung	T3
Hilar/mediastinal lymph node enlargement	N1, N2, or N3
Nodule(s) in ipsilateral or contralateral lung	T3, T4, or M1b
Separate destructive bone lesions	M1b

* Refer to Tables 9.2–9.4 for stage classification.

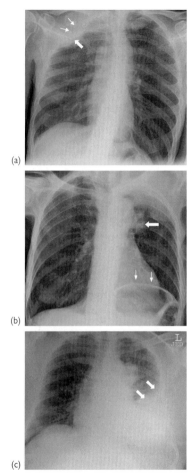

Fig. 9.11 Examples of CXR signs which have staging signficance. (a) CXR in a patient with a proven squamous lung cancer. There is an opacity in the right upper zones (thick arrow) associated with unequivocal signs of 1st and 2nd rib destruction (thin arrows), indicating T3 disease. (b) CXR in a patient with a Pancoast tumour of the left upper lobe. The upper ribs are destroyed but there is also a mass at the left hilum (thick arrow) and elevation of the left hemidiaphragm (thin arrows); the latter sign—which was not evident on earlier CXRs—strongly suggests phrenic nerve invasion and T3 status. (c) CXR in a patient with a central tumour occupying the aortopulmonary window and a large left pleural effusion (arrows); the presence of the latter, if malignant, indicates M1a disease.

Limitations of CXR staging (Fig. 9.12)

In the majority of patients and in the absence of overt signs, the CXR is of limited value for accurate staging. Importantly, CXR cannot reliably confirm/exclude the following:

- Subtle or 'early' chest wall/pleural or vertebral invasion.
- Invasion of the mediastinum and/or vital organs and/or major vessels.
- Relationship of tumour to the carina.
- Nodal or distal (i.e. small intrapulmonary or extrathoracic) metastases.

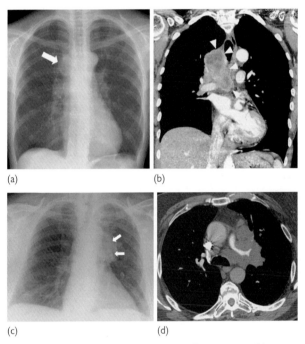

(a)　　　　　　　　　(b)

(c)　　　　　　　　　(d)

Fig. 9.12 Paired CXR and CT images in two patients illustrating some of the limitations of CXR staging. (a) CXR and (b) coronal CT in the same patient. The CXR shows a right paratracheal opacity (arrow). The extent of mediastinal invasion is underestimated on CXR but readily seen on the coronal CT (arrowheads) image. (c) CXR and (d) CT in another patient with a proven squamous lung cancer. The CXR demonstrates a large central mass (arrows) but the extent of mediastinal involvement is only evident on CT.

CT in staging:

CT is the principal radiological investigation for staging. The morphological features which have a potential impact on staging are listed (Table 9.6; Fig. 9.13).

Table 9.6 CT features of staging significance

CT feature	Potential stage*
Tumour size (1 to >7cm)	T1–T3
Nodule(s) in ipsilateral lobe or ipsilateral/contralateral lung	T3 or T4/M1a
Contiguous chest wall invasion/rib destruction	T3
Relationship to carina (<2cms or ≥2cms)	T2 or T3
Invasion of mediastinum or major organs/vessels	T3 or T4
Direct extension into vertebrae	T4
Lobar atelectasis/consolidation	T2b
Collapse of whole lung	T3
Hilar/mediastinal lymph node enlargement	N1, N2, or N3
Pleural/pericardial effusion	M1a
(Recent) elevation of diaphragm	T3
Remote destructive bone lesions	M1b
Extrathoracic metastases (e.g. adrenal, hepatic, CNS, bone)	M1b

* Refer to Tables 9.2–9.4 for stage classification.

Limitations of CT staging

Lung cancer is incorrectly staged (over- or understaging) on CT in around 40% of cases when compared to the final surgical/pathological findings (Fig. 9.14).

Difficulties in predicting the 'T' stage on CT

- Assessing tumour size—the distinction between T1 and T2 tumours (based on the longest visible dimension) is generally straightforward. However, problems may arise with central tumours especially where these are associated with significant collapse of the distal lung: the distinction between collapsed lung and obstructing tumour may then be difficult.
- Assessing relationship to carina—the distinction between a T2 and T3 tumour based on its distance from the carina (i.e. <2 or ≥2cms), is important for the decision about which operation (i.e. lobectomy, pneumonectomy or other surgery) is most appropriate. Accurate evaluation may be difficult to judge on standard axial CT images—the use of multiplanar MDCT reconstructions may be of value.

- Assessing mediastinal invasion—the identification of mediastinal invasion is crucially important as it represents the rough 'dividing-line' between surgical and non-surgical disease. Signs thought to indicate resectable tumour include a) <3cm of total contact with the mediastinum, b) a preserved fat plane between the tumour and the mediastinum and, c) <90° of contact circumferentially around mediastinal structures. However, the reliable identification of irresectable tumour—important for lowering 'open-and-close' thoracotomy rates—is difficult because of the poor sensitivity and specificity of CT.
- Assessing chest wall invasion—the presence of tumour abutting the chest wall or evidence of adjacent pleural thickening is insufficient evidence of pleural/chest wall invasion (i.e. T3 disease). Indeed, a history of pain may be a more sensitive marker of chest wall invasion than CT.

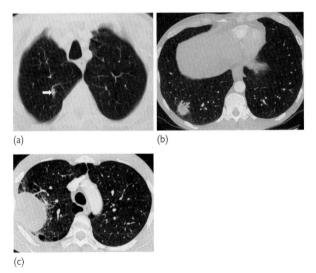

(a)

(b)

(c)

Fig. 9.13 CT staging of the primary tumour ('T' status) based on maximum dimensions. (a) CT through the upper lobes demonstrates a 1cm diameter (T1a) proven adenocarcinoma (arrow). (b) Image through the lower zones shows a spiculated 3.5cm diameter (T2a) adenocarcinoma and (c) large (>7cm diameter) right upper lobe lesion, with a provisional T3 staging.

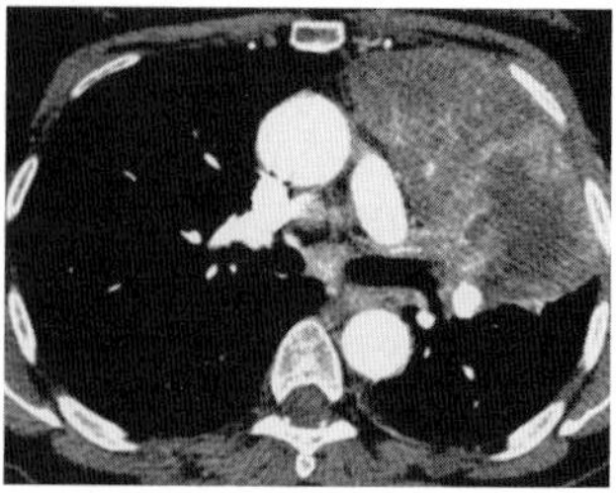

(a)

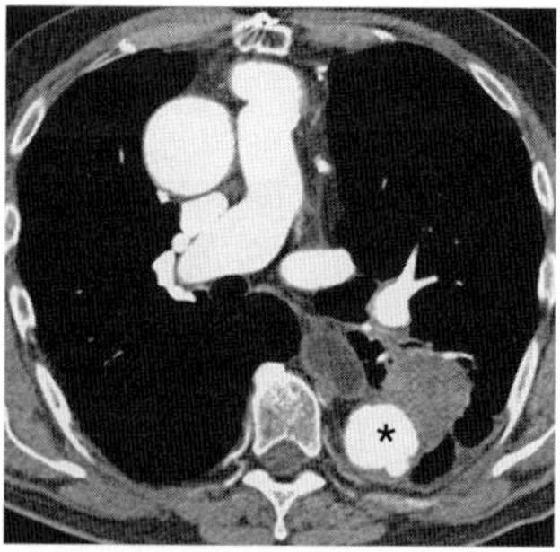

(b)

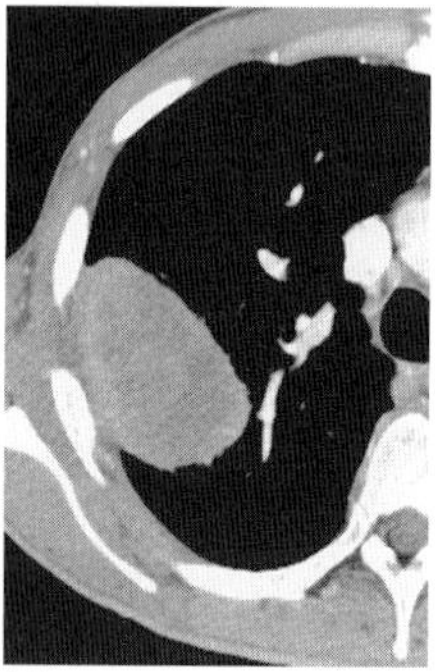

(c)

Fig. 9.14 Difficulties in CT staging. (a) CT just below the level of the carina in a patient with a central tumour. There is collapse of the left upper lobe and the demarcation between collapsed lung and tumour is lost. (b) Tumour in the left lower lobe adjacent to the descending thoracic aorta (asterisk). There is no fat plane between the tumour and aorta but there is just under 90° of contact; whether the tumour is adherent to or invading the aortic wall cannot be determined from these CT appearances. (c) Large right upper lobe lesion (in same patient as in Fig. 9.13c); there are no overt CT signs to indicate invasion of the chest wall. However, the patient reported chest wall pain and invasion was confirmed at surgery.

Difficulties in predicting the 'N' stage on CT

The reliable diagnosis of nodal metastases is a crucial aspect of staging: confirmed metastases in contralateral (N3) nodes indicates inoperable tumour. Tumour in mediastinal nodes (denoting N2 disease) may render surgery inappropriate in some patients. However, the CT staging of lymph node metastases is not straightforward (Fig. 9.15). An increase in the short axis diameter exceeding 1cm was the traditional yardstick for identifying nodal metastases. However, problems with reliance on nodal size include:

- Variations in the size of normal mediastinal and hilar nodes (ranging from 0.7–1.5cm).
- Nodes with a short axis diameter exceeding 1cm may be reactive or caused by other (non-malignant) disease.
- Nodes with a short axis diameter <1cm may harbour metastases (e.g. typically with adenocarcinoma).
- Pathologically confirmed metastases in nodes may be entirely 'invisible' on CT.

Difficulties in predicting the 'M' stage on CT

The demonstration of metastases at distant sites (most commonly the liver, adrenal glands, bones, and CNS) indicates stage IV inoperable disease. Overt metastases (e.g. destructive bone lesions, ring-enhancing masses in the brain or liver) generally pose no problems. Specific difficulties arise in the following circumstances:

- Occult distant metastases may not be detected on CT.
- The distinction between benign and metastatic masses in distant organs is not always straightforward (e.g. an enlarged adrenal may be a benign adenoma).

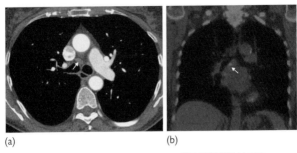

(a)   (b)

Fig. 9.15 Nodal disease in lung cancer: CT versus ^{18}FDG-PET/CT. (a) CT just below the level of the carina in a patient with a right lower lobe tumour (not shown). There is a small (<1cm) node (arrow); other nodes of similar dimensions were seen in the mediastinum. (b) Coronal PET-CT image confirms the presence of increased ^{18}FDG uptake (arrow) suggesting nodal metastasis and potential N2 disease.

^{18}FDG-PET in staging

The ability to image 'function' has had a significant impact on the staging of lung cancer. The problems associated with the relatively poor spatial resolution of early generation PET scanners have been overcome by the development of hybrid PET-CT scanners. The key aspects of whole body PET-CT and its value in the staging of lung cancer are listed below (Fig. 9.16):

- Data from PET-CT frequently alters (up- or down-grading) the staging according to CT.
- The staging of metastatic mediastinal and hilar nodal disease is significantly better on PET-CT than other imaging modalities (including CT alone or PET alone).
- The negative predictive value of PET-CT for metastatic nodal disease is particularly high.
- Standardized uptake values (SUVs), which reflect metabolic activity of a lesion, are linked to outcome: higher SUVs in the primary tumour and in regional lymph are associated with higher mortality.
- Distant metastases (including metastatic lesions in bones) not identified by other modalities, may be identified at PET-CT.

Limitations of ^{18}FDG-PET in staging
- There is a resolution limit (roughly 1cm diameter) below which PET-CT gives rise to false-negative results. As with CT, some nodes containing metastatic disease may be 'invisible'.
- Tumours with low metabolic activity may be negative on PET-CT.
- Inflammatory processes, particularly granulomatous, are associated with increased ^{18}FDG-PET uptake and lead to false-positive diagnoses.

Other imaging techniques used in staging
CT and PET-CT usually suffices for the pre-treatment staging of patients with lung cancer. Other tests are occasionally brought to bear and the imaging investigations which may be of value in specific scenarios include:

MRI in staging
- There are no convincing data that, in the majority of patients, MRI provides any superior staging information to CT.
- MRI may be of value in the further evaluation of suspicious lesions in the adrenal glands, liver, or bone.
- MRI will provide superior information about possible involvement of neurological structures (e.g. invasion of the brachial plexus by a superior sulcus (Pancoast) tumour; direct invasion of the spinal canal and cord).

Radionuclide scintigraphy in staging
- A radionuclide bone scan may confirm the presence of bone metastases (as can ^{18}FDG-PET/CT scanning).

Ultrasound and Endoscopic Ultrasound in staging
See comments on 📖 Lung tumours/Lung cancer, p328.

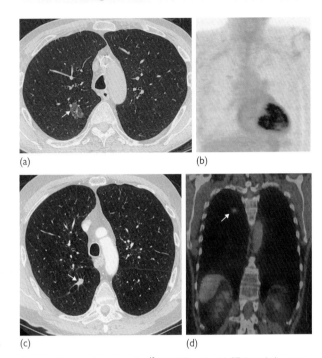

(a) (b)

(c) (d)

Fig. 9.16 False negative and positive [18]FDG-PET results. (a) CT through the upper lobes shows a non-solid nodule (arrow) in the right upper lobe which at biopsy was an adenocarcinoma. (b) 'Non-fused' coronal PET image in the same patient as in (a) showing no [18]FDG uptake in the right upper lobe. (c) Spiculated right upper lobe lesion (arrow) in a 65 year-old smoker and (d) corresponding fused PET-CT image demonstrating moderate [18]FDG uptake (arrow). The lesion was excised and the histopathological diagnosis was of a tuberculous granuloma.

Other malignant lung tumours

In contrast to lung cancer, all other primary malignant tumours are rare.

Malignant lung tumours

- Carcinoid tumour
- Lymphoma
- Sarcomas
  - Pulmonary artery sarcoma
  - Fibrosarcoma
  - Leiomyosarcoma
  - Liposarcoma
  - Rhabdomyosarcoma
  - Kaposi's sarcoma
- Carcinosarcomas
- Haemangiopericytoma
- Blastoma
- Plasmacytoma
- Pulmonary blastoma
- Pleuro-pulmonary blastoma
- Epithelioid haemangioendothelioma

Imaging

In the majority of cases, there are no specific features on 'routine' tests which will allow an accurate diagnosis of a malignant lung tumour to be made. The imaging features (typically a solitary intrapulmonary or endo-bronchial mass of soft tissue density ± calcification, ± cavitation) are non-specific and biopsy confirmation of the diagnosis is usually needed. Occasionally specific radiological features, ancillary imaging findings, and/or clinical data may point to a specific diagnosis:

Specific features of potential diagnostic value

Radiological features

- Low attenuation—indicating fat may be seen in liposarcoma.
- Consolidation (± air bronchogram/bronchiologram)—is a feature of primary pulmonary lymphoma (typically of non-Hodgkin's type). May be single or multiple foci and these may be combined with multiple intrapulmonary nodules.
- Intraluminal or part-intraluminal/part-extraluminal (bronchial) mass—a finding seen in carcinoid tumours.
- Intra-arterial mass—a feature of pulmonary artery sarcoma.

Ancillary imaging findings

- Hypertrophic (pulmonary) osteoarthropathy—a finding in some patients with haemangiopericytoma.

Carcinoid tumour

The imaging of pulmonary carcinoid tumours is also considered in benign pulmonary tumours (see 📖 Lung tumours/Bronchial carcinoid, p324).

Primary pulmonary lymphoma

- The majority are of non-Hodgkin's type (most commonly marginal zone lymphoma derived from bronchial mucosa-associated lymphoid tissue (MALT) and less frequently, diffuse large B-cell lymphoma). True primary pulmonary Hodgkin's lymphoma is rare. There are recognized associations with Sjögren's syndrome, dysgammaglobulinaemias, and acquired immunodeficiency syndrome.
- ♂:♀ ≈ 1:1. Occurring at any age (median ≈ 60 years).

CXR findings (Fig. 9.17)

- Multiple nodules.
- Multiple focal areas of consolidation.
- Hilar/mediastinal lymph node enlargement.
- Pleural effusions (seen in around 20% of patients).

CT findings (Fig. 9.17)

- Multiple nodules—may have a centrilobular distribution.
- Multiple areas of consolidation often with an air bronchogram/bronchiologram. Cavitation is uncommon.
- Multiple foci of ground-glass opacification.
- Thickening of interlobular septa.
- Pleural effusions.

Other imaging tests

- ^{18}FDG-PET scanning demonstrates heterogeneous or homogeneous uptake in pulmonary lesions. However, the differentiation between lymphoma and other malignant/non-malignant (but metabolically-active) pathology is impossible.

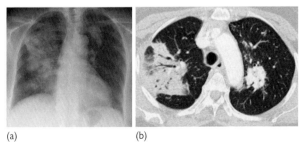

(a)   (b)

Fig. 9.17 (a) CXR and (b) CT in a patient with biopsy-confirmed MALToma. There are multifocal, bilateral areas of consolidation.

Solitary pulmonary nodule or mass

An isolated lung nodule (measuring up to 3cm in diameter) or mass (>3cm diameter) on CXR or CT is a relatively common finding. Imaging evaluation is an important aspect of the multidisciplinary approach to the management of solitary lung lesions. The list of possible causes is long (Table 9.7). However, in clinical practice, granulomatous lesions and lung cancer account for the vast majority.

Table 9.7 Causes of a solitary pulmonary nodule or mass

- **Inflammatory/infective**
  - Granulomatous (post-tuberculosis or fungal infection (e.g. histoplasmosis))
  - Infectious (e.g. lung abscess)
  - Necrobiotic (rheumatoid) nodules
  - Bronchocentric granulomatosis
  - Mucous impaction/bronchocoele
  - Wegener's granulomatosis
  - Sarcoidosis
- **Neoplastic**
  - Malignant (lung cancer and other malignant lung tumours, solitary metastasis)
  - Benign (hamartoma, benign carcinoid)
- **Congenital**
  - (Extra-lobar) pulmonary sequestration
  - Intrapulmonary cyst
  - Bronchial atresia with mucus impaction
- **Vascular**
  - Pulmonary infarct
  - Haematoma/contused lung
  - Pulmonary artery aneurysm
  - Pulmonary vein varix
- **Miscellaneous causes**
  - Amyloid
  - Organizing pneumonia
  - Intrapulmonary lymph node

Adapted from *Imaging of Diseases of the Chest*, Hansell DM, Lynch DA, McAdams HP, Bankier AA (eds). 5th edition (2010) Mosby-Elsevier.

Investigation of the solitary pulmonary nodule/mass

The following sections deal with the radiological aspects of the solitary pulmonary nodule. However, the importance of clinical data needs to be remembered. Specific aspects of the clinical information which may influence the interpretation of the imaging are listed in Table 9.8.

Table 9.8 Important clinical factors when evaluating a solitary pulmonary nodule or mass

- **Age**
  - In general, there is an increased prevalence of malignant tumours with age; lung cancer is rare in patients aged <40 years.
- **Ethnic/geographical origin**
  - Higher prevalence of tuberculosis in patients from certain regions (e.g. sub-Saharan Africa, South East Asia).
  - Higher prevalence of histoplasmosis in mid-western North America.
  - High prevalence of hydatid in Southern America, Northern Africa, Australia, and Greece.
- **Smoking history**
  - A smoking history is of importance when assessing the significance of a solitary pulmonary nodule/mass.
- **History of extra-thoracic malignancy**
  - A solitary nodule/mass in the context of certain cancers (head and neck, bladder, breast, cervix, ovarian, oesophageal, gastric and prostate) is more likely to represent a lung cancer than metastasis; NB the smoking history is important in this regard.
  - A solitary nodule/mass in patients with melanoma, sarcomas and testicular tumours is more likely to represent a metastasis than lung cancer.

The radiological evaluation of the solitary pulmonary nodule/mass

In patients with a solitary pulmonary nodule or mass, the main question which radiological tests seek to answer is whether the lesion is benign or malignant. The radiological features which suggest benignity or malignancy are discussed below and are compared in Table 9.9. However, a confident diagnosis of one or the other is often not forthcoming and histopathological confirmation may then be necessary.

Size

In general, the larger the nodule/mass (i.e. >3cm) on CXR or CT, the greater the likelihood that the lesion represents lung cancer, particularly if there is a smoking history. A nodule smaller than 1cm that is visible on CXR usually implies the presence of calcification and hence benignity (NB non-calcified subcentimetre diameter lesions are generally not resolved on CXR).

Shape

The outline of a lesion may provide clues about the likelihood of malignancy. Features that suggest a malignant cause (see also 📖 'Imaging tests used in lung cancer' Pulmonary tumours/Lung cancer, p328) include:

- Spiculation or a corona radiata
- Lobulation
- Notched outline

By contrast, a completely smooth outline is more often associated with a benign nodule/mass.

Density characteristics (Figs. 9.18 and 9.19)

Most lung nodules/masses tend to be of soft-tissue attenuation on CXR or CT. Careful attention should be paid to the presence of differential densities within lesions and the changes in density seen following the injection of IV contrast:

- Calcification—calcification within a lesion usually suggests a benign aetiology. This is particularly true for smaller lesions (measuring <3cm in diameter) with smooth outlines and when the calcification is uniform, laminated, or where the calcification has a 'popcorn' type configuration. However, calcification may be seen in primary or secondary malignant tumours (e.g. where calcification in pre-existing benign granuloma is 'engulfed' by lung cancer or calcification in metastases from bone/cartilage forming tumours (osteosarcoma or chondrosarcoma)).
- Fat—the presence of fat (low) attenuation in a solitary pulmonary lesion indicates a benign hamartoma or lipoma (see 📖 Lung tumours/ Benign pulmonary lesions, p322).
- Ground-glass or mixed ground-glass/solid nodules—(also termed non-solid and part-solid respectively). A focal nodule of ground-glass attenuation or a nodule with ground-glass and solid elements should be viewed with suspicion. There is a higher likelihood that part-solid nodules (as opposed to solid and non-solid lesions) represent adenocarcinoma.
- Contrast enhancement—most malignant lesions demonstrate an increase in attenuation (>15HU), over a period of minutes, following the injection of IV contrast—probably because of neovascularization— whereas benign lesions do not; the caveat is that benign inflammatory nodules may also demonstrate some post-contrast density increase.

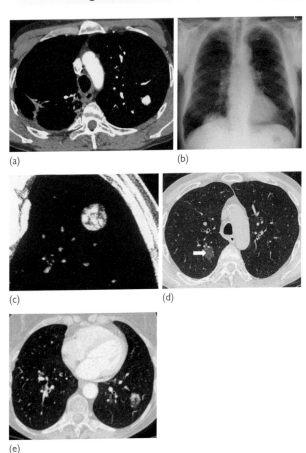

(a)

(b)

(c)

(d)

(e)

Fig. 9.18 Density characteristics of diagnostic value. (a) CT through the upper lobes in a patient with previous tuberculosis. There is a well-defined nodule in the left upper lobe with dense homogeneous calcification. The appearances are those of a tuberculoma. (b) Large right lower lobe mass (partly obscured by the right hemidiaphragm) on CXR with amorphous ('popcorn') calcification in a benign hamartoma. (c) Prone targeted CT image through the left lower lobe demonstrates a lesion of mixed attenuation; there are areas of lower attenuation indicating fat within the lesion. The appearances are those of another benign hamartoma. (d) CT through the upper lobes showing a non-solid nodule in the right upper lobe (arrow); biopsy confirmed the diagnosis of adenocarcinoma. (e) Part-solid nodule (high density admixed with ground-glass attenuation)—another adenocarcinoma.

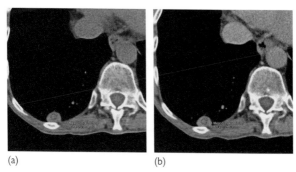

(a)   (b)

Fig. 9.19 Effect of contrast enhancement in a benign solitary pulmonary nodule. (a) Targeted CT image through the right lower lobe demonstrating a well-defined peripheral nodule; mean pre-contrast attenuation = 42HU. (b) CT through the same lesion following the injection of IV contrast; maximum contrast enhancement (at 2 min) = 47HU; this is below the threshold normally seen in malignant nodules (i.e. >15HU).

Growth (Fig. 9.20)

Growth rate is a key aspect of radiological evaluation and is usually measured in terms of the time taken for a lesion to double in volume (termed the 'volume doubling time'). As a general rule, malignant lung tumours double in volume in anywhere between 1 month and 1.5 years; a nodule or mass that doubles in volume at a rate faster or slower than this usually (but not always) excludes a malignancy. Leading on from this, the absence of any growth over 2 years is the traditional 'end-point' for declaring that a nodule or mass is benign. However, against this, some malignant nodules/masses (typically adenocarcinoma) may grow very slowly. Lesions which reduce in size can be considered benign.

Table 9.9 Comparison of radiological features which may distinguish between benign and malignant solitary nodules

	Benign	Malignant
Cavitation	Yes (uniform wall)	Yes (irregular wall thickness)
Outline	Completely smooth	Spiculated, lobulated, or umbilicated
Density	Calcification	Non-calcified (usually)
	Fat density	Soft-tissue density ± low attenuation (necrosis)
		Non-solid or part-solid
Growth	No/slow growth or a reduction in size	Volume doubling time: 1 month–1.5 years
Density increase following contrast	<15HU	>15HU

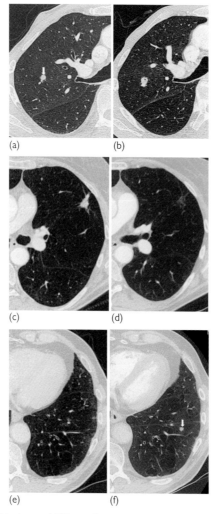

Fig. 9.20 Paired targeted CT images demonstrating serial changes of different solitary pulmonary nodules over time. (a) and (b) CT images through the right upper lobe 8 months apart demonstrating growth—and cavitation—in a squamous lung cancer (arrow). (c) and (d) CT through the left upper lobe taken 2 months apart confirming almost complete resolution of an irregular opacity. (e) and (f) CT through the left lower lobe in a patient with colon cancer under follow-up; CT performed 8 months apart shows a 'new' nodule in the left lower lobe (arrow).

Pleural diseases

Pleural anatomy

Pleural anatomy has also been covered earlier in this book (see 📖 Key radiological anatomy/Pleura, p40). What follows is a more detailed review of the important aspects of pleural anatomy.

- The visceral pleura covers the lung and extends into underlying lung to form the fissures.
- The parietal pleura lines the chest wall, diaphragm, and mediastinal surfaces; the inferior extent reaches the level of the xiphoid process/8th costochondral junction anteriorly to the 10th rib in the mid-axillary line and to the level of the first lumbar vertebra posteriorly.
- The parietal and visceral layers meet at the hila.
- The pleural space separates parietal and visceral pleura and contains a small physiological volume of fluid (~20ml).
- The combined thickness of visceral and parietal layers and the pleural space is ~0.2mm.
  NB Intercostal arteries may be tortuous and not covered by the rib phalange for a short distance from their origin from the aorta to the angle of the rib; this is an important consideration when undertaking pleural intervention.

Imaging tests in the investigation of pleural disease

The CXR and CT are the principal tests but ultrasonography deserves special mention: the widespread availability of ultrasound, the capacity for 'real-time' imaging, relative speed, the absence of any ionizing radiation and the ability to undertake 'guided' intervention are the key advantages of ultrasound. Other tests such as MRI may have a role in selected cases and there is increasing interest in the use of [18]FDG-PET imaging.

CXR

- The normal pleura, apart from the fissures, is not normally visible.
- A lateral decubitus projection may be used in the detection of small pleural effusions (this projection is not often requested since ultrasonography is capable of identifying small effusions with relative ease).
- Uniform pleural thickening is only seen over the lateral aspects of the lung on a frontal CXR (i.e. not mediastinal or diaphragmatic surface).

CT (Fig. 10.1)

- The optimum technique comprises contiguous image acquisition following IV contrast injection but with an approximately 40–60 second delay since pleural thickening may enhance relatively late.
- The normal pleura is seen as a 1–2mm soft tissue attenuation line at the chest wall/lung interface and consists of innermost intercostal muscle, the parietal and visceral pleura, and the endothoracic fascia (the 'intercostal stripe').
- Thin density line of the pleura is normally visible between ribs but not internal to ribs. Exceptions to this include: i) the presence of fat internal to rib (fat attenuation); ii) the presence of subcostal muscle in ~15% (in the paravertebral region); iii) transverse thoracic muscle (parasternal) and iv) intercostal vessels (paravertebral).
- CT may distinguish benign from malignant pleural thickening and is of value for guiding aspiration (where ultrasound may have failed).

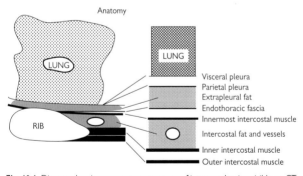

Fig. 10.1 Diagram showing component structures of intercostal stripe visible on CT. Reproduced with permission from eds WR Webb, NL Müller, and DP Naidich *High Resolution CT of the Lung, 3rd Edition* (2001) Lippincott, Williams & Wilkins.

Ultrasound
- The normal pleura may be identified on ultrasound as a thin, bright ('shimmering') line which, in real-time, moves with breathing.
- Characteristic 'comet-tails' (hyperechoic reverberation artefacts) is a normal feature on ultrasound.
- Small pleural effusions and pneumothoraces may be identified more readily than on CXR; moreover, the distinction between solid and predominantly fluid lesions may be made with ultrasound.
- Ultrasound is ideally suited to guiding percutaneous intervention of not only pleural but also chest wall and peripheral pulmonary lesions.

MRI
- In general, MRI offers no significant advantage over other imaging techniques in the investigation of pleural disease.
- On occasion, MRI is of value in the staging of malignant pleural mesothelioma but then, only in a 'problem-solving' capacity (e.g. when there is equivocal diaphragmatic involvement on other imaging tests).

[18]FDG-PET
The role of PET imaging is principally in the evaluation of malignant pleural disease. Some of the specific applications for [18]FDG-PET include:
- Detection of pleural metastases.
- Assessment of unsuspected nodal and extra-thoracic disease in patients with malignant pleural mesothelioma.
- To guide percutaneous or surgical (video assisted thoracoscopic) biopsy in patients with suspected malignant pleural disease.
- In differentiating between benign and malignant pleural disease. NB false positive [18]FDG uptake may occur with benign pleural plaques and infective pleuritis; false negative [18]FDG-PET is seen in patients with epithelioid-type mesothelioma, malignant solitary fibrous tumour, prostatic cancer metastases and lymphoma.

Pleural effusion

The presence of a small amount (~20ml) of fluid is physiological and permits the free movement of the pleural surfaces. Increased production or decreased absorption leads to the accumulation of excess pleural fluid. In general, if the protein level within the fluid is normal in comparison to serum levels (i.e a transudative effusion) the pleura itself tends to be normal. In contrast, a high pleural fluid protein content (an exudate), generally indicates that the pleura is, for whatever reason, abnormal. See Table 10.1 for the causes of pleural effusion.

Table 10.1 Causes of a pleural effusion

Transudative effusions
- **Raised vascular pressure**—cardiac failure, constrictive pericarditis, fluid overload
- **Reduced oncotic pressure**—hepatic cirrhosis, nephrotic syndrome, hypoalbuminemia
- **Reduced pleural pressure**—lung atelectasis (e.g. total lung collapse)

Exudative effusions
- **Trauma**
- **Infections**—NB including extrapleural infections (e.g. subphrenic abscess)
- **Inflammatory**—rheumatoid arthritis, systemic lupus erythematosus, Wegener's granulomatosis
- **Neoplasms**—benign and malignant
- **Vascular/cardiac**—pulmonary thromboembolism, SVC obstruction, post-cardiac injury (Dressler's syndrome)
- **Renal**—uraemia, renal tract obstruction, renal infection/nephritis
- **Hepatic**—cirrhosis, hepatitis, liver abscess
- **Pancreatic**—acute/chronic pancreatitis
- **Ascitic**—benign or malignant ascites, peritoneal dialysis
- **Splenic**—infarction, haematoma, abscess
- **Inhalation**—asbestos-related
- **Drug-induced**—phenytoin, ergotamine, β-blockers
- **Miscellaneous**—hypothyroidism, sarcoidosis, yellow-nail syndrome, ovarian hyperstimulation syndrome

Imaging of pleural effusions

- The usual appearance of a moderately large pleural effusion on an erect frontal CXR is homogeneous lower zone opacification with a well-defined curvilinear upper border; complex effusions are also well demonstrated on CXR.
- The lateral CXR is more sensitive than the frontal projection for the detection of small amounts of pleural fluid because the posterior costophrenic angle is more inferior than the lateral costophrenic angle.

- A lateral decubitus CXR may be more sensitive still for the detection of small amounts of pleural fluid (NB ~175ml of fluid are required to cause blunting of the costophrenic angle—often the earliest sign of a pleural effusion on a frontal CXR). However, ultrasound is the optimal test for the diagnosis of small pleural effusions.

CXR findings (Figs. 10.2–10.7)
The different CXR manifestations of pleural fluid are summarized below:
- Lower zone opacity with a linear upper margin and a lateral 'meniscus'—the typical sign on erect CXR in patients with uncomplicated pleural effusion.
- Apparent elevation of the hemidiaphragm—indicating subpulmonary effusion; the radiological clue with differentiates fluid from true hemidiaphragmatic elevation is that the apparent peak is more lateral in the former.
- Increased density with preservation of bronchovascular markings—in supine patients.
- Complete 'white-out'—with a large pleural effusion and usually with contralateral mediastinal displacement (NB the absence of significant contralateral shift in the presence of a large effusion indicates either that there is major collapse of the underlying lung or that there may be 'fixation' of the mediastinum possibly by tumour)
- Air-fluid level (hydropneumothorax)—results in an unusually straight upper border; may indicate that there has been intervention or the presence of a broncho-pleural fistula.
- Bizarre shapes—if there is inflammation/infection leading to loculation, fluid may become encysted.
- Subpleural fluid (e.g. oedema, lymph) may mimic a pleural effusion and this appearance has been termed a 'lamellar effusion'. This type of fluid collection may be distinguished from a true pleural effusion by the unusually sharp lateral border and the preservation of the sharp costophrenic angle.

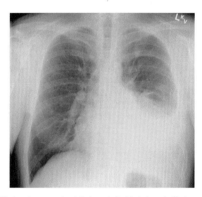

Fig. 10.2 CXR showing a moderately large left-sided pleural effusion with a meniscus-shaped upper border.

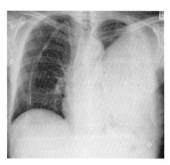

Fig. 10.3 CXR in a patient undergoing chemotherapy showing a large loculated left pleural effusion caused by empyema.

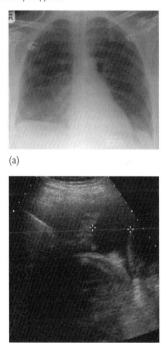

(a)

(b)

Fig. 10.4 (a) CXR in a patient with a right subpulmonic pleural effusion. The hemidiaphragm appears elevated but note the relatively lateral position of the highest portion of the apparent hemidiaphragm. (b) Ultrasound in the same individual demonstrates the hypoechoic fluid above the diaphragm. The calipers measure the distance between the atelectatic right lower lobe and the hemidiaphragm.

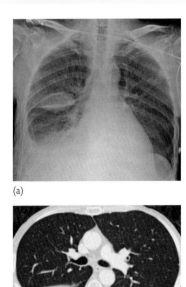

(a)

(b)

Fig. 10.5 Radiological appearances of encysted pleural fluid. (a) A 'pseudotumour' on CXR in the right mid zone caused by fluid encysted in the horizontal fissure and (b) CT in another patient with post-operative fluid in the right oblique fissure.

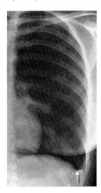

Fig. 10.6 CXR showing a left hydropneumothorax. Note the subtle air-fluid level (arrow) on the left.

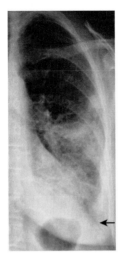

Fig. 10.7 CXR showing a lamellar 'effusion' (arrow) in a patient with lymphangitis carcinomatosis caused by breast cancer.

Ultrasound findings (Fig. 10.8)

Ultrasonography readily confirms the presence of pleural fluid. Additional findings (e.g. septation, internal echoes, pleural thickening), which may be of diagnostic value are also demonstrated. The features of a pleural effusion on US imaging include:

- Low reflectivity around the lungs—there may be internal echoes depending on the composition of pleural fluid (e.g. blood, fibrinous strands).
- Septations—US is superior to CT in this regard.
- Ancillary findings: in patients with malignant effusions, US may demonstrate features of malignant infiltration (e.g. irregular nodular thickening).

CT findings

- Fluid density—uncomplicated effusions will be seen in the dependent pleural space. Complex collections (for instance, secondary to infection or inflammation), may become loculated with apparently separate 'pockets', not necessarily in the dependent regions.
- Pleural thickening ± enhancement (following IV contrast)—smooth or irregular thickening in inflammatory or malignant disease respectively.
- Linear (pulmonary) bands ± volume loss—may be evident in association with inflammatory effusions.
- Ancillary findings: the underlying cause of effusion (e.g. pneumonia, lung cancer) may be identified on CT.

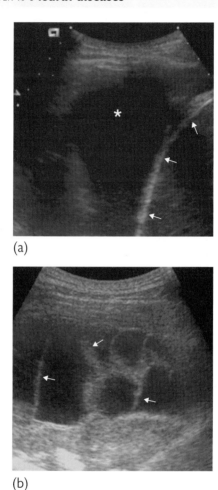

(a)

(b)

Fig. 10.8 Variable appearances of pleural fluid on US. (a) Uncomplicated pleural effusion in the right hemithorax seen as hypoechoic region (asterisk). The normal curvilinear high reflectivity of the hemidiaphragm (arrows) is clearly depicted. (b) Complicated (parapneumonic) pleural effusion with multiple septa of variable thickness (arrows).

Miscellaneous causes of pleural effusion

Some of the different causes of a pleural effusion listed in Table 10.1 are briefly considered below. Infective (parapneumonic) effusions, an important category of pleural fluid, is considered in more detail.

Cardiac failure

- One of the commonest causes of pleural effusions in clinical practice.
- The majority of effusions related to cardiac dysfunction are bilateral but purely right-sided effusions and, less often, isolated left-sided effusions occur.

Nephrotic syndrome

- The majority of pleural effusions in patients with nephrotic syndrome are bilateral
- Pleural effusions are transudative.
- Effusions may be recurrent and subpulmonary.

Hepatic cirrhosis ('hepatic hydrothorax')

- Pleural effusions are common in patients with cirrhosis and may be a consequence of low plasma oncotic pressure. NB Transdiaphragmatic spread of ascitic fluid through diaphragmatic defects (in the tendinous portion of the diaphragm) may also account for pleural fluid in patients with chronic liver disease.
- Effusions are usually right-sided (less commonly left-sided or bilateral) and may vary in volume.

Traumatic (haemothorax) (Fig. 10.9)

- Both open and closed thoracic trauma may cause pleural effusions.
- A haemothorax may be rapidly progressive because of the absence of a tamponade effect; a tension haemothorax may ensue and constitute a medical emergency. NB Other causes of rapidly accumulating pleural effusions, in the context of trauma, include a ruptured oesophagus, thoracic duct/venous injury.
- The presence of blood in the pleural space may be suspected on CT when fluid of higher than expected attenuation is seen in the pleural space.

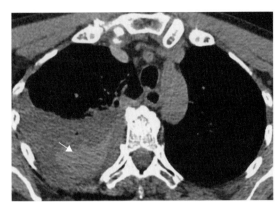

Fig. 10.9 Unenhanced CT in an individual demonstrating increased attenuation (arrow) in a large pleural effusion due to active haemorrhage following chest trauma.

Inflammatory

- Inflammatory pleural effusions are common in patients with connective tissue disease (e.g. rheumatoid arthritis, systemic lupus erythematosus (SLE)), asbestos exposure, and following cardiac surgery:
  - A pleural effusion is the commonest thoracic manifestation of rheumatoid arthritis; an effusion may predate overt joint manifestations. ♂ > ♀; effusions are often asymptomatic but may persist or occur ~20 years after presentation. There may be residual pleural thickening and folded lung.
  - SLE may present with a pleuritis ± pleural effusion. Unlike rheumatoid arthritis, pleuritic pain is common. Pleural fluid aspiration often shows elevated neutrophil or lymphocyte levels with a normal glucose levels; fluid may be positive for anti-neutrophil antibody (ANA).
  - A benign haemorrhagic exudate may be a complication of asbestos exposure that may occur anywhere between 15–40 years after exposure. Effusions may be asymptomatic, recurrent, and/or persistent. Diffuse pleural thickening may result.
  - The post-cardiac injury (Dressler's) syndrome may occur days or weeks following myocardial infarction or cardiac surgery and is a diagnosis of exclusion. Patients generally present with fever and pleuritic chest pain. There are pleural and pericardial effusions (bilateral or unilateral and, if the latter, commoner on the left) ± parenchymal consolidation. Effusions may be haemorrhagic or serosanguinous.

Neoplastic

- Most commonly due to metastasis (adenocarcinoma) to the pleura.
- Common tumours that metastasize to the pleura include lung, breast, lymphoma, ovary, stomach, and pancreas.
- Putative mechanisms for the development of malignant pleural effusions include lymphatic or thoracic duct obstruction or increased pleural permeability.
- The diagnosis of a malignant pleural effusion is made by cytological examination of pleural fluid or biopsy.

Uraemic

- A fibrinous pleuritis is common in uraemia and may be associated with a pericardial effusion.
- Uraemic effusions may occur despite haemodialysis and are often blood-stained.
- Effusions are unilateral in ~80% and may cause diffuse and significant pleural thickening.

Drug-induced

- Drugs known to cause pleural effusions include phenytoin, ergot derivatives, β-adrenergic blockers, methotrexate, and nitrofurantoin.
- A full list is available on the website: www.pneumotox.com.

Chylous

- A chylous effusion contains lymphatic fluid (chyle) from the intestine, liver, or lower limbs and is classically 'milky' in appearance.
- The principal causes of chylothorax are: thoracic duct rupture, venous obstruction, leakage from pleural lymphatics, and extension of subdiaphragmatic chylous ascites. The majority are due to malignancy but other recognized causes include trauma and surgery. In some patients chylous effusions are idiopathic. Miscellaneous rare causes include thoracic duct atresia, tuberous sclerosis, lymphangioleiomyomatosis, congenital lymphangiectasia, and lymphangiomatosis.

Infectious/parapneumonic effusions and empyema

- Pleural effusions secondary to pulmonary infections are common; primary infection of the pleural space (empyema) is less common.
- The commonest non-tuberculous organisms causing infectious effusions are *Streptococcus pneumoniae*, *Staphylococcus aureus*, anaerobic, and gram-negative bacteria.
- The response of the pleura to bacterial pulmonary infection may be considered in three broad stages:
  - **Exudative stage:** an initial outpouring of sterile fluid in which there is a low white blood cell count, low lactate dehydrogenase (LDH) levels, a normal pH and normal glucose levels. If appropriate antibiotic therapy is started promptly, the pleural fluid usually resolves spontaneously.
  - **Fibropurulent stage:** caused by bacterial invasion from the adjacent lung; polymorphonuclear leucocytes, bacteria, and debris accumulate in the pleural space. With the development of fibrin sheets, the pleural fluid begins to loculate and septate. At this stage, the pleural pH and glucose are typically low with an increased LDH level; pH may vary in different pockets. The presence of loculations may make intercostal tube drainage more difficult; however, internal septations do not predict unsuccessful tube drainage.
  - **Organization stage:** this phase develops in the absence of treatment. There is pleural fibrosis and thickening which, if severe may cause physiological impairment, necessitating surgical decortication. Occasionally in tuberculous empyema, a condition called *empyema necessitans* may develop where pus drains spontaneously through the chest wall.

Imaging of parapneumonic effusions/empyema

CXR and US are mainstays of radiological investigation both for diagnosis and follow-up; US is also of value in patients in whom intervention is being considered. CT is generally reserved for more complex cases.

CXR findings

- Pleural effusion—in the early stages (see 📖 Pleural diseases/Pleural effusion, p361).
- Loculations—as the pleural fluid becomes more complex.

Ultrasound findings (Fig. 10.10)

The US appearances vary and depend on the timing:

- Pleural fluid—anechoic and non-septated or with the presence of internal echoes and septa.
- Pleural thickening.
- Collapsed and/or consolidated lung.

CT findings (Figs. 10.11–10.12)

- Pleural fluid—the extent and location of separate locules of fluid are well demonstrated at CT. Separate locules have a 'lenticular' configuration. In contrast to US, septations are not readily apparent on CT.
- Pleural thickening ± enhancement following IV contrast.
- 'Split pleura' sign—thickening and 'separation' of the pleura.
- Hypertrophy/increased attenuation of extrapleural fat.

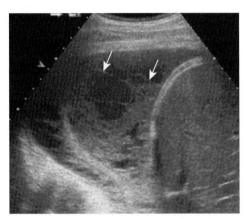

Fig. 10.10 Ultrasound in a patient with an empyema showing multiple thin septations anteriorly (arrows) and echogenic debris in the more dependent part of the hemithorax.

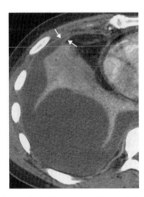

Fig. 10.11 CT in another patient with empyema demonstrating enhancement of the parietal and visceral pleura post IV contrast resulting in the 'split pleura sign' (arrows). There is loculated pleural fluid but septa are not shown.

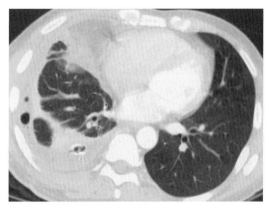

Fig. 10.12 CT on lung window settings in the same patient in Fig. 10.10 showing locules of gas caused by internal septations within the pleura after drain insertion.

Radiological management of parapneumonic effusions/empyema

- CXR supplemented by US are the initial investigations of choice in patients with parapneumonic effusion and empyema.
- On diagnostic aspiration, if there is frank pus, chest tube drainage under imaging guidance is generally indicated. Fine bore intercostal drains inserted with a guidewire (i.e. the Seldinger technique) are often safer and better tolerated by patients than large calibre drains.
- In the absence of frank pus, measurement of pleural fluid pH is recommended and is a useful to guide further management: a pleural pH of <7.2 mandates drainage (the caveat being that different pleural fluid locules may have different pH values).
- The role of intrapleural fibrinolytics is still debated: a large randomized-controlled trial has shown no advantages with streptokinase although newer agents such as recombinant tissue plasminogen activator are currently being evaluated in patients with parapneumonic effusions/empyema.
- Failure to improve with intercostal chest tube drainage is a good indication for CT to visualize drain position or exclude underlying parenchymal (e.g. lung abscess) or airway abnormalities (such as aspirated foreign bodies).

Benign pleural thickening

- Benign pleural thickening caused by pleural fibrosis may be localized or diffuse.
- The common causes of pleural thickening are listed in Table 10.2. Any exudative pleural effusion may lead to benign pleural thickening.
- The development of fibrosis is dependent on the degree of mesothelial cell and basement membrane injury; exudative effusions are more likely to result in fibrin deposition.
- When pleural thickening is diffuse there may be significant functional impairment and, rarely, respiratory failure. Thoracic pain is a worrying feature and should prompt rigorous exclusion of mesothelioma.

Table 10.2 Common causes of benign pleural thickening

- Post-infectious/empyema (including tuberculosis)
- Post-traumatic/haemothorax
- Surgery or pleurodesis (usually unilateral)
- Radiation or drug-induced
- Asbestos-related
- Connective tissue diseases
  - Rheumatoid arthritis
  - Systemic lupus erythematosus
- Uraemia
- Cryptogenic fibrosing pleuritis

Imaging of benign pleural thickening

The imaging features of benign pleural thickening (irrespective of cause) are described and illustrated below:

CXR findings (Figs. 10.13–10.15)

- Smooth thickening—soft tissue density without overt nodularity seen internal to ribs and associated with blunting of the costophrenic angles ± volume loss. On the right, thickening may extend into the horizontal fissure. Extrapleural fat may mimic diffuse pleural thickening but costophrenic angles are spared.
- Apical 'cap'—caused by pleural thickening at the apices; may be associated with TB, emphysema, diffuse parenchymal lung disease, or advancing age.
- Veil-like density—if pleural thickening is seen *en face*.

Ultrasound findings

- Pleural thickening—homogeneously dense echogenic layer if >1cm thick ± calcification.

CT findings (Figs. 10.15–10.18)

CT is of value in differentiating between benign and malignant pleural thickening; the typical CT appearances which indicate benignity are summarized below. However, it must be stressed that CT has a relatively low negative predictive value for malignancy. Thus, further investigations are often necessary, particularly when clinical suspicion is high.

- Pleural thickening—smooth (i.e. non-nodular) soft tissue density; typically occurring postero-basally with 'tapering' lateral margins. The maximum thickness of the pleura is usually <1cm and there is little if any extension to the mediastinal surfaces.
- Calcification—may or may not be present (calcification is a feature of thickening caused by a tuberculous empyema or haemothorax). NB Following talc pleurodesis, the appearances are similar to other causes of calcified pleural thickening.
- Prominent extrapleural fat.
- Pleuro-parenchymal bands ± folded lung—see 📖 Pleural diseases/ 'Folded' lung and pleuro-parenchymal bands, p383.

MRI findings

The morphological appearances of benign pleural thickening mirror those seen on CT. On T2-weighted images there is a hypointense signal and there is typically no enhancement after gadolinium injection on T1-weighted sequences.

^{18}FDG-PET findings

- Benign pleural thickening is associated with moderate ^{18}FDG uptake.
- Following talc pleurodesis there may be markedly increased uptake leading to a potentially false positive diagnosis of malignancy.

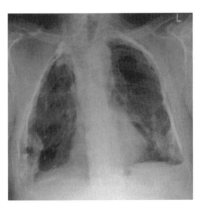

Fig. 10.13 CXR of an individual with bilateral densely calcified pleural thickening due to previous tuberculous infection. Note the previous right thoracoplasty.

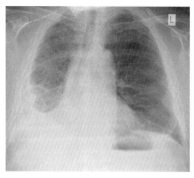

Fig. 10.14 CXR of a patient with smooth benign diffuse pleural thickening in the right hemithorax caused by previous asbestos exposure. There is blunting of the costophrenic angle and limited pleural fluid.

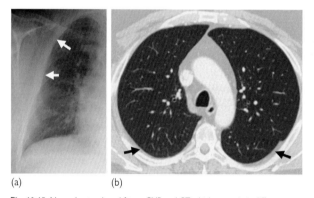

(a)   (b)

Fig. 10.15 Normal extrapleural fat on CXR and CT which may mimic diffuse pleural thickening. (a) CXR showing smooth density internal to the ribs (arrows). Importantly, there is no blunting of the costophrenic angles. (b) CT in the same patient demonstrating the typical (low) density characteristics of normal extrapleural fat (arrows).

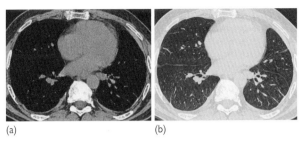

(a)   (b)

Fig. 10.16 CT of bilateral diffuse pleural thickening caused by asbestos exposure on (a) mediastinal and (b) lung windows settings showing linear pleuro-parenchymal bands.

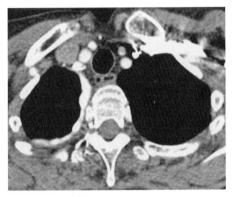

Fig. 10.17 CT in a patient with pleural thickening following talc pleurodesis. Note the hyperdense pleura on the right.

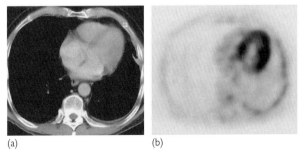

(a)   (b)

Fig. 10.18 (a) CT and (b) ^{18}FDG-PET/CT study showing moderate uptake of ^{18}FDG tracer (SUV = 3.5) in a patient with benign diffuse pleural thickening caused by asbestos exposure. There was no change at 2 year follow-up.

Asbestos-related pleural disease

Exposure to asbestos is associated with benign and malignant pleural disease.

Asbestos-related pleural diseases

- Benign
  - Effusion
  - Pleural plaques
  - Diffuse pleural thickening
  - 'Folded' lung and pleuro-parenchymal bands
- Malignant
  - Malignant pleural mesothelioma

Pleural plaques

- Discrete areas of hyaline fibrosis, arising from the parietal pleura caused by occupational or environmental exposure to asbestos; plaques do not appear until at least 20–30 years after first exposure have elapsed.
- Histopathologically, plaques consist of raised areas of smooth hyaline fibrosis, giving a characteristic thoracoscopic appearance likened to 'icing on a cake'. Usually bilateral, under the anterior and lateral surfaces of the ribs, in the paravertebral regions, on the hemidiaphragmatic pleural surface. May or may not be calcified.
- Pathogenesis of plaque formation is not fully understood but is likely to be related to mechanical effects of asbestos fibres on the parietal pleura.
- Plaques do not predispose to mesothelioma and are not associated with functional impairment or symptoms.
- Plaques may slowly increase in size, as may the degree of calcification over time.

Imaging of pleural plaques

CXR findings (Fig. 10.19)

Detection of plaques on CXR is dependent on their size, position, presence/absence of calcification, and technical factors.

- Multiple opacities—well-defined and typically bilateral (NB post-mortem studies show 10% are unilateral).
- Plaques oriented tangential to the x-ray beam appear as discrete areas of pleural thickening with well-demarcated edges whereas lesions that are *en face* have a 'holly leaf' configuration.
- Conspicuity of plaques is increased when calcified.
- Plaques are most apparent in the region of the 6th–9th ribs laterally or on the diaphragmatic surface; costophrenic angles are characteristically spared.

CT findings (Figs. 10.20–10.23)

CT is more sensitive than CXR, particularly for the detection of small non-calcified plaques under ribs and in the paravertebral region. The CT signs of asbestos-related plaques are:

- Focal (discontinuous) foci of soft-tissue thickening of the pleura ± calcification. Usually bilateral and well-circumscribed with well-demarcated (squared-off) edges.
- Usually involve parietal pleura (occasionally on visceral pleura with plaques in fissures).

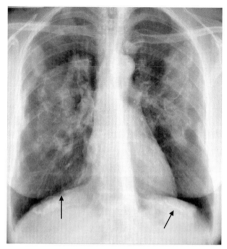

Fig. 10.19 CXR in a patient with calcified bilateral pleural plaques. Note the diaphragmatic pleural plaques (arrows). Reproduced with permission from *Self-assessment Colour Review of Thoracic Imaging*, SJ Copley, DM Hansell and NL Müller. Manson Publishing Ltd, 2005.

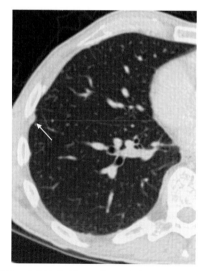

Fig. 10.20 CT in an individual with a small non-calcified asbestos-induced pleural plaque (arrow), not identified on CXR.

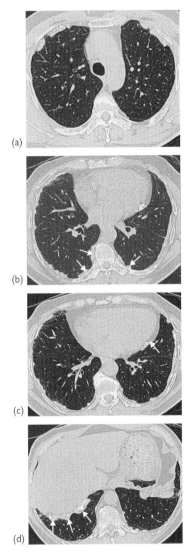

(a)

(b)

(c)

(d)

Fig. 10.21 CT in an patient with extensive calcified pleural plaques (a) under the anterior upper ribs, (b) in the paravertebral regions (arrows), (c) on the mediastinal and (d) the diaphragmatic pleura (arrows).

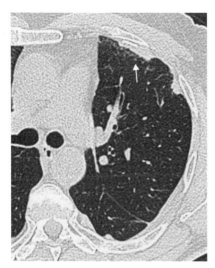

Fig. 10.22 CT in an individual with calcified pleural plaques and a subtle subpleural reticular pattern (arrow) possibly due to mechanical effects on the underlying lung rather than asbestosis.

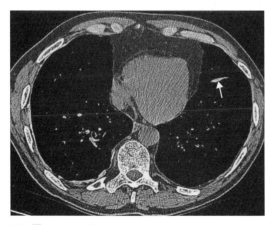

Fig. 10.23 CT on mediastinal window settings in an asbestos-exposed individual demonstrating a pleural plaque in the oblique fissure (arrow).

Diffuse pleural thickening

Diffuse pleural thickening in asbestos-exposed individuals is a consequence of haemorrhagic exudates resulting in visceral pleural fibrosis. The radiological features of diffuse pleural thickening are not specific and similar to any other cause of diffuse pleural thickening; a noteworthy exception is the finding of pleural plaques which can coexist. Encysted pleural fluid may also be evident. Occasionally, it may be difficult to differentiate between extensive pleural plaques and diffuse pleural thickening.

'Folded' lung and pleuro-parenchymal bands

- Folded lung (synonyms: 'rounded atelectasis', pulmonary pseudotumour, or atelectatic pseudotumour) refers to peripheral atelectatic lung adjacent to an area of pleural thickening. Pleuro-parenchymal bands (also termed 'crows feet') are thought to be a *forme fruste* of folded lung.
- First recognized in asbestos-exposed individuals but known to occur as a consequence of any exudative pleural effusion (e.g. following thoracic trauma or surgery).
- The pathogenesis is not clear but thought to be due to compression and atelectasis of lung parenchyma by pleural fluid which results in adherence of the parenchyma.
- Pleuro-parenchymal bands are a useful ancillary feature of subtle diffuse pleural thickening affecting the visceral pleura. Such bands may be functionally significant but in medicolegal terms, it is important to differentiate bands from asbestosis.

Imaging of folded lung

The radiological features which confirm the benign nature of this abnormality are not always identified on CXR. The distinction between folded lung and a mass, such as lung cancer, cannot always be made with confidence on CXR. In contrast, the CT appearances of folded lung are usually characteristic.

CXR findings (Fig. 10.24)
- Rounded mass—typically 3–5cm in diameter, abutting an area of pleural thickening.
- Bilateral or unilateral.
- The lingula and right middle lobe (followed by the lower lobes) are the most commonly affected sites.

CT findings (Fig. 10.24)
- Rounded/wedge-shaped mass—with swirling bronchovascular structures (likened to a 'comet-tail') leading into mass.
- Localized pleural thickening—in contact with the peripheral mass.
- Volume loss—in affected lobe.

US findings
- Rounded mass.
- Thickening of adjacent pleura.
- Highly echogenic line—extending from the pleura into the mass.

MRI findings
The appearances are similar to those seen at CT. The specific features on MR images are:
- Low signal on T1-weighted and high signal on T2-weighted images but with areas of hypointensity.
- Enhancement following IV gadolinium.

[18]FDG-PET findings
- Folded lung may demonstrate low grade [18]FDG uptake.

Imaging of pleuro-parenchymal bands

CXR findings (Fig. 10.25)
- Linear bands—generally measuring ~2–3cm in length and associated with pleural thickening; may be single or multiple.

CT findings (Fig. 10.25)
- Linear bands—making contact with diffusely thickened visceral pleura. Bands may be single or multiple, radiating either from a focal point (giving rise to a 'crow's foot' appearance) or multiple points from the thickened pleura.
- Parenchymal distortion/volume loss.

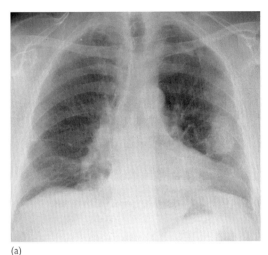

(a)

(b)

Fig. 10.24 CXR and CT of folded lung. (a) CXR in an individual with folded lung in the left midzone. The appearances simulate lung cancer. (b) CT demonstrating the characteristic swirling ('comet tail') of bronchovascular structures arising from the peripheral mass which makes contact with the thickened pleural surface; there is volume loss (note the position of the oblique fissure [arrow]) by comparison with the fissure on the right.

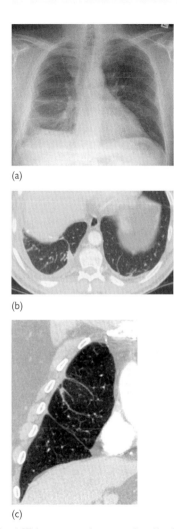

(a)

(b)

(c)

Fig. 10.25 CXR and CT demonstrating pleuro-parenchymal bands. (a) CXR shows multiple pleuro-parenchymal bands in association with right diffuse pleural thickening. (b) CT in another patient with diffuse pleural thickening and bilateral pleuro-parenchymal bands. (c) Targeted coronal CT through the right lung shows smooth pleural thickening and multiple linear bands arising from a focal point.

Malignant pleural mesothelioma

- An inexorably progressive primary tumour of the pleura which is strongly (but not invariably) linked to previous asbestos exposure.
- The incidence of malignant pleural mesothelioma (MPM) is increasing and likely to peak in around 2020 in the UK and Europe; ♂ > ♀. Long latency (~20–40 years) between exposure and development of mesothelioma. The outlook remains poor with a median survival of ≤12 months.
- Mesothelioma occurs with exposure to any type of asbestos fibre but amphiboles (such as crocicolite ('blue' asbestos) with its needle-shaped fibres) are most carcinogenic.
- Three histopathological subtypes of MPM are recognized: epithelioid (most frequent), sarcomatoid, and mixed (biphasic).
- Differentiation between metastatic pleural adenocarcinoma, mesothelioma, and reactive mesothelial hyperplasia can be difficult but has improved with the development of antibody-based and immunohistochemical (e.g. calretinin and cytokeratin) tests.
- Macroscopically, the tumour forms plaques, nodules, or sheet-like thickening on the visceral and parietal pleura which result in lung encasement.

Imaging of malignant pleural mesothelioma

CXR findings (Figs. 10.26 and 10.27)

- Pleural thickening—typically lobulated (nodular), circumferential, and restricted to one hemithorax; a localized mass is uncommon.
- Pleural effusion—of variable volume. However, even with a large volume of pleural fluid there may be relatively little contralateral mediastinal shift (a pointer to the diagnosis). With progression, the volume of pleural fluid generally decreases as tumour volume increases.
- Volume loss—even with apparently limited disease.
- Rib destruction or pneumothorax—rare.

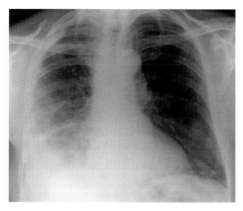

Fig. 10.26 CXR in a patient with proven mesothelioma. There is subtle right-sided volume loss and a small pleural effusion.

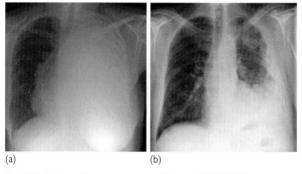

(a)   (b)

Fig. 10.27 Radiographic progression in mesothelioma (a) Initial CXR in a patient with a large pleural effusion due to MPM with contralateral mediastinal shift. (b) Subsequent CXR taken several months later shows reduction in the volume of pleural fluid after drainage but conspicuous lobulated pleural thickening.

CT findings (Fig. 10.28)

Typical CT features

The CT features described here are relatively specific but far less sensitive for malignancy. Therefore, these signs have a high positive predictive value but a low negative predictive value. CT features do not reliably distinguish between MPM and metastatic pleural adenocarcinoma.

- Pleural thickening—generally exceeding 1cm in thickness, circumferential or involving the mediastinal pleura (mediastinal pleural thickening may be subtle but is highly suggestive of malignancy).
- Thickening may involve the fissures.
- Pleural nodularity
- Pleural effusion—see also 'CXR findings'.

Less common CT features

- Chest wall invasion—less common; may occur along the track of a previous percutaneous biopsy or chest drain insertion (in the absence of 'prophylactic' local radiotherapy).
- Focal mass ± rib destruction
- Calcification—may be due to coexisting pleural plaques or (rarely) as a manifestation of osteoblastic stromal calcification in patients with mixed-type mesothelioma.

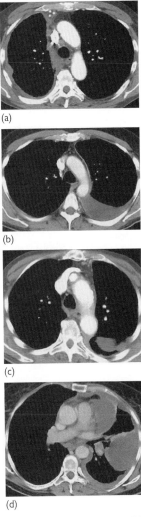

(a)

(b)

(c)

(d)

Fig. 10.28 CT appearances of MPM (a) Contrast-enhanced CT in MPM demonstrating circumferential and nodular malignant pleural thickening in the right hemithorax. (b) CT in another patient shows subtle pleural thickening of the mediastinal pleural surface on the left. (c) CT image demonstrating tumour nodularity extending along the oblique fissure. (d) CT in a patient with biopsy-proven MPM; there is loculated pleural fluid resembling an empyema (but note the marked volume loss within the left hemithorax).

Ultrasound findings (Fig. 10.29)

- May be useful to demonstrate pleural thickening/nodularity) in patients with an otherwise undiagnosed pleural effusion. Ultrasound may also be useful for guiding biopsy (NB colour Doppler ultrasonography may be then used to avoid intercostal vessels).

MRI findings (Fig. 10.30)

- Pleural thickening/nodularity—on T1-weighted images MPM has a slightly greater signal intensity than muscle and moderately greater than muscle on T2-weighted sequences; there is enhancement following IV gadolinium.
- Contrast-enhanced fat-saturation T1-weighted images may distinguish benign from malignant disease.

[18]FDG-PET findings

- Different patterns of radioisotope uptake are recognized including an encircling pattern and focal pleural uptake.
- Useful for demonstrating unsuspected nodal or extrathoracic metastases.
- Comparable accuracy to CT and MR for differentiating benign from malignant disease (NB false negatives = epitheloid-type MPM, false positives = pleural plaques).
- May be useful to guide biopsy to metabolically active areas of disease in selected cases.
- [18]FDG uptake is broadly correlated inversely with survival.

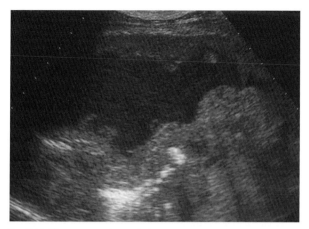

Fig. 10.29 US in a patient with mesothelioma demonstrating nodular pleural thickening.

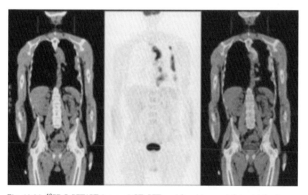

Fig. 10.30 ^{18}FDG-PET/CT (coronal CT, PET, and fused images left to right) of a patient with mesothelioma showing left pleural uptake of tracer. Reprinted from *Clinical Radiology* 2005:**60**;1237–47 Benamore R. O'Doherty MJ, Entwistle JJ. Use of imaging in the management of malignant pleural mesothelioma, with permission from Elsevier.

Benign pleural tumours

Benign pleural tumours are rare and only two (localized fibrous tumour (fibroma) and pleural lipoma) are considered here. The majority of patients are asymptomatic and such lesions are often discovered incidentally.

Imaging features of pleural vs pulmonary lesions

It is important to distinguish between lung and pleural masses, which, when large, may be suprisingly difficult. A careful analysis of the imaging findings may permit such a distinction. The features on CXR and CT which may favour one over the other are summarized below (Table 10.3; Figs. 10.31 and 10.32).

Table 10.3 CXR/CT features of pleural and pulmonary lesions

- **Pleural lesions**
  - Broadest at base
  - Obtuse angle of contact with pleural surface/chest wall
  - Well-defined medial margin but more ill-defined laterally
- **Pulmonary lesions**
  - Narrower at base
  - Acute angle of contact with pleural surface/chest wall
  - Well-defined around non-pleurally based margins of the lesion

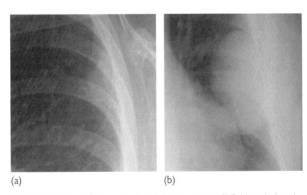

(a)   (b)

Fig. 10.31 (a) Magnified view of a pleurally-based lesion on CXR. Note the broad base and obtuse angle in relation to the pleural surface/chest wall. (b) Magnified view in a patient with a peripheral lung lesion abutting the pleura showing a narrow base and an acute angle where the lesion makes contact with the pleural surface/chest wall.

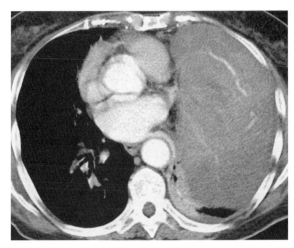

Fig. 10.32 CT in a patient with a large localized fibrous tumour occupying much of the left hemithorax. Determining whether the mass originates in the lung or from the pleura is not straightforward for a tumour of this size. Note the enhancement of vessels within the mass following IV contrast.

Pneumothorax

- Pneumothorax is an abnormal collection of air in the pleural space.
- Pneumothoraces may broadly be categorized as being spontaneous (primary or secondary) or traumatic (Tables 10.4 and 10.5).
- Primary spontaneous pneumothorax occurs in otherwise healthy individuals with an approximate incidence of 10/100,000 population. There is an association with smoking; most commonly occur in males aged between 20–40 years. The typical cause is rupture of an apical subpleural bleb. Pneumothoraces may be bilateral but are not usually synchronous.
- Secondary pneumothoraces generally occur in individuals with underlying lung disease (Table 10.4) and are less common than primary pneumothoraces.

Table 10.4 Causes of a spontaneous pneumothorax

- **Primary**
  - Primary spontaneous
  - Familial (rare)
- **Secondary**
  - Airflow obstruction (e.g. COPD)
  - Infection (e.g. subpleural cavitating pneumonia, pneumatocoeles)
  - Infarction
  - Neoplasms (primary or secondary)
  - Diffuse lung disease (e.g. Langerhans' cell histiocytosis, tuberous sclerosis, lymphangioleiomyomatosis, idiopathic pulmonary fibrosis, sarcoidosis)
  - Catamenial pneumothorax (endometriosis)
  - Inherited connective tissue disorders (e.g. Marfan's syndrome)

Table 10.5 Causes of traumatic pneumothoraces

- **Iatrogenic**
  - Mechanical ventilation
  - Thoracotomy or thoracocentesis
  - Percutaneous biopsy or drainage (e.g. lung, renal, biliary)
  - Tracheostomy
  - Central venous catheter insertion
- **Non-iatrogenic**
  - Closed injuries (ruptured oesophagus or trachea)
  - Penetrating injuries

Imaging of pneumothorax

In uncomplicated cases, the CXR is the only imaging test required for the diagnosis and follow-up of patients presenting with a pneumothorax.

CXR findings (Figs. 10.33–10.36)
Erect CXR
- A visible visceral pleural edge—parallel to the chest wall with absence of vascular markings in pneumothorax space. NB Prominent skin folds, clothing, and hair projected on the chest wall occasionally mimic the appearance of a visceral pleural edge.
- Pleural effusion—usually of limited volume due to blood in the pleural space; this is an almost invariable finding.
- Contralateral mediastinal shift and/or diaphragmatic depression—indicating increased pressure in the pleural cavity and a potential medical emergency (tension pneumothorax).

Lateral CXR
- Visibility of the anterior/posterior visceral pleural edge. NB A lateral 'shoot-through' projection is sometimes of value for the detection of pneumothoraces in critically-ill supine patients.

Supine CXR
- Increased (hypochondrial or hemithoracic) transradiancy—this may be more readily apparent when serial CXRs are reviewed.
- Increased clarity of mediastinal, cardiac, or diaphragmatic margins.
- Deep costophrenic sulcus (the 'deep sulcus sign') or depression of the hemidiaphragm.
- Lucency (air) in the major or minor fissures, in the subpulmonic space.

Ultrasound findings (Fig. 10.37)
Ultrasound may be of value in detecting pneumothoraces particularly in situations where the CXR appearances are complex and difficult to interpret (e.g. in critically-ill patients on ICU). Ultrasound features which may identify a pneumothorax are:
- The absence of comet tail artefacts at chest wall/lung interface
- The lack of pleural 'gliding' on real-time ultrasound imaging.

NB COPD and emphysematous bullae may mimic the appearances of a pneumothorax on US.

CT findings
CT is not usually indicated for the diagnosis of pneumothoraces. However, it may be useful in specific circumstances (e.g. on ICU) where CXR appearances may be difficult to interpret, if a loculated pneumothorax (or another complication) is suspected or if intervention is being considered. The CT appearances of a pneumothorax generally pose no problems in interpretation. However, occasionally, the differentiation of a large bulla from a pneumothorax may be difficult, even on CT.

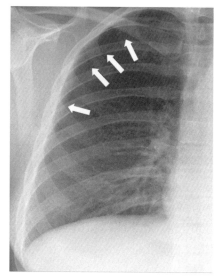

Fig. 10.33 CXR in a young female patient with a subtle right pneumothorax. Note the visceral pleural/lung edge (arrows).

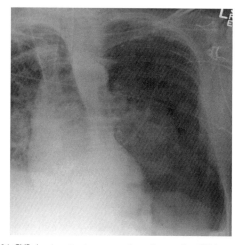

Fig. 10.34 CXR showing a tension pneumothorax in a ventilated ICU patient, requiring immediate treatment. There is mediastinal deviation to the contralateral side and a 'deep sulcus' sign.

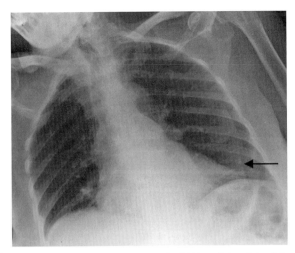

Fig. 10.35 CXR in a patient with a prominent skin fold (arrow) that mimics a left pneumothorax. Note how the line does not extend to the apex and that lung markings are visible lateral to this line.

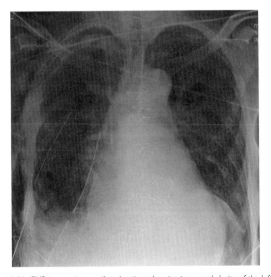

Fig. 10.36 CXR in a supine ventilated patient showing increased clarity of the left heart border because of air in the antero-medial pleural space.

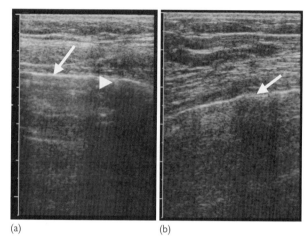

(a)   (b)

Fig. 10.37 Ultrasound showing (a) normal 'comet-tail' artefact (arrowhead) below the pleural-chest wall interface (arrow). (b) Ultrasound in another patient with a pneumothorax: there is an absence of any comet-tails. The arrow again shows the pleural-chest wall interface.

Localized fibrous tumour (fibroma)

- A tumour derived from the submesenchymal cells of the visceral pleura; the tumour is benign in the majority of patients but there is a spectrum of aggressiveness.
- Presents in adults (aged 45–65 years); ♂:♀ ≈ 1:1.
- Not linked with previous asbestos exposure or smoking but there is an association with previous thoracic irradiation.
- The tumour is commonly attached to the pleura via a vascular pedicle (accounting for a characteristic 'mobile mass').
- Usually indolent and may be present for >20 years.
- Rare sites include the paraspinal, paramediastinal, intra-fissural, and intraparenchymal regions.

Imaging of localized fibrous tumour

CXR findings (Fig. 10.38)

- Rounded or oval mass—in contact with pleural surface; variable size (1–40 cm in diameter; the majority are >7cm in diameter).
- Generally arise in lower portion of thorax and slow-growing.
- Depending on position, the appearances may mimic a raised hemidiaphragm. Obtuse angle with the pleural surface/chest wall (NB rarely an acute angle due to the vascular pedicle).
- Change in shape/position—demonstrated with different patient positioning (e.g. supine versus prone) or with different levels of inspiratory effort (e.g. inspiratory and expiratory).

CT findings (Fig. 10.39)

- Rounded or oval mass—pleurally-based (when the lesion is large this may be difficult to appreciate even on CT). Well-defined and of soft tissue attenuation (NB low attenuation may indicate necrosis (particularly in larger tumours)).
- Acute angle with pleural surface at some point (due to the vascular pedicle).
- Enhancement following IV contrast (this may be heterogeneous in both benign and malignant lesions) with prominent vessels.
- Change in shape/position.
- Calcification—uncommon.
- Pleural effusions—rare.

Ultrasound findings
- Hypoechoic mass ± cystic areas.

MRI findings
- Rounded or oval mass—heterogeneous signal on T1- and T2-weighted images; there are no differentiating features between benign and malignant lesions.
- Enhancement following IV gadolinium.

¹⁸FDG-PET findings
- Few reports in the literature. May demonstrate low to moderate ¹⁸FDG uptake but avid uptake if malignant degeneration present.

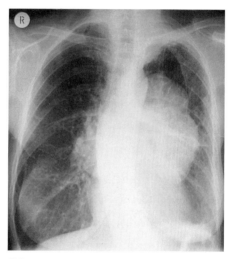

Fig. 10.38 CXR in a patient with a large left pleural fibroma.

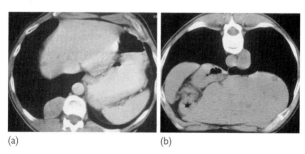

(a)   (b)

Fig. 10.39 CT of a pleural solitary fibrous tumour in (a) supine and (b) prone positions showing a characteristic change in shape because of a vascular pedicle.

Pleural lipoma

- A benign pleural lesion arising from subpleural fat; NB malignant liposarcomas are extremely rare.

Imaging of pleural lipomas

CXR findings (Fig. 10.40)
- Pleurally-based mass—smooth and well-defined with a rounded or lenticular shape.
- Pliable so may change in shape with different phases of breathing.

CT findings (Fig. 10.41)
- Pleurally-based mass—density characteristics (uniform fat attenuation (−70HU to −130HU)) are obvious on CT. Minor soft tissue stranding may be visible but admixed fat and soft tissue attenuation should raise suspicions of a malignant liposarcoma. May change shape with respiration

MRI findings
- Pleurally-based mass—'fat' signal (high signal on T1- and intermediate signal on T2-weighted images).

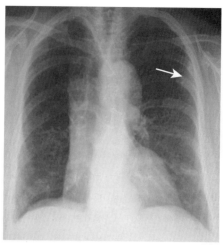

Fig. 10.40 CXR in a patient with a pleural lipoma (arrow). There is a subtle broad-based lesion in the left upper zone.

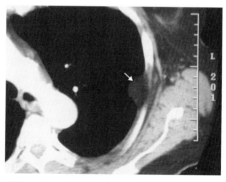

Fig. 10.41 CT in a patient with a pleural lipoma (arrow). Note the fat density, similar to subcutaneous fat.

Mediastinal diseases

Mediastinal masses

Mediastinal masses are frequently detected as incidental findings on CXR or CT and the list of possible causes is wide (Tables 11.1 and 11.2; Figs. 11.1 and 11.2). A systematic approach, paying particular attention to the age of the patient, the anatomical localization of the lesion and the morphological/density characteristics will allow the observer to suggest the correct diagnosis or, at the very least, a manageably short list of differential diagnoses.

Radiological considerations

Confirming the mediastinal origin of a mass

Making the distinction between a mass which originates in the mediastinum from one that is primarily within lung is not usually a problem on CT or MRI. However, interpretative difficulties may arise on CXR. Thus, a knowledge of radiographic anatomy and, specifically, on the normal lines, interfaces and recesses that are usually visible on a CXR is helpful (see also 📖 Key radiological anatomy/Mediastinal anatomy, p27).

CXR findings

Signs on CXR that may indicate the presence of a mediastinal abnormality include:
- Absence or bulging of the azygo-oesophageal line
- Increased opacification in the retro-sternal space on a lateral CXR
- Splaying of the carina
- Filling-in of the aortopulmonary window
- Loss of the paravertebral or the paratracheal stripes.

CT findings

Difficulties may occasionally arise on CT when a pulmonary mass makes contact with the mediastinum or when a large mediastinal mass appears to protrude beyond the confines of the mediastinum. The CT signs which favour one over the other are:
- Spiculated or irregular margin (lung > mediastinal)
- Well-defined margins (mediastinal > lung)
- Broad-base on the mediastinum (mediastinal > lung)
- Obtuse angle at the edges of the lesion (mediastinal > lung).

The influence of age

The relative prevalence of different mediastinal masses varies with age. Some of the causes of mediastinal masses in children and adults are listed in Table 11.1.

Table 11.1 Variable causes of mediastinal masses in children and adults

Paediatric	Adult
Neurogenic tumours	Metastatic nodal enlargement
Germ cell tumours	Goitre
Thymic hyperplasia	Thymoma
Lymphoma	Lymphoma
Developmental cysts	Neurogenic tumours

The anatomical location in the mediastinum

The location of lesions in the mediastinum is based on arbitrary and ultimately non-anatomical compartments of the mediastinum (e.g. anterior, posterior and superior mediastinum). A more practical system—which has relevance for CT—describes the location as related to readily recognizable anatomical landmarks (e.g. paracardiac, paravertebral, or paratracheal). See Table 11.2.

Table 11.2 Causes of a mediastinal mass predicted by anatomical location

- **Pre-vascular**
  Lymph node enlargement (benign or malignant)
  Thymic enlargement/masses or cyst (except thymolipoma)
  Germ cell tumours
  Aneurysms
  Parathyroid cyst
  Lymphangioma (cystic hygroma)
- **Pre-tracheal, subcarinal, and paraoesophageal**
  Lymph node enlargement
  Developmental cysts—bronchogenic and oesophageal
  Thyroid enlargement/masses
  Hiatus hernia
- **Paracardiac/juxtadiaphragmatic**
  Developmental cysts—pericardial
  Fat pad
  Lymph node enlargement
  Thymolipoma
  Diaphragmatic hernia
- **Paravertebral**
  Neurogenic tumours
  Lymph node enlargement
  Developmental cysts—neurenteric and gastroenteric
  Abscess
  Extramedullary haemopoeisis

Adapted from *Imaging of Diseases of the Chest*. Hansell DM, Lynch DA, McAdams HP, Bankier AA (Eds) 5th Edition (2010). Mosby– Elsevier.

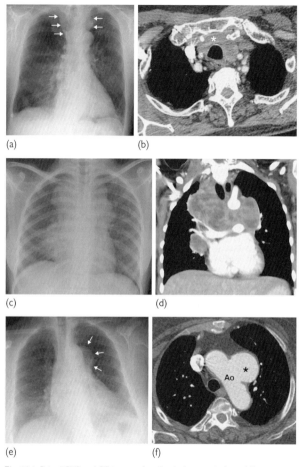

Fig. 11.1 Paired CXR and CT images of mediastinal masses in three different patients. (a) Thyroid enlargement: there is a well-defined opacity in the upper mediastinum (arrows) whose lateral margins can be 'traced' in their entirety. (b) Corresponding CT confirms the presence of a mass that straddles the trachea anterior and laterally (asterisk). (c) CXR shows bilateral lobulated soft-tissue density masses caused by tuberculous lymph nodes. (d) Coronal CT shows extensive (necrotic) mediastinal lymph node enlargement. (e) CXR with a mediastinal mass adjacent to (but not obscuring) the aortic arch with well-defined lateral margins (arrows). (f) CT at the level of the aortic arch (Ao) confirms the diagnosis of a saccular aortic aneurysm (black asterisk).

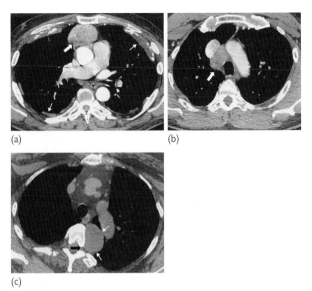

Fig. 11.2 Three examples of masses in different mediastinal locations. (a) CT below the carina shows a well-defined nodal mass in the pre-vascular space (thick arrow); incidental asbestos-related plaques (thin arrows) are noted. (b) Right paratracheal nodal mass (arrow) in a patient with lymphoma. (c) CT through the upper zone shows a well-defined mass (white arrows)—a neurofibroma; note the close proximity to the intervertebral foramen (black arrow).

Density characteristics

The evaluation of differential densities within a mediastinal mass is important (Fig. 11.3). Because of the superior contrast resolution and the absence of any anatomical superimposition, the density characteristics of a mediastinal lesion are readily judged on CT. Magnetic resonance imaging (MRI) may have a role in some patients. The important density changes of diagnostic value include:

- Calcification: typically occurs in lymph nodes but also goitres and in a variety of mediastinal neoplasms including thymoma, germ cell tumours, duplication cysts, neurogenic tumours.
- Fluid: seen in lesions that are composed predominantly of water such as developmental cysts.
- Fat: lesions which contain fat include pericardial fat pad, germ cell tumours, and a number of thymic tumours (e.g. thymolipoma, thymic liposarcoma).

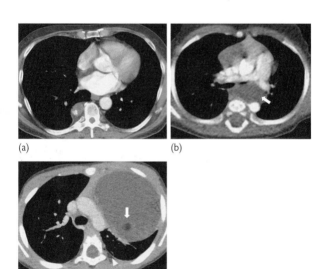

(a)　　　　　　　　　　　　　(b)

(c)

Fig. 11.3 Differential density in mediastinal masses. (a) Amorphous calcification in a biopsy-proven paravertebral neurogenic tumour (b) Fluid density in a duplication cyst; the attenuation (arrow) is lower than the density of soft-tissue as highlighted by the normal thymus (in the prevascular space) (c) Fat density (arrow) in a mediastinal germ cell tumour, roughly comparable to normal fat attenuation in the chest wall (arrowhead).

Lymph node enlargement

Enlargement of mediastinal lymph nodes (often accompanied by enlarged hilar nodes), is a manifestation of many diseases. The list of causes of intrathoracic nodal enlargement is given in Table 11.3; the term 'lymph node enlargement' is preferred to the often used 'lymphadenopathy' because size criteria alone do not discriminate between (normal) 'reactive hyperplasia' and important disease. In specific circumstances, a confident diagnosis may be suggested on the basis of radiological findings. However, in many cases, the appearances are non-specific and a diagnosis may only be established by histopathological examination.

Table 11.3 Causes of intrathoracic lymph node enlargement

- **Reactive**
- **Neoplastic**
  - Lymphoproliferative diseases
  - Metastatic disease
- **Infections**
  - Mycobacterial (tuberculous, non-tuberculous)
  - Bacterial
  - Fungal
  - Viral
- **Inflammatory**
  - Sarcoidosis
  - Suppurative airways disease (e.g. bronchiectasis)
  - Idiopathic interstitial pneumonias and other diffuse interstitial lung diseases
  - Occupational lung disease (e.g. silicosis, coal worker's pneumoconiosis, chronic berylliosis, asbestosis)
  - Connective tissue diseases (e.g. rheumatoid arthritis)
  - Amyloid
- **Miscellaneous**
  - Drug-induced
  - Left ventricular failure with pulmonary oedema

Radiological features of diagnostic value in patients with intrathoracic lymph node enlargement

In patients with enlarged mediastinal lymph nodes, close analysis (Figs. 11.4 and 11.5) will, in some instances, allow refinement of the differential diagnoses.

Nodal calcification

The identification of calcification within enlarged lymph nodes generally (but not always) excludes malignant disease. The commonest benign causes of lymph node calcification are:

- Post-tuberculous infection.
- Sarcoidosis.
- Occupational lung diseases—silicosis, coal worker's pneumoconiosis.

Malignant tumours in which nodal calcification is known to occur include:
- Lymphoma following treatment—lymph node calcification prior to treatment occurs in <1% of cases.
- Metastases from osteogenic sarcoma, chondrosarcoma, and mucinous adenocarcinoma.

The pattern/distribution of calcification in lymph nodes
The manner in which calcification is deposited in lymph nodes may be of diagnostic value. For example, the distribution of calcification within enlarged nodes differs between sarcoidosis and tuberculosis: calcification tends to be more focal within lymph nodes in sarcoidosis but more often occupies the entire node in tuberculosis. Nodal calcification is also more often bilateral and 'softer' (resembling icing sugar) in sarcoidosis.

Another example of calcium deposition in lymph nodes is the well-known 'egg-shell' pattern. This occurs most commonly in silicosis and coal worker's pneumoconiosis but is also encountered in sarcoidosis, treated Hodgkin's lymphoma, blastomycosis, histoplasmosis, and amyloidosis.

Low density within enlarged lymph nodes
Low attenuation at the hila of lymph nodes represents normal fat in the sinus. More extensive and central low attenuation with a rim of high attenuation in enlarged nodes indicates necrosis which is most commonly seen in mycobacterial (tuberculous or non-tuberculous) infections or in metastatic lymph nodes. Necrosis in lymphomatous nodes is recognized but is uncommon.

Distribution of nodal enlargement
The distribution of intrathoracic lymph node enlargement may favour one diagnosis over another. The combination of mediastinal, particularly sub-carinal, and symmetrical hilar lymph node enlargement is typical of sarcoidosis (see also 📖 Diffuse parenchymal lung diseases/Granulomatous DPLD: sarcoidosis, p190). By contrast, bilateral but asymmetrical hilar nodal enlargement with mediastinal lymph nodes raises the possibility of lymphoma. In tuberculosis, nodal enlargement is determined by lymphatic drainage pathways and tends to be on the side of any intrapulmonary disease. Isolated paracardiac or paravertebral lymph nodes are unlikely to be due to sarcoidosis and should prompt consideration of alternative diagnoses (e.g. lymphoma, metastatic disease).

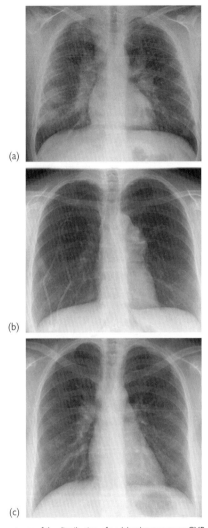

(a)

(b)

(c)

Fig. 11.4 Importance of the distribution of nodal enlargement on CXR.
(a) Symmetrical hilar and right paratracheal nodal enlargement in sarcoidosis; there
are also multiple nodules in the right lung. (b) Abnormal enlargement of lymph
nodes in the aortopulmonary window in lymphoma and (c) unilateral enlargement
of right hilar and tracheobronchial lymph nodes in a young TB-contact with a
positive Mantoux test.

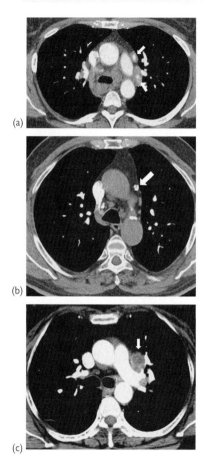

Fig. 11.5 Importance of the density characteristics of enlarged lymph nodes on CT. (a) Nodal enlargement in sarcoidosis the calcification (arrows) is focal, central and has a 'soft' quality. (b) Unilateral nodal calcification caused by tuberculosis; calcification (arrow) occupies almost the whole node and is 'harder' than in sarcoidosis. (c) Low central attenuation (necrosis) in an enlarged tuberculous lymph node (arrow).

Mediastinal cystic lesions

Cystic lesions of the mediastinum are uncommon and often incidental findings on imaging tests. The causes of cystic mediastinal lesions are listed in Table 11.4 and the imaging findings of specific causes are given below. Of the various causes of mediastinal cysts, the developmental (foregut duplication) cysts are the most frequent.

Table 11.4 Causes of mediastinal cystic lesions

- **Developmental (foregut duplication) cysts**
- **Thymic cyst**
- **Cystic degeneration in mediastinal tumours**
  - Thymoma
  - Lymphoma
  - Germ cell tumours
- **Hydatid cyst**
- **Mediastinal abscess**
- **Thoracic duct cyst**
- **Parathyroid cyst/carcinoma**
- **Pancreatic pseudocyst**
- **Lymphangioma (cystic hygroma)**
- **Lateral thoracic meningocoele**

Imaging of mediastinal cysts

Mediasinal cysts have relatively stereotypical features which will depend, to a greater or lesser degree on size, location and composition of the lesion.

Most cystic or cyst-like lesions have a homogeneous soft tissue density on CXR whereas CT will demonstrate the predominant fluid composition (an attenuation value of <20HU). The thickness of the cyst wall, the presence of solid components and enhancement (if any) following IV contrast will be readily demonstrated on CT and MRI. In some cysts a high protein content, calcium, or haemorrhage increases the density of the cyst contents. MRI may also be of value: a cyst containing water will give low signal on T1-weighted and high signal on T2-weighted images. Lesions with proteinaceous material or blood are associated with high signal on both T1- and T2-weighted MR sequences.

Miscellaneous cystic mediastinal lesions

Bronchogenic cyst

- Rare congenital lesion caused by anomalous branching of the foregut in the embryo. Cysts are lined by pseudostratified columnar epithelium and contain cartilage, smooth muscle, and mucous glands in their walls.
- Majority present <40 years.
- Majority (65–80%) of bronchogenic cysts are mediastinal but extra-mediastinal (intrapulmonary, pleural) and even extra-thoracic (intra-abdominal, cutaneous, cervical) sites are recognized.

CXR findings (Figs. 11.6 and 11.7)

- Well-defined mediastinal mass.
- Usually in contact with a central airway (trachea, right/left main bronchi).
- Uncomplicated cysts have a homogeneous density; pockets of air may be seen if infected.
- Calcification in the wall or in suspension 'milk of calcium' is less common.
- Features related to compression of adjacent structures are uncommon because the contents are not usually under tension.

CT findings (Figs. 11.6 and 11.7)

- Well-defined (smooth or lobulated mediastinal mass with a uniform thin wall.
- Most commonly related to tracheal carina or central bonchi.
- Homogeneous fluid density (<20HU) is the norm but cyst contents may appear 'solid'. Higher attenuation may also be seen if the contents become infected, there is haemorrhage, or there is milk of calcium. Low (air) density within the cyst is rare but implies fistulation and/or infection.

Other imaging tests

- In some cases, MRI may demonstrate the fluid composition of a cyst more accurately than CT: signal characteristic generally mirror those of CSF (i.e. on T1-weighted sequences there is homogeneous low signal whereas there is uniform high signal on T2-weighted sequences).
- Endoscopic ultrasound may demonstrate a well-defined mass devoid of internal echoes but with posterior acoustic enhancement; dependent echogenic material may be present.

Oesophageal cyst

- Rare developmental lesions derived from the embryonic foregut.

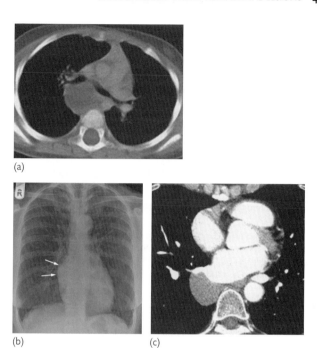

Fig. 11.6 Bronchogenic cyst. (a) A well-defined lesion of low (fluid) attenuation is present in the subcarinal region—a typical location for a bronchogenic cyst. (b) CXR in a different patient, demonstrating an abnormal contour of the right heart border (arrows). (c) CT in the same patient as in (b) confirms a fluid-filled cyst posterior to the right pulmonary venous confluence.

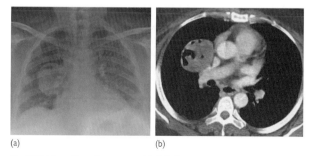

Fig. 11.7 Infected bronchogenic cyst. (a) CXR demonstrates a well-defined lesion in the right mid zone containing an air-fluid level. (b) CT confirms the presence of a complex cystic lesion containing air. Surgical excision confirmed the diagnosis of an infected bronchogenic cyst.

- May be diagnosed at any age but typically in childhood; can cause dysphagia and chest pain.

CXR features (Fig. 11.8)
- Well-defined mass—adjacent to the oesophagus; rounded or tubular.
- Homogeneous density.

CT findings (Fig. 11.8)
- Well defined para-oesophageal mass.
- Fluid or soft-tissue attenuation.

Other imaging tests
- MRI will confirm the fluid nature of cyst contents: there is low signal on T1-weighted and high signal on T2-weighted sequences. In cysts with a high protein content high signal on T1- and T2-wieghted sequences will be seen.
- Radionuclide scanning with [99m]technetium-labelled sodium pertechnetate may confirm the presence of gastric mucosa in some cysts.

Pericardial cyst
- Rare lesions caused by abnormal outpouching of the parietal pericardium during embryological development.

CXR findings (Fig. 11.9)
- Well-defined rounded or ovoid mass adjacent to the heart. In some patients there may be a pointed superior margin on a lateral CXR; this feature is thought to be due to 'drooping' of the cyst from a high attachment to the pericardium.
- Most commonly seen on the right and typically in the cardiophrenic recess but can be found at other sites adjacent to the pericardium.
- Can slowly enlarge over time.

CT findings (Fig. 11.9)
- Well-defined rounded or ovoid mass adjacent to the heart; may have a triangular shape.
- Fluid attenuation in the majority but the density of the lesion may be higher, simulating a solid mediastinal mass.
- Change in size/shape with different levels of inspiratory effort or patient position is of diagnostic value.

Other imaging tests
- MRI will reveal the typical signal characteristics (low on T1- and high on T2-weighted images) of a fluid-containing lesion: high T1 signal is seen in cysts with high proteinaceous content.
- Echocardiography may be of value in diagnosis and surveillance.

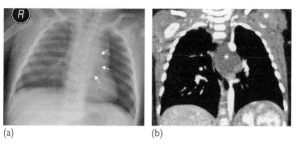

Fig. 11.8 Oesophageal duplication cyst on CXR and CT in a 4-month-old child. (a) CXR demonstrates a subtle but definite mediastinal opacity with a well-defined left lateral border (arrows). (b) Coronal CT showing a well-defined fluid attenuation mass (asterisk).

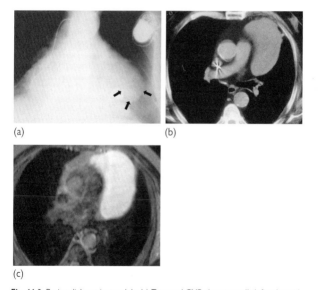

Fig. 11.9 Pericardial cyst in an adult. (a) Targeted CXR shows a well-defined ovoid mass adjacent to the enlarged heart (arrows). (b) CT at the level of the pulmonary trunk shows a well-demarcated mass with a homogeneous density. (c) MR image at the same anatomical level as the CT demonstrates a homogeneous mass with high signal on T1-weighted sequences indicating proteinaceous contents.

Hydatid cyst

- Infection due to *Echinococcus granulosus* most commonly involves the liver. Mediastinal lesions are very uncommon even in endemic regions (e.g. Turkey, North Africa, South America).

CXR findings

- Well-defined mediastinal mass.
- Homogeneous fluid density unless there is cyst rupture or communication with an airway: an air-fluid level and collapsed cyst membranes (the exocyst and endocyst) may be seen producing the 'water lily' sign.

CT findings (Fig. 11.10)

- Well-demarcated lesions; may be seen at various sites in the mediastinum (pre-vascular, pre/paratracheal, paravertebral). In rare instances, a hydatid cyst may be intramyocardial.
- Fluid attenuation ± calcification. In complex cysts, an air-fluid level and/ or membranous layers of the exo- and endocyst may be seen.

Cystic hygroma/cystic lymphangioma

- A rare congenital anomaly representing remnants of lymphatic tissue from the embryological period (arising because of a failure to establish normal communication or abnormal sequestration); an acquired (adult) form also occurs secondary to chronic lymphatic obstruction.
- Typical presentation is in childhood (majority in first 2 years) and young adults: macroscopically, there are cavernous or cystic, endothelium-lined, lymphatic spaces. The majority are found in the neck and axillae. 10% extend into the mediastinum; only 1% are confined to the mediastinum.

CXR findings

- Mass of soft tissue density in the neck and/or mediastinum.

CT findings

CT is usually not indicated and the diagnosis of cystic hygroma is often made with US and/or MRI. CT features include:
- Smooth mediastinal mass with a variable location (i.e. pre-vascular, pre-tracheal, sub-carinal, paracardiac, or para-vertebral).
- Fluid attenuation (<20HU) in the majority but may be of higher density ± enhancement following IV contrast.
- Internal septa may be visible in the cavernous-type of cystic hygroma.

Other imaging tests (Fig. 11.11)

- On MRI, there is low or intermediate/heterogeneous signal on T1-weighted and uniform high or heterogeneous signal on T2-weighted sequences. Multiples locules or septa may be seen in the mass.
- Pre-natal diagnosis of neck and chest wall cystic hygromas is possible with US.

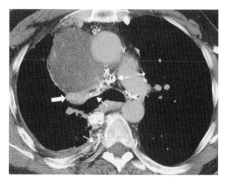

Fig. 11.10 Hydatid cyst in an adult. There is a well-defined mediastinal mass of mixed, but predominantly fluid, attenuation. The cyst is causing compression of the superior vena cava (thick arrow) and there are dilated venous mediastinal and chest wall collaterals (thin arrows).

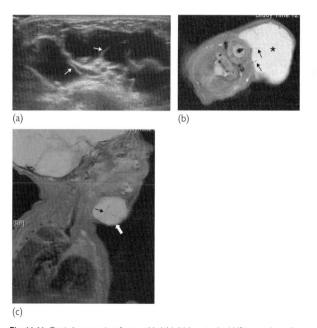

(a)

(b)

(c)

Fig. 11.11 Cystic hygroma in a 3-year-old child. (a) Longitudinal US image through the left antero-lateral neck demonstrating a septated (arrows) cystic lesion. (b) Axial STIR image shows the cystic lesion (asterisk) which contains internal septa (arrows) and (c) sagittal STIR images through the cervical cystic hygroma (white arrow) again demonstrating high signal and internal septa (black arrow).

Lateral thoracic meningocoele

- An outpouching of the spinal meninges commonly associated with neurofibromatosis.

CXR findings

- Well-defined para-vertebral mass of soft tissue density.
- Scalloping of adjacent vertebral bodies and ribs (indicating relative chronicity).
- Thoracic kyphoscoliosis and other stigmata of neurofibromatosis.

CT findings

- Well-defined para-vertebral mass which is typically unilateral; fluid attenuation.
- Communication with the spinal canal through the intervertebral foramen may be seen; pre-CT injection of intrathecal contrast may be of value in confirming communication with CSF in spinal canal.

Other imaging tests

- MRI is the investigation of choice for evaluation of lateral thoracic meningocoeles; MRI signal characteristics are those of fluid (low signal on T1-weighted and high signal on T2-weighted images).
- Communication with the subarachnoid space is readily demonstrated.

Mediastinal fat-containing lesions

The causes of lesions in the mediastinum which are composed predominantly of fatty elements is listed in Table 11.5.

Table 11.5 Mediastinal fat-containing lesions

- **Mediastinal lipomatosis**
  - Corticosteroid therapy
  - Obesity
  - Cushing's disease
- **Tumours of mediastinal fat**
  - Lipoma
  - Liposarcoma
  - Lipoblastoma
- **Tumours containing fat**
  - Thymolipoma
  - Germ cell tumour
- **Herniation of subdiaphragmatic fat**
- **Extramedullary haematopoiesis**

Mediastinal lipomatosis

Mediastinal lipomatosis is synonymous with excessive mediastinal fat and is frequently associated with corticosteroid therapy. The imaging features of mediastinal lipomatosis on CXR and CT are described below.

Imaging of mediastinal lipomatosis

CXR findings (Fig. 11.12)

- Smooth mediastinal widening—no mass effect on adjacent tracheal or vascular structures. Usually associated with excessive extrapleural fat and prominent epicardial fat pads.

CT findings (Fig. 11.12)

- Excessive mediastinal fat—Uniform low attenuation (−70 to −130 HU). Fat deposition may be focal.

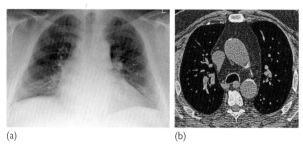

(a)   (b)

Fig. 11.12 Mediastinal lipomatosis. (a) CXR shows a widened superior mediastinum. (b) CT in the same patient with excess fat causing mediastinal widening.

Tumours of mediastinal fat

Tumours originating in mediastinal fat are rare and account for less than 1% of mediastinal masses. The subtypes include benign lipomas and lipoblastomas in children and malignant liposarcomas which occur in middle age.

Imaging tumours of mediastinal fat

CXR findings
- Well-defined, rounded mediastinal masses (benign and malignant).
- Benign lipomas do not compress adjacent structures unless very large.
- Large mediastinal lipomas may simulate cardiomegaly.

CT/MRI findings
- Benign lipomas demonstrate homogeneous fat attenuation or signal intensity; soft tissue strands are a minor component.
- Liposarcomas, angiolipomas, myelolipomas, and lipoblastomas demonstrate variable amounts of fat and soft tissue attenuation or signal intensity.
- Liposarcomas usually occur in the anterior mediastinum and show diffuse infiltration.
- Low-grade liposarcomas may have a large fat component, whereas high-grade liposarcomas typically have a minor fat component and consist of mainly heterogeneous soft tissue.

Subdiaphragmatic fat herniation

Intra-abdominal fat may herniate through a variety of diaphragmatic defects including the foramina of Morgagni or Bochdalek and the oesophageal hiatus.

Imaging subdiaphragmatic fat herniation

CXR findings (Fig. 11.13)

● Soft-tissue density 'mass'—smooth outline; the location of herniation is often characteristic on frontal and lateral CXR.

CT findings (Fig. 11.13)

● 'Mass'—fat attenuation (−70 to −130 HU); omental vessels can sometimes be traced.

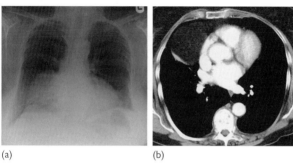

(a)   (b)

Fig. 11.13 (a) CXR showing a right-sided paracardiac mass and (b) CT in the same patient with a Morgagni hernia containing intraperitoneal fat.

Thymus

The thymus is the site of differentiation and maturation of T-lymphocytes. Derived from the branchial pouches in the neck, the thymus descends into the pre-vascular mediastinal space during embryological development. The normal thymus reaches its maximum weight (relative to the body) just before birth, and its greatest absolute weight at puberty, following which there is steady involution.

Normal thymus

Recognizing the normal imaging appearances of the thymus and the changes which occur with age is important when thymic disease is considered (Fig. 11.14). Except in neonates and infants—when the thymus can manifest as a unilateral 'sail-shaped' opacity of soft tissue density—the normal thymus is not visible on CXR. The normal thymus is readily visible on CT and MRI.

Frequency of a visible, normal thymus with respect to age

The frequency with which the normal thymus is seen on CT or MRI varies with age (Table 11.6).

Table 11.6 Identification of normal thymus on CT: variation with age

Age group (years)	Frequency (%)
6–19	100%
20–29	100%
30–39	72%
40–49	74%
>49	17%

Reproduced with permission from Baron RL et al. Computed tomography of the normal thymus. *Radiology* 1982; **142**:121–125. Copyright RSNA Publications.

Location of the normal thymus

The normal thymus is most often centred anterior to the aortic arch. The normal gland may extend caudally to the level of the heart.

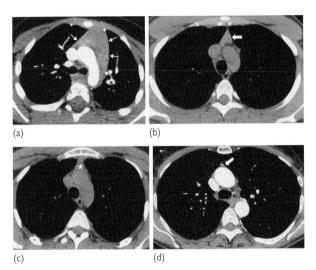

(a)   (b)

(c)   (d)

Fig. 11.14 Normal CT appearances (size and shape) of the thymus at different ages. (a) 1-year-old child with a normal thymus anterior to the aortic arch (arrows). (b) 20-year-old with a normal but smaller thymus. (c) 35-year-old patient with an 'arrowhead' configuration (asterisk) and d) 69-year-old patient with minute residual thymic tissue (arrow).

Shape of the normal thymus

The outline of the normal thymus varies on axial imaging.

Variations in shape of the normal thymus

Shape	Frequency (%)
Arrowhead configuration	> 60%
Two separate lobes*	> 30%
'Single' lobe*	~6%

*Each lobe may be ovoid, elliptical, triangular, or semilunar in outline.

Reproduced with permission from Baron RL et al. Computed tomography of the normal thymus. *Radiology* 1982; **142**:121–125. Copyright RSNA Publications.

Size of the normal thymus and changes with age

At all ages (<49 years), the longitudinal length of the left lobe exceeds that of the right. The maximum thickness of both lobes decreases with age with the greatest decline occurring between ages 6–19 and 20–29 years.

Density characteristics of the normal thymus and changes with age

The attenuation characteristics of the normal thymus change with age: fatty replacement occurs with age and leads to a progressive decrease in density. Under 19 years, the thymus is of soft-tissue attenuation (>30HU) and usually isodense or slightly higher than the muscles of the chest wall. Over 40 years, the density of the thymus tends to approximate that of fat (i.e. < −10HU).

Thymic enlargement/masses

Thymic neoplasms (e.g. thymoma, germ cell tumours, thymic lymphoma) and thymic hyperplasia are the common causes of generalized enlargement (Table 11.7). An enlarged thymus may be discovered as an incidental imaging finding in a patient undergoing investigation for other reasons (e.g. staging tests for a known malignancy or in patients on corticosteroid therapy) or during evaluation of a patient with a condition known to be associated with a thymic enlargement (e.g. myasthenia gravis).

Table 11.7 Causes of thymic enlargement or a thymic mass

- **Thymic neoplasms (benign and malignant)**
  - Thymoma
  - Carcinoma
  - Lymphoma
  - Carcinoid
  - Thymolipoma
- **Thymic hyperplasia ('true' or lymphoid)**
- **Thymic cyst**

Thymoma

- Most common primary epithelial tumour of the thymus. Biological behaviour ranges from a benign encapsulated tumour to locally invasive masses; extrathoracic metastases are uncommon.
- ♂ : ♀ ≈ 1:1, most commonly occurring in 5th–6th decades (uncommon in childhood).

Important associations of thymoma

- **Myasthenia gravis (in 35–50% of patients with thymoma)**
- **Hypogammaglobulinaemia (~10%)**
- **Red blood cell aplasias (~5%)**
- **Other associations**:
  - Connective tissue diseases (rheumatoid arthritis, SLE, Sjögren's syndrome, polymyositis).
  - Autoimmune endocrine disorders (Addison's disease, Cushing's syndrome, Hashimoto's thyroiditis).
  - Neurological disorders (Lambert-Eaton myasthenic syndrome, limbic encephalomyelitis).

Adapted from Rosado-de-Christenson ML et al. Thymoma: radiologic-pathologic correlation. *RadioGraphics* 1992; **12**:151–168 and Nishino M et al. The thymus: a comprehensive review. *RadioGraphics* 2006: **26**:335–348.

Imaging of thymoma
CXR findings (Fig. 11.15)
- Mediastinal mass—smooth outline; unilateral on a frontal CXR. An opacity filling the normal retrosternal lucency on a lateral CXR. Most common in the pre-vascular space but may be seen adjacent to the heart.
- Punctate or peripheral curvilinear calcification.
- Features suggestive of malignancy include an irregular interface of the mass with lung, unilateral pleural nodularity/irregular pleural thickening ± pleural effusion.

CT findings (Fig. 11.15)
- Unilateral rounded or ovoid mediastinal mass with a smooth or lobulated outline; diffuse enlargement is less common (cf. thymic hyperplasia).
- Homogeneous or heterogeneous soft-tissue density with variable enhancement following IV contrast. Foci of low attenuation (reflecting haemorrhage, necrosis, or cystic degeneration) may be present.
- Calcifications may be amorphous and curvilinear.
- Most common in the pre-vascular space; with enlargement a thymoma tends to spread caudally along a mediastinal surface ('glacial' growth).
- Features suggesting invasive thymoma on CT are not reliable but include irregular interfaces with or invasion of adjacent structures (lung, mediastinal fat, chest wall, or major vessels or pericardium/heart). Metastatic spread into the pleural space is manifest as pleural nodularity or irregular/circumferential pleural thickening and a pleural effusion.

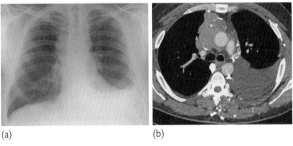

(a)   (b)

Fig. 11.15 CXR and CT in a 42-year-old patient with a malignant thymoma. (a) CXR shows a lobulated mediastinal mass and a left pleural effusion. (b) CT in the same patient showing a predominantly right-sided mass of soft-tissue density. There is some localized curvilinear calcification anteriorly. The SVC is occluded and there are dilated venous collaterals in the posterior chest wall.

MRI findings
- Unilateral rounded or ovoid mediastinal mass with a smooth or lobulated outline.
- Intermediate signal on T1- and high signal on T2-weighted image sequences; signal intensity may heterogeneous. Fibrous septa may be seen.
- Features indicating invasion are similar to those seen at CT but equally insensitive.

Thymic carcinoma
- Rare epithelial tumour (distinct from thymoma).
- ♂:♀ ≈ 1:1. Usually presenting in 5th–6th decades and associated with a poor prognosis.

CXR findings
- Lobulated mediastinal mass of soft tissue density ± calcification.

CT findings (Fig. 11.16)
- Lobulated or irregular mass—most commonly in the pre-vascular space but also in other mediastinal compartments.
- Homogeneous (isodense with skeletal muscles) or heterogeneous attenuation. Focal areas of low attenuation indicating necrosis or cystic degeneration may be present.
- Nodular or stippled areas of calcification.
- Enlargement of regional lymph nodes.

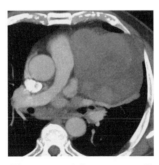

Fig. 11.16 Targeted CT in a patient with thymic carcinoma. There is a large lobulated mediastinal mass of heterogeneous soft tissue attenuation. The mass makes contact with the left anterolateral pleural surface/chest wall but there are no obvious CT signs of transgression.

MRI findings
- Lobulated or irregular mass in the pre-vascular space.
- Homogeneous T1- and heterogeneous (iso- or hyperintense relative to chest wall muscles) T2-weighted signal.
- Foci of cystic degeneration manifest as lesions of low signal on T1- and high signal on T2-weighted images.

Thymic lymphoma
- Lymphomatous involvement of the thymus is usually of Hodgkin's type and generally occurs as part of generalized disease.

CXR findings
- Well-defined lobulated mass or masses.
- Unilateral or bilateral.

CT findings
- Diffuse enlargement of the thymus with well-defined, lobulated margins or multiple masses.
- Homogeneous or heterogeneous attenuation (the latter occurs when there is necrosis, cyst formation, or as a consequence of treatment).

Thymolipoma
- Rare, slow-growing benign tumour of the thymus composed of otherwise normal fatty and thymic tissue.
- Occasionally associated with other diseases (e.g. myasthenia gravis, aplastic anaemia, Graves' thyrotoxicosis).
- Thymolipomas can grow to a large size and typically presents in young adulthood as an asymptomatic mediastinal mass.

CXR findings
- Large lobulated mass of homogeneous density, most commonly adjacent to the heart/diaphragm (rarely in the pre-vascular space). Because it is soft, the mass often 'moulds' itself to adjacent structures.
- Thymolipomas may be mistaken for cardiac enlargement, lower lobe consolidation or elevation of the hemidiaphragm.

CT findings
- Large, unilateral well-defined mass adjacent to the heart/hemidiaphragm.
- Heterogeneous attenuation consisting of fat (typically < −10HU) and soft-tissue (>20–30HU) elements; the latter are thought to represent residual (normal) thymus or fibrous septa.

MRI findings
- Large unilateral para-cardiac or juxtadiaphragmatic mass.
- High signal (related to fat) interspersed with bands of low signal on T1-weighted images.

Thymic hyperplasia

- Enlargement of the thymus may occur, particularly in children, under conditions of 'stress' (true thymic hyperplasia) or in the context of autoimmune disease (lymphoid hyperplasia) (Table 11.8).

Table 11.8 Causes and associations of thymic hyperplasia

- **True thymic hyperplasia**
  - Recovery from 'stress' (e.g. post-chemotherapy, severe burns, radiotherapy). NB The thymus initially atrophies but then increases in volume after the stressful episode.
  - 'Rebound hyperplasia' refers to an excessive increase in thymic volume (x2–3 normal size).
- **Lymphoid (follicular) hyperplasia**
  - Myasthenia gravis (thymic hyperplasia present in 65–70%).
  - Other autoimmune diseases (SLE, rheumatoid arthritis, Sjögren's syndrome, Hashimoto's thyroiditis, Addison's disease, Graves' disease, autoimmune haemolytic anaemia).
  - HIV infection.

Adapted from Nishino M et al. The thymus: a comprehensive review. *RadioGraphics* 2006; **26**:335–348.

Imaging of thymic hyperplasia

CXR findings

- CXR has a limited role in the detection of thymic hyperplasia.

CT findings (Fig 11.17)

- Diffuse enlargement of both lobes but with preservation of the normal shape of the thymus.
- A focal rounded or ovoid mass—less common.
- Homogeneous soft-tissue density.
- Thymic hyperplasia following chemotherapy occurs on average five months (range 1–11 months) after cessation of treatment and the gland may remain enlarged for up to four years.

MRI findings

- Diffuse enlargement of both lobes or occasionally a focal mass.
- Signal intensity is similar to that of normal thymus.
- Chemical shift imaging (which detects small amounts of fat) may distinguish between hyperplastic and neoplastic enlargement: a drop in signal on the 'opposed phase' images indicates the presence of fat and favours the diagnosis of hyperplasia over a neoplasm.

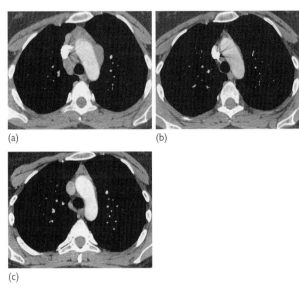

(a)   (b)

(c)

Fig. 11.17 Rebound thymic hyperplasia following treatment for lymphoma. (a) Staging CT study demonstrates enlarged mediastinal nodes. (b) CT performed 7 months later shows complete radiological remission. (c) CT undertaken 4 months after (b) demonstrates the presence rebound thymic hyperplasia. The normal thymic tissue, anterior to the aortic arch, has an 'arrowhead' configuration.

Thymic cysts
- May be congenital or acquired.
- Congenital cysts are rare, originate from the 4th branchial arch and usually present in childhood.
- Acquired cysts are found in a variety of contexts:
  - Malignancy: Hodgkin's disease (with or without previous radiotherapy), thymoma, thymic carcinoma, germ cell tumours, and seminoma.
  - Infections: tuberculosis, HIV.

CXR findings
- Similar to other thymic masses.

CT findings
- Congenital cysts tend to be thin-walled and unilocular whereas acquired lesions may have an identifiable wall and internal locules.
- Cyst contents tend to be of fluid attenuation (<20HU; as with other cystic mediastinal lesions) but may have higher attenuation if there has been bleeding into the cyst.

MRI findings
- The fluid and solid components and the presence of protein or haemorrhage in cysts may be more easily differentiated on MRI.

Germ cell tumours

Germ cell tumours are derived from primordial cells which, in the embryo, migrate to the gonadal ridge. These tumours occur most commonly in the testes and ovary but the mediastinum is the most common extragonadal site. The histopathological features and classification (but not the prevalence) of individual types of mediastinal germ cell tumours is identical to that in the gonads (Table 11.9).

Table 11.9 Subtypes of mediastinal germ cell tumours

- **Teratoma**—most common germ cell tumour of mediastinum
  - Mature teratoma (accounts for 60–70%)
  - Immature teratoma
  - Teratoma with malignant transformation
- **Seminoma**—accounting for up to 40%
- **Non-seminomatous**
  - Embryonal carcinoma
  - Yolk sac tumour
  - Chorioncarcinoma
- **Mixed**

Adapted from Ueno T et al. Spectrum of germ cell tumors: from head to toe. *RadioGraphics* 2004; **24**:387–404.

Mature teratoma

- Most common mediastinal germ cell tumour containing elements derived from at least two but usually all three germ cell layers (mesoderm, endoderm, and ectoderm).
- ♂ > ♀; typically in young adults (i.e. 20–40 years).

CXR findings (Fig. 11.18)

- Well-defined (smooth or lobulated) mediastinal mass—typically unilateral.
- Calcification or ossification—amorphous calcification or identifiable bony elements/formed teeth may be seen.
- Relative radiolucency or the presence of a fat-fluid level—may be present but rarely appreciated on CXR.

CT findings (Fig. 11.18)

- Well-defined mass—with a smooth/lobulated contour; varying size. Most (70%) are unilateral but ~30% may cross the midline and rarely the tumour may be confined to the midline.
- Differential densities—readily identified on CT and include soft-tissue (in all cases), fluid (in >85%), fat (>75%), and calcification/ossification (~50%); some combination of all four densities is seen in just over one third of cases. Fluid attenuation is most often the dominant component.
- A fat-fluid level is highly suggestive of the diagnosis but only occurs in ~10% of cases.
- Ancillary findings include: mass effect (especially with large tumours), lung atelectasis, consolidation, pleural and pericardial effusions.

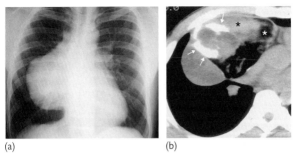

(a)   (b)

Fig. 11.18 CXR and CT in an adult patient with a mature teratoma. (a) CXR shows a large mass arising from the mediastinum and protruding into the right hemithorax. The mass is of soft tissue density with no obvious differential densities. (b) CT in the same patient shows curvilinear calcification (arrows), soft tissue (black asterisk), and fat (white asterisk) densities.

MRI findings
- Well-defined (smooth or lobulated) mediastinal mass. Heterogeneous signal reflecting the different histopathological components of soft-tissue, fat, and fluid; soft-tissue components are isointense with skeletal muscle. Fluid is of low signal on T1- and high signal on T2-weighted sequences. Fat is of high signal on both T1- and T2 weighted images.

Seminoma
- Most common malignant germ cell tumour of the mediastinum.
- ♂ > ♀. Usually presenting in 3rd–4th decades.

CXR findings (Fig. 11.19)
- Anterior mediastinal mass of soft tissue density with lobulated or irregular outlines; may extend across the midline.

CT findings (Fig. 11.19)
- Anterior mediastinal mass—lobulated or irregular outline; often asymmetric. Heterogeneous attenuation with foci of reduced density reflecting cystic degeneration or necrosis; some enhancement of soft-tissue elements following IV contrast.
- Invasion of mediastinal fat/other mediastinal structures.
- Calcification—significantly less common than in mature teratomas.

MRI findings
- Anterior mediastinal mass—homogeneous signal on T1-weighted images. Foci of low signal on T1-weighted sequences may indicate areas of necrosis or cystic degeneration.

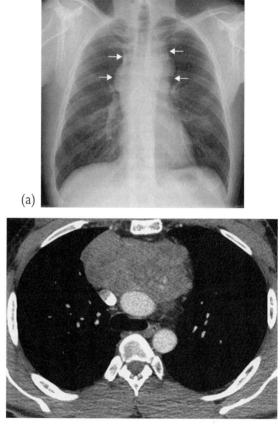

Fig. 11.19 CXR and CT of a patient with a malignant seminoma. (a) CXR shows a lobulated mass extending on both side of the mediastinum (arrows) (b) CT through the upper zones shows a lobulated mediastinal mass in the pre-vascular space. The mass is of heterogeneous but predominantly soft tissue attenuation.

Fibrosing mediastinitis

- Abnormal proliferation of acellular collagen and dense hyaline fibrosis in the mediastinum. The causes of fibrosing mediastinitis are given in Table 11.10.
- Rare condition (even in areas where histoplasmosis and tuberculosis are endemic); fibrosing mediastinitis may be an abnormal immunological response to 'injury' in susceptible individuals.
- ♂:♀ ≈ 1:1. Occurring over a wide age range (10–70 years).
- Macroscopically, fibrosing mediastinitis manifests either as a localized mass or is diffusely infiltrative.

Table 11.10 Recognized causes and associations of fibrosing mediastinitis[1]

- **Idiopathic**
- **Infections**[2]—*Histoplasma capsulatum*, *Aspergillus* sp. (and other fungal infections), tuberculosis, *Wuchereria bancrofti*
- **Trauma**
- **Following mediastinal irradiation**
- **Sarcoidosis**
- **Drugs**
- **Miscellaneous**—Langerhans' cell histiocytosis, Riedel's thyroiditis, rupture of bronchogenic cyst, post-radiofrequency ablation for atrial fibrillation, retroperitoneal fibrosis, orbital pseudotumour, sclerosing cholangitis

[1]The diagnosis of 'benign' fibrosing mediastinitis must be distinguished from mediastinal fibrosis which occurs in the context of other malignancies (e.g. (nodular sclerosing) Hodgkin's lymphoma, non-Hodgkin's lymphoma, malignant pleural mesothelioma, thymic carcinoid, and thymoma). [2] Of the infectious causes, histoplasmosis and tuberculosis are the most common worldwide.

Imaging of fibrosing mediastinitis

CXR findings

- Mediastinal widening—seen in 50–90% of patients; may be very subtle.
- Thickening, loss of clarity, or obliteration of mediastinal interfaces/stripes (e.g. thickening of the right paratracheal stripe).
- Hilar, right paratracheal, or subcarinal mass—calcification may be seen in the localized form of fibrosing mediastinitis but less common in the diffuse infiltrative type.
- Tracheal or central airway narrowing—may be associated with segmental/lobar atelectasis or 'obstructive' pneumonia.
- Pulmonary oligaemia ± peripheral 'wedge-shaped' consolidation (the latter denoting infarcted lung)—caused by arterial occlusion.
- Pulmonary oedema (see 📖 Air space diseases/Pulmonary oedema, p126)—due to venous occlusion; oedema may be unilateral or even localized to one lobe.

CT findings (Fig. 11.20)

- Localized mass or diffuse soft-tissue infiltration—the localized variety is typically in the right paratracheal, right hilar, or sub-carinal regions.
- Calcification—more common in the localized than in the diffuse form of fibrosing mediastinitis.
- Pulmonary arterial/venous narrowing or obliteration.
- Coronary arterial narrowing or obliteration.
- Superior vena caval (or other mediastinal venous) narrowing or obliteration.
- Central airway narrowing or occlusion.
- Left atrial compression.
- Pulmonary parenchymal signs: veno-occlusive oedema, peripheral infarcts.
- Signs of the underlying cause (e.g. sarcoidosis, previous tuberculosis).

MRI findings

- Localized or diffusely infiltrating mediastinal mass.
- Heterogeneous (low-to-intermediate) signal on T1-weighted images; variable regions of high and low signal on T2-weighted sequences.
- Regions of low signal reflect either fibrosis or foci of calcification. Extensive areas of low signal on T2-weighted images are more suggestive of fibrosing mediastinitis than an infiltrative malignancy.

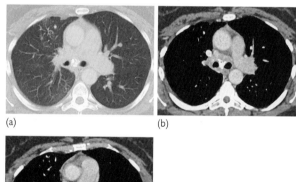

(a)

(b)

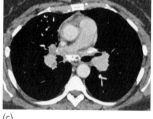

(c)

Fig. 11.20 CT in a 42-year-old patient with fibrosing mediastinitis caused by histoplasmosis. (a) CT on lung window settings shows very localized oedema in the right upper lobe. (b) CT just below the level of the carina shows a calcified subcarinal mass and abnormal soft tissue around the central airways. (c) CT at a slightly lower level than b) showing contiguous involvement of structures at the right hilum.

Pneumomediastinum

- The abnormal presence of air/gas in the mediastinum.
- Pneumomediastinum occurs as a result of perforation of respiratory or alimentary tracts; the possible causes of a pneumomediastinum are summarized in Table 11.11.

Table 11.11 Causes of a pneumomediastinum

- **Alveolar rupture**
  - Spontaneous (e.g. asthma, pulmonary fibrosis, childbirth)
  - Mechanical ventilation
  - Lung rupture by rib fracture
  - Compressive thoracic trauma
- **Laceration of central bronchus or trachea**
- **Spontaneous or iatrogenic perforation**—e.g. oesophagus, pharynx, duodenum, colon, or rectum (NB air tracks into mediastinum)
- **Iatrogenic**—e.g. following mediastinoscopy or sternotomy

Imaging of pneumomediastinum
CXR findings (Fig. 11.21)
- Lucencies, bubbles, or streaks of gas—superimposed on the mediastinum. NB Air may track extra-pleurally at the lung apex (simulating a pneumothorax) or along the diaphragm (the 'continuous diaphragm' sign). A pneumomediastinum may be differentiated from a pneumopericardium by the demonstration of air extending around and above aortic arch in the former.

CT findings (Fig. 11.22)
- Linear/curvilinear gaseous mediastinal densities—may be associated with pneumothoraces and subcutaneous/surgical emphysema.

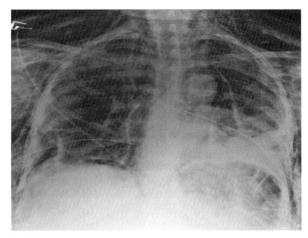

Fig. 11.21 CXR showing a mediastinum, bilateral chest drains, and extensive subcutaneous surgical emphysema.

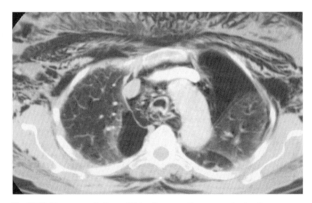

Fig. 11.22 Pneumomediastinum, bilateral pneumothoraces, and extensive subcutaneous emphysema.

Recommendations for Further Reading

Reference books:

Hansell DM, Lynch DA, McAdams HP, Bankier AA. *Imaging of diseases of the chest.* 5th edition. Mosby-Elsevier (2010).

Webb WR, Müller NL, Naidich DP. *HRCT of the lung.* 4th edition. Wolters Kluwer/Lippincott Williams & Wilkins (2008).

Guidelines and position statements:

ATS/ERS international multidisciplinary consensus classification of the idiopathic interstitial pneumonias. *Am J Respir Crit Care Med* 2002;165:277–304.

British Thoracic Society guidelines for the management of suspected acute pulmonary embolism. *Thorax* 2003;58:470–484.

Havelock T et al. Pleural procedures and thoracic ultrasound: British Thoracic Society pleural disease guideline 2010. *Thorax* 2010;65 (Suppl 2):ii61–ii76.

MacMahon H et al. Guidelines for management of small pulmonary nodules detected on CT scans: a statement from the Fleischner Society. *Radiology* 2005;237:395–400.

Mayo JR et al. Radiation dose at chest CT: a statement of the Fleischner Society. *Radiology* 2003:228:15–21.

Raghu G et al. An official ATS/ERS/JRS/ALAT statement: idiopathic pulmonary fibrosis – evidence-based guidelines for diagnosis and management. *Am J Respir Crit Care Med* 2011;183:788–824.

Remy-Jardin M et al. Management of suspected pulmonary embolism in the era of CT angiography: a statement from the Fleischner society. *Radiology* 2007;245:315–326.

Wells AU et al. Interstitial lung disease guideline: the British Thoracic Society in collaboration with the Thoracic Society of Australia and New Zealand and the Irish Thoracic Society. *Thorax* 2008;63 (Suppl V):v1–v58.

Selected papers:

Goldstraw P et al. The IASLC lung cancer staging project: proposals for the revision of the TNM stage groupings in the forthcoming (seventh) edition of the TNM classification of malignant tumours. *J Thorac Oncol* 2007;2:706–714.

Godoy MCB, Naidich DP. Subsolid pulmonary nodules and the spectrum of peripheral adenocarcinomas of the lung: recommended interim guidelines and management. *Radiology* 2009;253:606–622.

Hansell DM et al. Fleischner Society: glossary of terms for thoracic imaging. *Radiology* 2008;246:697–722.

Travis WD. Classification of lung cancer. *Semin Roentgenol* 2011;46:178–186.

Webb WR. Thin-section CT of the secondary pulmonary lobule: anatomy and the image – the 2004 Fleischner Lecture. *Radiology* 2006;239:322–338.

Index